AF449293

LIFE HISTORY RESEARCH IN
Psychopathology

VOLUME 3

Life History Research in Psychopathology

VOLUME 3

DAVID F. RICKS, ALEXANDER THOMAS, AND
MERRILL ROFF, EDITORS

The University of Minnesota Press, Minneapolis

Library of Congress Catalog Card Number: 77-98098

ISBN 0-8166-0702-8

"Life Events and Psychiatric Symptomatology" by Jerome K. Myers, Jacob J. Lindenthal, and Max P. Pepper was published in slightly different form as "Life Events and Mental Status: A Longitudinal Study," by the same authors and D. R. Ostrander, in *The Journal of Health and Social Behavior*, 1972, 13, 398–406, and is reprinted here by permission of the American Sociological Association.

to
Herbert G. Birch
1918–1973

LIFE HISTORIES fascinate everyone, and life history research, which is concerned with the changes and developments that take place in people over time, provides a common focus of interest for a diverse group of scientists and practitioners. In an ongoing series of conferences on the scientific study of lives, the Society for Life History Research in Psychopathology has provided a meeting place for people studying many different influences on life spans and trajectories. The influences described in volumes 1 and 2, and further developed in this volume, range from genetics, early nutrition, and intimate family relationships to large-scale sociological and cultural patterns of life and work.

The major theme in our previous two volumes has been the description of the antecedents and outcomes of contrasting forms of deviance: schizophrenia, neuroses, depression, character disorders, alcoholism, delinquency, psychosomatic illness, and so on. Comparing antecedents of these various disorders showed that a few variables, such as disturbed parents, low intelligence, and poor relationships with peers, were antecedents of a wide range of behavioral difficulties. Other variables are quite specific, indicating, for instance, that a child or adolescent who was extremely anxious, felt vulnerable and overwhelmed, was not sure of the reality of his daily experiences, and felt isolated from others was a distinct risk for a later schizophrenic outcome.

This volume continues our long-term major concern, but it adds three new elements. The first is a thorough critical discussion of the merits and problems in high-risk research, an area of work currently enjoying a deserved burst of popularity. Careful readers of section 1 are likely to come away with a new appreciation of high-risk research, together with a new understanding of its possible pitfalls.

The second new emphasis in this book is not so much a birth as it is a wedding. One of the sources of the systematic study of developmental psychopathology is developmental psychology, including longitudinal studies of children and the work of people like Havighurst and Neugarten, who see human development as the study of the whole life cycle. Knowing when a life crisis is a normal, predictable reorganization preceding a new level of development, and being able to differentiate such crises from disintegrative or regressive reactions to stress, remains a tremendous challenge. This volume brings together studies of normal and deviant lines of development, allowing some systematic comparisons.

Our first volume dealt with drug intervention in relation to background factors, and the second volume continued a concern with treatment, but this volume moves much further in the direction of constructing a life history framework for the interpretation of intervention and outcome studies. The effect of any intervention is relative to what would have happened if no intervention had taken place. Life history research provides the developmental models and the research designs for making such comparisons. In this volume we consider outcomes of various treatments for a particular group of schizophrenics, residential work with several groups of boys, and psychotherapy with depressed and anxious adult women. Such a sampling just begins the process of looking at intervention in a life history framework. Our aim is not to provide a general review of intervention studies, a task already done with admirable scope by Allen Bergin, one of our participants, but to show that intervention can be interpreted in a more comprehensive and systematic way than it has been in the past.

A reader who is new to studies of developmental psychopathology may be helped by mention of other antecedents in this field. Where did this lusty, demanding newcomer originate, and who are his ancestors? His nourishing mothers have certainly been the developmental psychologists, who have provided the research methods and the most general conceptual models with which he has furnished his shop. The father, though, must be acknowledged to have been the scientist turned reluctant clinician, Freud, who initiated an intellectual tradition of case studies that continued down through Jung and Morton Prince to Henry Murray (an honored participant in this meeting), Robert White, and Erik Erikson. Medicine, long before Freud, had discovered that the key to prevention, or at least effective intervention, lay in careful investigation of the natural history of disease processes, and of the history of the person: "Psychiatric processes do not lend themselves to consideration as disease processes relatively divorced from the normal constitution and development of the individual. They are to be understood only in the context of the life history of the individual, and the personal biography becomes an essential facilitative device in the process of treatment" (S. Novey, *The Second Look* [Baltimore: Johns Hopkins University Press, 1968], p. 3).

If developmental psychology is the mother, and clinical case study the father, the older brother of life history research in psychopathology has been psychometrics and the study of individual differences over time by the use of structured instruments. Like many older brothers, this one has set a standard of excellence that has been hard for his younger sibling to match. The work of Terman, E. L. Thorndike, Robert Thorndike, and their associates on the adult significance of ability levels in children, and the early work on the inheritance of intelligence rapidly developed a quality of measurement and statistical sophistication not yet approached in most research on psychopathology.

Why are methods of research so important, and why do we spend so much time on them in all three volumes? Simply because shortcut solutions, dictated by a hasty practical resolve to get on with solving immediate problems, rarely provide lasting answers. Our leading paper is an effective demonstration of the ongoing mutual influence of clear conceptualization of problems and inventive methods for solving them. Herbert Birch died a few months after presenting this paper, but he will continue to be an important part of life history research, as model, mentor, and critic for us all.

One main method of life history research in psychopathology has come to be a combination of clinical case study over time with careful construction of rating scales and other measuring techniques, the case studies either coming from existing records (child guidance clinics, schools, courts, probation departments, state hospitals, etc.) or developed out of longitudinal designs for work with high-risk groups. It is this synthesis of clinical data, psychometric method, and developmental conceptualization that gives life history research in psychopathology its unique identity.

The reader will not find in this volume some of the locusts that plague much current work in psychology, psychiatry, and related fields. We offer no quickie techniques of research or of psychotherapy, no screams, no panaceas. We have kept our concerns to major problems of real-life significance, and we have tried to give due importance to the major influences on life, beginning with genetic endowment and the intrauterine environment and proceeding through family, school, and peer influences to adult work and the stresses that come from both the external environment and internal transformations through mid-life.

The papers were presented in a two-day invitational conference at Teachers College, Columbia University. The participants included persons expert in genetics, pediatrics, psychiatry, psychology, and sociology. Each author was asked to present his paper in nontechnical language, so that it could be understood by everyone present, and when an author found it necessary to use technical terms from his particular shop, the editors have asked for explanations.

The book can be read by students in medicine and in psychology, psychiatrists, psychologists, sociologists, and others. We believe that life history research has something to contribute to each. Our aim of providing a useful life history framework for both research and practice was well expressed by one of the reviewers of the first volume, who said he wished that he could have read it when he was starting his career as an internist, and that if he had a son starting to practice now, this would be a book that he would give him. We hope that we have provided another such book.

A focus on research does prevent us from presenting a systematic textbook description of the varieties of disordered lives. Readers interested in such a presentation might read one of the excellent textbooks available (e.g., Lidz's *The Person* and White and Watt's *The Abnormal Personality*) along with this book. Students interested in further study of the lives on which these reports are based should consider reading both autobiographical reports of mental illness and case histories gathered at various times in the lives of disturbed persons. *Developmental Abnormal Psychology*, by Roff, Mink, and Hinrichs, presents raw material on lives over time, and so challenges the reader to try his own integrations.

The clinics, schools, child guidance centers, residential treatment centers, and hospitals that provided data for many of these studies deserve our special gratitude. It is not easy to tolerate curious and skeptical researchers when one is busy solving immediate and pressing problems.

We are also indebted to Jessica Schairer and David Josiah Ricks, who helped plan and coordinate the conference, and to Teachers College, which supported it. The University of Minnesota Press edited the papers with a rare combination of tact, gentleness, and intelligence.

D. F.

A. T.

M. R.

X

❧ *Table of Contents*

LIFE HISTORY RESEARCH IN
Psychopathology

VOLUME 3

HERBERT G. BIRCH] *Methodological Issues in the Longitudinal Study of Malnutrition*

I WOULD like to share with you some of the problems that my colleagues and I have encountered over a period of about ten to fifteen years in our concern with the problem of the relation of malnutrition to mental and physical development. I suggested that we discuss this because it seems to me that all of the issues that are raised in other areas of longitudinal research with respect to so-called genetic, sociological, familial, and other environmental factors and their interaction as they affect behavior and development come into very sharp focus in this area of research. I think that we have begun to develop some ways to cope with some of these complexities and have developed a useful model system for consideration.

Let me start with a little bit of autobiography in a sense. About a decade ago when I first began to decide that I wanted to work on problems of nutrition and mental development, various of my students and friends and colleagues said, "What are you, mad? You're working on interesting things right now; the object of scientific research is to work in areas that are potentially productive. I can't think of a more dismal area in which to work than this one." And I said, "Well, why do you think it's dismal?" One of my friends answered, "After all, back in the 1940's a whole series of people here at Columbia and elsewhere began to say that if we gave food of particular kinds to children who were mentally retarded, like glutamic acid supplements, they would become

NOTE: This study received support from the National Institute of Child Health and Human Development, grant NICHHD 00719, and from the Association for the Aid of Crippled Children.

This paper was prepared from the tapes of an address given by the late Dr. Birch. The tapes have been edited and prepared for publication by Dr. Margaret E. Hertzig, who assumes full responsibility for any inaccuracies in or misinterpretation of the material.

very smart indeed, and these people reported that such children did become smarter. At the time of that research Lauretta Bender made some rather caustic remarks about one of the principal investigators. She said that if this thing really works he ought to take it himself. However, that stuff just went down the drain and it's really a quite unpromising area to work with altogether. It's in a class with folklore like 'fish is brain food' and so on." I replied, "Just because some people have done poor work in a given area doesn't mean that the area is not important. What else is there that bothers you?" He said, "Look at the very good work that was done during the war on starvation — for example, the work done by people like Keys, Brozek, and their colleagues (1950) in Minnesota. We know that the conscientious objectors who volunteered for medical research rather than bear arms in a given period were starved to the brink of death, and although their mental functions were abysmal at the time that they were acutely malnourished and severely starved, by the time they had been nutritionally rehabilitated and had physically recovered, they were functioning just as well as they were at the start. So that there really is no good reason to think that this area is a productive area." I asked, "Who told you about the Keys and Brozek study?" And he answered, "You did."

So I said, "Why do you think you are giving me some new information then? The problem is that the Keys and Brozek study and all the other studies of adult malnutrition and its effect on mental development represent the study of the effects of a particular stress or condition on a brain that is already mature, on an organism that is already developed and whose functional capacities are already manifest. What you are saying is that we can come to conclusions about important influences on development on the basis of information that we obtain from individuals at the adult level. This would be just as bad as saying we could conclude what the consequences of traumatic damage to the brain are in children from our studies of traumatic damage to the brain in adults. We know, for example, that lateralized damage in adults may very often be reflected in particular disturbances in language and speech, but if we have similar lateralizing damage in young children, this is *not* reflected in the same kind of disturbance of function. Therefore, even when we have localized anatomic damage, we have no basis for generalizing from the consequences of this damage in the mature and developed organism to the consequences of this damage for the developmental period. What I'm interested in is the question of the effects of malnutrition upon development, upon the development of brain, upon the development of behavior. And there are good reasons for thinking, first, that the developing brain has certain metabolic requirements for proteins, for fats, for minerals, for calories, and that if these requirements are not met, real threats to the normal development of brain and behavior will occur. Second, malnutrition has as its first effect a change in the behavioral style of a child. The child becomes apathetic, he becomes irritable, he becomes environmentally unresponsive, he becomes an organism who is incapable of profiting from the environment that surrounds him. Consequently, one has good bases for hypothesizing that malnutrition in a developing individual may indeed affect developmental course with respect to brain and behavior."

I didn't convince anybody and nobody convinced me. This is one of the features of discussions generally that was recognized by Omar Khayyam many years ago — you say your piece and other people say their piece, and then you go on and do what you wanted to do anyhow. So, various of us decided that we would enter this unpromising area and begin to study the relation of brain and behavior to malnutrition experienced early in the life of individuals. The first studies were follow-ups of children who had been victims of cataclasms of a social kind — war, famine, revolution, and so on. So, for example, Cabak and her colleagues (1965) in Yugoslavia followed up, in a poorly designed study of children who had been severely malnourished as a consequence of the immediate postwar dislocations in Yugoslavia, the functioning of these children at school age some 4–6 years after recovery. She compared these children with a group of children who had not been hospitalized for severe malnutrition and found that the children who had been malnourished were smaller and had lower IQ's than did the comparison group. The comparison group was poorly defined; it simply drew children from generally similar social class circumstances in Yugoslavia. This kind of study was the first of the nutritional studies using as the model situation a crisis affecting the nutritional status of the child — that is, this child was severely malnourished, he was at the brink of death, he recovered, and does his recovery now represent recovery without developmental sequelae or does it have developmental sequelae? That is a crisis model.

A second kind of model was developed by Cravioto and Birch (1966). We argued that when children are malnourished, they tend more frequently on a world scale to be chronically malnourished. The acutely malnourished children hospitalized with diseases like marasmus and kwashiorkor represent only the dramatic and visible tip of an iceberg, underneath which is a much larger group with chronic subnutrition. This affects millions of children all over the world and is reflected in a stunting and diminution of their development. This kind of thinking emphasizes a chronic model rather than a crisis model as the basis for looking at the problem. Instead of looking at cases of marasmus and kwashiorkor as dramatic instances of severe malnutrition, and studying their developmental consequences, one has the responsibility of looking at individuals and populations of children who have been chronically subnourished and then studying the nature of their development.

This chronic model from a social point of view is probably the more important because it is the model that characterizes the generality of conditions for development of something like 50 to 60 per cent of the children in the world today. Recognizing that this is the chronic state of affairs for children in the world is hardly new. As a matter of fact, one of the first pieces of published research by the then young and thereafter distinguished anthropologist, Franz Boaz (1910), the father of modern anthropology in the United States, was a study to determine whether living in America with opportunities for better health care and better nutrition resulted in changes in stature in immigrant groups. Boaz selected Sicilian and Jewish immigrants, who tended to breed within their own groups, so as to maintain a common gene pool, and he looked at the height of successive generations of such immigrants. He found that there were successive increments in height with successive generations living in the United States.

Boyd Orr in England in the 1930's returned to this problem and reported that the social class differences in Great Britain were reflected by intergenerational differences in relative stunting in different subsections of the population. In a magnificent monograph called *Food, Health and Income* (1936), he established a totally new basis for public health and views of social medicine at that time. What he pointed out was that in Britain the upper class is tall and the lower class is short, and that the shortness and tallness has been a historical progression continuing throughout the nineteenth century and culminating in gross height differences in the twentieth century. I can remember standing in the streets of Glasgow in 1937 and, though I am not particularly tall, looking over the heads and shakos of the Gordon Highlanders as they paraded down the street.

A view of sports introduces you to the same problem. Each generation of stunted nationalities produces the flyweight champions of the world. These are stunted lightweights, not individuals who are midgets. The studies of Greulich (1958) on the West Coast with respect to the effect of living in America upon the heights of Japanese immigrants again indicates the shift in stature and in growth with nutritional change. And the changes in Japan in the postwar period ape the situation he found on the West Coast. However, Japanese orphanages have not made the dietary changes introduced into postwar Japan by the armies of occupation. They have retained the traditional prewar diet, and children growing up in orphanages have growth achievements which are the same as the children in the prewar Japanese generation.

Thus, there is abundant evidence from all over the world, in advanced as well as in newly developing countries, that subnutrition, inadequacies of intake on a chronic basis, is registered in growth retardation in children and that this growth retardation reflects their chronic exposure to conditions of subnutrition. Looking at that kind of chronic model, we decided to study those children in a population characterized by nutritional risk who were the best grown children in the community and those who were the least well grown. We went to the Guatemalan highlands to study ethnically homogeneous tribes of people in communities of nutritional risk. Among these Cakchiquel-speaking tribes, in looking at age groups of children one is struck by marked differences in height at the same age and in the same grade in the school. We then asked two questions. Do these children of different stature differ in their abilities to process environmental information? Do they differ in their neuro-integrative capacities and organizations? We already knew that they differed in their school learning and in whatever kinds of modified IQ tests we could give them in that region. We decided to use a relatively culturally unaffected instrument and to look at the differences in their ability to process normal amounts of environmental information. Birch and Lefford (1963) had demonstrated that in normal children there is a clearly defined developmental course for the development of the capacity to process information across the different sensory systems. We demonstrated, for example, a clear developmental course in the child's ability to tell whether a figure that he saw was the same or different from a figure that he felt behind a screen, to tell whether what he saw and the path through which you moved his arm were the same or different, and to tell whether what he felt and what his kinesthetic organizations were were the same or different.

When we applied these measures to children in the Guatemalan highlands, we found that the shorter children lagged 2–3 years behind the taller children in the same community, that they were exhibiting profound lags in neuro-integrative competence. Cravioto and I looked at each other (neither of us is tall), and we said, What do you mean, shorties are dumb and tallies are smart? I said, "Joaquin, that's impossible. All right, what do we do about it? You and I are not stunted. We are familially short. We are not at risk. If anything, we have both been overnourished and overfed." To answer this question, we had to go to an ethnically identical Guatemalan group living under conditions in which there is not nutritional risk. There are such affluent groups. We predicted that in these groups two things would differ: first, in the affluent groups, children's heights would correlate positively and significantly with parents' heights in contrast with the absence of such a significant correlation in our community at nutritional risk; and second, shorter and taller children would not differ in their neuro-integrative capacities in the village in the affluent group. Both hypotheses were confirmed. In contrast with the village at nutritional risk and the people at nutritional risk, shortness and tallness in the community not at such risk were not associated with dysfunctions in the processing of environmental information.

Publication of these findings created a good deal of interest (Cravioto, Delicardie, & Birch, 1966). Questions of course began to arise, most of which we had anticipated in a rather extensive critical discussion in our own monograph — if you try to be your own severest critic, it gives you a jump on the situation after a while. You can be a critic of your own work by standing aside and asking, What rubbish is this? We asked, How do we know that the shorter children in this nutritionally deprived community are not *backward* because they are stunted, but are children who, though stunted, also come from social backgrounds which are less stimulating, come from larger families, from worse conditions with less opportunities for learning, and so forth? In other words, conditions of health disadvantage are rarely, if ever, separate from conditions more ubiquitous, such as social disadvantage.

So we did an ecologic study of taller and shorter children in communities at nutritional risk, concerned now with the nature of the family circumstances, the general stimulating value of the environments, and so on. And what we found, as you would expect, was that the shorter children came from homes with larger families, ones that had less contact with the broader culture (for example, less radio listening), lesser degrees of partial literacy upon the part of the parents, more children more closely spaced, smaller amounts of cash income, poorer housing. So, one might ask, How can you state that nutrition is making such a contribution to their maldevelopment when all of these other circumstances are also associated with it? And if one goes a step further, he may argue as some people do—as did Karl Pearson, the brilliant statistician who moved from a socialist to an establishment figure in the period from 1900 to 1925—that in a free society genetically endowed individuals seek their natural level. How do you know that these individuals who are functioning less well in the community are not simply familially, polygenically if you will, less competent in an intellectual sense? All of these questions have a familiar ring, don't they? They in fact raise the issues that dominate phases of the discussion throughout the first section of this volume. Let's add one more to this family of questions: How do you know that the children who are malnourished and chronically malnourished were not children who were initially defective children, who were behaving poorly from birth onward, who were poor stimuli to their mothers, who as a consequence were relatively neglected, and who now owe their stunting and their incapacity to initial incapacity?

What issues do we have now? We have genetics, we have condition at birth and the nature of the child as a stimulus, we have the problem of the relationship of the interaction of social circumstances and developmental circumstances to the level of functioning in children who have differential nutritional experiences. These are the questions at issue. How do you answer them? The point is that it is almost impossible to fell such a series of questions at one blow. You have to develop a series of research strategies that systematically begins to take these issues into account.

Let us take as our first issue, then, the question of whether these children who become malnourished were children who were deviant as neonates and who were therefore inadequate stimuli for their mothers and poorly cared for. The only way to answer this question is by an anterospective study of a total cohort of births in a community characterized by nutritional risk. This we did. In a village in southwest Mexico (Cravioto, Birch, DeLicardie, Rosales, & Vega, 1969), we identified risk rates for malnutrition; we identified all demographic aspects of the total population in the community; we enrolled all pregnant women in a given 12-month period in the study, maintained their cooperation, and studied all pregnancies and all deliveries. We further evaluated all infants at 2 days of age, at 2 weeks of age, at biweekly intervals thereafter for the first year, at bimonthly intervals in the second year, and at trimonthly intervals in all succeeding years. The children are now 6 years of age, and we are continuing to evaluate them.

This community of approximately 6,000 people had a birth rate of 50/1000 and one could have predicted an annual birth cohort of 300. Sexual behavior was cooperative, gestations were maintained, and precisely 300 children were born in this community in the 12-month period. All have been enrolled in the study, and all survivors have been followed continuously since. With regard to the first question of initial differences, we had the primary data on the characteristics of the children at birth, their weight on the second day of life, their neurologic characteristics on the basis of pediatric neurologic examination at birth and at biweekly intervals thereafter, pediatric and social monitoring of development, and psychological monitoring of the development of the child in the first periods of life. By 2 years of age, 22 children became severely enough malnourished to require hospitalization if they were to survive; 22 of 300 gives a risk rate of approximately 6 per cent for severe malnutrition. These children did not differ in any of their characteristics at birth or as neonates from the group as a whole. They were representative children within the group, so the first question then is answered. It is not the child who is abnormal at birth and then pursues an abnormal course who becomes malnourished. Rather, it is a child whose mother's milk fails (and when I say mother, I mean mother; in these communities, the food source of the child is the mother). If the milk fails, the mother, following traditional practice, substitutes a cornstarch and water mix called atolé, which has about as much value for growth as any such mix, which is nil. The children raised on atolé become severely malnourished and ill. Thus, the children who become malnourished are not the ones who are initially defective, at least on the basis of any measure that we can have.

Now let's turn to the next questions, How about genetics, how about family environments in which the children live? To approach this problem, a second kind of model is required, one comparing children who are nutritionally abnormal with sibs who have not been exposed to the condition of nutritional risk. These sibs have been reared in the same household, and they in general at least share one parent. We began to look at this problem first in a study in Mexico, where we looked at all children who in a given period of time had been hospitalized for severe malnutrition in the pediatrics wards of the army hospital (Birch, Piñeiro, Alcalde, Toca, & Cravioto, 1971). In field research and epidemiologic research, the most important thing is to be able to find cases on follow-up. The army hospital in Mexico provides care for the extended families of recruits, and furthermore, the recruit and his family can be traced for follow-up because he is army registered or has been army registered. We were able to locate 37 out of an initial base of 54 such children and families, and that's very good indeed in these communities. The ones that we couldn't locate had at the time of illness not been distinguishably different from the ones that we did locate. We paired the 37 children with a sib in the same family within a close age range who was not school age. These 37 were all children who had been in a hospital with marasmus or kwashiorkor before 30 months of age and who were between 6 and 12 years of age at follow-up, 4–10 years from the time of hospitalization. The IQ of the sibs was 14 points higher than the IQ of the previously malnourished cases. Similar differences existed across other variables.

This appears to suggest that even when you compare malnourished individuals after a long period following the acute illness with their sibs who have not experienced this illness, you end up with significant differences between the cases and their sib comparisons.

What's wrong with this study? First of all, the sib, unless a twin, is either younger or older than the index case. Because we had taken only sibs within the 6–12 year age range, they would tend to be older than the index cases, and they are, so differences may be the product of developmental lags and slowness in development of the index cases, who might catch up at a later point. They should really be compared not only with their sibs, but with an age-matched comparison group of children deriving from the same social circumstances. Second, the sibs that we were able to obtain were either brothers or sisters of the index cases, so that the sibs were not all of the same sex as the index cases. The possibility exists that this contributed to the severe difference. This is unlikely because the sibs were more heavily weighted with girls than boys and in slowly developing and newly developing countries, girls are always stupider than boys on every test that you give. Don't get excited. Girls are less valued, they do less well in school, and they do less well on most psychological tests. They are a depressed portion of the population. That's true not only in Latin America, it's true in New York City. For example, the monograph by Lesser, Fifer, and Clark (1965) is worth looking at. It compares different ethnic groups and different social classes. If you look at the Puerto Rican subsegment of their study population, you will find that whereas middle-class Puerto Rican boys perform far better than do lower-class Puerto Rican boys in school subjects, middle-class Puerto Rican girls perform at the same level as lower-class Puerto Rican girls on the same subjects. And both do less well in their schoolwork than the lower-class boys. So that these tendencies against girls are carried forward into the first generation in the new community, and this should be borne in mind. This is true in Latin America generally.

Well, once you complete a study you can't just do it again. Either you summon the energy to do another study or you're left with the limitations of the one you have. Fortunately we still had enough energy, so Hertzig, Tizard, Richardson, and I, in a collaboration with the British Medical Research Council Tropical Metabolism Research Unit in Jamaica, then carried out a second sibship follow-up study of cases with marasmus and kwashiorkor (Birch & Richardson, 1972; Hertzig, Birch, Richardson, & Tizard, 1972; Richardson, Birch, Grabie, & Yoder, 1972; Richardson, Birch, & Hertzig, 1973). We compared only same-sex sibs and also compared all index cases and all sibs with matched comparison cases drawn from the same school class. The comparison case was defined as the child of the same sex in that class having a birth date closest to the birth date of the index child or sib. This gives a comparison general population group that comes from the same general circumstances as the index cases and their sibs. We found that at school age, children who had been hospitalized for severe malnutrition before two years of age were shorter, lighter, and had smaller head circumferences than did their sibs and than did the comparison children. The comparison children and the sibs did not differ significantly from one another. The index cases had lower IQ scores than the sibs and the comparison cases, but the sibs did not differ significantly from the comparison cases except for a slight difference in the performance portions of IQ tests. The index cases had more findings of neurologic abnormality than their sibs or the comparison group. In schoolwork, every child's ability to read and write was examined. The index cases were significantly worse than their comparisons, and worse than their sibs, whereas the sibs were not worse than their comparisons.

What about school behavior? Most investigators have restricted themselves to the study of cognitive and perceptual functions in previously malnourished children, though in fact in the communities in which they live, their social behavior and their general adaptations are probably more important determiners of later function than whether they have a 10- or 12-point difference in IQ. Therefore, we decided to look at behavior at home and at school. Every teacher of every child was interviewed with respect to the behavior of all male children in her class, so that she did not know that we were interested in any particular case and did not know that we were interested in the relation of behavior to nutrition. The index children, the previously malnourished children, were consistently as a group judged by the teacher to have more behavioral problems and more difficulties in school and social adaptation than did their sibs or the comparison group. The behavioral difficulties related to reduced attentiveness, less cooperation in social behavior in classroom, increased distractability, lower resistance levels to fatigue, and a tendency to be socially isolated and withdrawn and less forthcoming and less volunteering in classwork. Wondering whether the teacher's judgment reflected a halo effect stemming from the fact that these children were in fact duller than the comparison children or than the sibs, we decided to get a judgment of social behavior and social attachment from the children's peers as well as from their teacher. We did a sociometric examination of every classroom on the island. This was a 100 per cent follow-up, and it covered the entire island from Kingston all the way to Negril, a distance of 125 miles. We asked members of the class to list the three boys they most liked to play with. The sibs were chosen by their classmates as frequently as were the comparison cases, but the index children were chosen very infrequently indeed and significantly less often than their siblings who had not been malnourished.

These are some of the findings of our studies, and they leave us convinced that malnutrition is making a contribution above and beyond the child's familial circumstances, above and beyond the particular environmental opportunities that he experiences. However, whenever you do these studies there is a nagging, nagging problem. It runs like this: Whenever we look at risk conditions and make comparisons, we find what we call a condition of risk if children exposed to it emerge with significantly more frequent negative outcomes than do children in a group that has not been exposed to this condition. This is true for low birth weight, for example. In her paper (pp. 42–52), Dr. Hertzig indicates that some 44 per cent of the children in a particular birth weight range and without social disadvantage were neurologically impaired at the end of a particular follow-up period. But I'd like to emphasize the other side: namely, that 56 per cent of the children are not impaired. Why is it that 44 percent are impaired and 56 per cent are not impaired? Let's look at our malnutrition cases. Are all the children who were seriously malnourished now functioning less well than their sibs who were not malnourished? Of course not. The trend is in this direction, but there are a number of the children who were malnourished and yet who function as well as their sibs and as well as the comparison cases. The intriguing problem, if we move from risk condition to mechanisms for the production of defective outcome, is to identify why some of these children exposed to the condition of risk turn out badly and others are spared. What is the basis for this? This is the problem that emerges in the risk condition work in any of our studies. Over the last several months, I must say I have been obsessed with this problem.

It's not the first time I have been obsessed with a problem, but this one really has its hooks into me. So I began to think about it. All of our risk condition work is from the point of view of a model design that could be called a critical event analysis — in other words, an episodic study which says that at a particular time in life, so-and-so was severely malnourished, or at the time of conception so-and-so's mother was schizophrenic, or at the time of birth, so-and-so was low birth weight, or at another point, so-and-so was anoxic. We deal with an episode in a developmental course. Can we approach the problem not from the point of view of an intermittent analysis, from episode to criterion, from episode to outcome as it were, but can we try to look at it developmentally?

Well, what I'm in the middle of doing in the nutritional area is just that. Some children who come to the hospital with severe malnutrition, with marasmus and kwashiorkor, were developing well before their hospitalization. Then their mother's milk failed, or they got some infection, or the mother got some infection, or there was a social dislocation; in turn, there was an abrupt, critical, and severe exposure to food lack with severe downward course, rapid weight loss, and the development of serious malnutrition with edema and depigmentation and a variety of other pathology, all requiring hospitalization if the child is to survive. Now that's one child. Another child has a different course. He starts out at the same point, same birth weight, as the first child, but where the other child is growing adequately, he is getting just enough to keep him alive. Surviving marginally, he is chronically stunted and ill, and at a given point he goes over the brink; he abruptly develops symptoms of severe malnutrition, and he is hospitalized. Should the consequences of the identifying hospitalization episode be the same for the acute and the chronic case? The work of Winick (1968; Winick & Rosso, 1969), for example, or Dobbing (1964) or Zamenhof (1968) would suggest that chronic subnutrition should result in a reduced number of brain cells, reduced myelination, and altered enzymatic organization to a considerable degree, all more than would be the case for an individual who was developing otherwise normally and then abruptly went downhill. This is fascinating, but how can you tell who was which, when the children come to the hospital from out of the bush? How can you, from the case history in a scale-less country, find out from the mother whether there was a normal weight gain or normal growth gain? When there has been no pediatrician, what pediatric record are you going to look at? You need not be helpless because nutritional inadequacy is registered in the growth of long bone. Chronic subnutrition is reflected in stunting. Abrupt malnutrition is reflected in acute disorganizations of electrolytes and other metabolites, but the child doesn't shrink. Therefore, you can identify two groups at hospitalization, shorties and tallies, both equally clinically ill, both equally severely sick, both at the same risk of death from malnutrition at this point, but one a case of chronic malnutrition and the other a case of acute malnutrition.

We have studied children 8–10 years later in school. What has happened in between? Is there a rehabilitation course? Can individuals recover when confronted with the mythology that there is no recovery? Just because brain and cell number don't recover, this does not mean that behavioral competence can't recover. We have little or no knowledge about the relation between the number of brain cells that need to be destroyed to have permanent impairment on a neurologic basis. The work of Lashley (1929) and others suggests strongly that the brain is redundant in its cell number and a considerable number of cells can be lost without any serious loss in functional capacity. We then have the post-illness period. Some children in the post-illness period get good nutrition and recover and grow rapidly during this period, so at school age they are relatively tall. Others over that 6–10 years do not have good nutritional conditions, and at school age they are stunted. So you have tallies and shorties at school age. Are they the same as tallies and shorties at the time of hospitalization? No. So you now have four groups: tall-talls, tall-shorts, short-talls, and short-shorts. Tall-talls were children who were growing well who were acutely sick. After they recovered from their illness, they functioned well. They would do splendidly. What about tall-shorts? They were doing well up to the time of hospitalization. Thereafter they were subjected not only to the acute episode, but to a chronic period of subnutrition. They should do less well. What about the short-talls? That's a fascinating group. It was chronically stunted in the pre-illness period, but in the post-illness period, it had relatively better conditions, and opportunities for recovery existed, so that hypothetically, if rehabilitation can be effective, they should do as well or almost as well as the tall-talls. And what about the short-shorts? They should be at the bottom of the barrel. They should be the ones who do not function well at all. What do we find? In every comparison tall-talls are not different from their controls. Tall-shorts in every comparison are significantly different from their controls; they do less well. Short-talls do almost as well as their controls and almost as well as the tall-talls. And the short-shorts are at the bottom of the barrel; they function worse on every measure that you can look at.

This suggests that the acute crisis model episode when viewed developmentally results in four developmentally definable subpopulations with different consequences attaching to the life experience of these individuals as it may affect subsequent development. I am in the middle of this analysis, and the more I work with this model, the more it seems to me that it begins to pose different questions for us in looking at risk conditions. In short, what we really have to begin to know is what were the antecedant circumstances to the exposure to risk — namely, what was the organism that came into the condition of risk? Second, to what extent were the conditions that preceded the risk event continued in the subsequent life of the individual or to what extent were compensatory opportunities present in his life circumstances? To the degree that we move from episodic analysis to longitudinal and linear analysis of the developmental course of the individual, we begin to define the risk conditions in more appropriate ways and to identify opportunities for appropriate intervention. If I had been asked six months ago whether I thought that nutritional and social rehabilitation could produce relatively full recovery in seriously malnourished children, on the basis of my then episodic analysis, I would have said no. Today I do not say that. I think that the evidence suggests strongly that the pessimistic picture of a malnourished child doomed to stupidity and ignorance with a nonrehabilitable permanent impairment is not borne out by developmental analysis of the data and that opportunities for intervention and rehabilitation do exist.

Well, those are a few of the highlights of a program of investigation in which we are looking at a variable that quite clearly is one that occurs in interaction with social conditions of relative advantage and disadvantage, of one that occurs in connection with different familial subgroupings, and so on. Within this framework, what I have tried to indicate is the degree to which a systematic family of inquiries addressing itself to questions which are identified can permit us to come to relatively firm answers with respect to these questions, and move us from what is essentially associative analysis between episode and its criterion, episode and outcome, to an analysis which leads us to developmental hypotheses. With such hypotheses we may move from the conditions of risk to the conditions or processes that relate this condition of risk to the family of outcomes with which it happens to have its associations.

COMMENTARY

ROFF. One problem I wonder if you've run into is taking 10 different babies and giving them what is objectively the same deprivation, none more deprived than others, and determining how each one turns out.

BIRCH. The general problem you raise is, of course, a problem that goes with a family of issues which the microbiologist and epidemiologist Theobold Smith pointed to many years ago. All ten members of his laboratory staff, including himself, volunteered to have their throats painted with a culture of streptococci. You see, heroism is not gone — Walter Reed rides again and all that. And in the Arrowsmith atmosphere that characterized that laboratory, what happened to the ten all smeared with the same culture of streptococci? Two got sore throats, seven had nothing happen to them, and one got a serious renal infection. In other words, the risk rate in this population was 30 per cent for negative or pathologic outcome, for exposure to the risk condition. This is fairly high, but obviously the not-risk rate was 70 per cent. One of the mechanisms is the existence of different numbers of phagocytes and effective eaters of bacteria in the blood streams of the different individuals. A second is the presence of different tissue resistances including different lysozymes and other enzymatic inhibitors of intracellular penetrants of the bacteria themselves. A third is a series of immune mechanisms — individual differences with respect to the levels of immunity. We are confronted then with individual differences in susceptibility, also involving numerous mechanisms. Among the mechanisms, for example, are those related to the nature of the endocrine response to stress, so that in certain strains of organisms that are nutritionally stressed you have profound effects upon adrenal and thyroid function, whereas in others this is minimal.

In other words, the host organism is one of the factors that contributes to the effectiveness of exposure to any particular condition of risk.

We know little about these host factors, although we have some hypotheses. One hypothesis is that when there are individual differences attributable to the host, they derive from differences in the ancestral history of the host — by which we mean in some instances the nature of selection, assortative matings, and gene pools that have contributed to the genetic endowment of this host, and in other instances we mean the intrauterine conditions that have characterized this individual and his ancestors over successive generations. Thus, one consequence of malnutrition in prior generations is to stunt the mother, to increase the likelihood of a stunted intrauterine growth, to increase the likelihood of defective functioning in the neonatal period, and to increase risk of subsequent functioning, in contrast to growing in another kind of uterus. So hypothetically, we have both acquired influences affecting the individual and transmitted and assorted genetic organizations affecting the individual. But we really don't know what these mechanisms are and what the mechanisms of individual difference are at this point in time.

A number of people have argued that it is relatively futile to attempt to define these sources for individual differences under conditions in which an enormous amount of nonorganismic variance exists. In other words, in a situation in which there can be either contributions from ancestral history in the sense of assortative genetic transmission or ancestral history and contemporary experience with respect to environment, the variance of the phenotype is the sum of the variances that can be attributed to environmental factors and to genetic factors. But that's only half the equation, because genetics is not even hypothetically democratic, and presumptively, particular gene pools are associated in particular environmental circumstances. The equation thus far reads: variance phenotype $=$ Variance G $+$ Variance E, to which must be added a term correlation between G and E, $+K$ or some constant times correlation of G and E. But that's not all. The phenotype is now the product of the environment. For example, the set of genes that define the shape of the milkweed plant produce a graceful leafy plant when the plant is growing in the lowlands, but when Haldane put it up on a mountain, he got a plant that looks like a cabbage. Thus, the fourth term in the equation becomes a function of G times E.

Our ability to handle these sources for variance is inadequate. And when we find low interaction terms in our analyses, these reflect not low interactions, but ignorance. In other words, they reflect, in Jensen's (1969) data, for example, absence of data, not absence of a process. Scarr-Salapatek (1971) has explored the interesting hypothesis that heritability coefficients among monozygotic twin pairs would be a reflection of the degree to which they were or were not in optimal environments. She argued that individuals in suboptimal environments would have enormous environmental contributions of a variable kind to the production of the phenotype. Consequently, phenotypic differences across twin pairs could be quite great, whereas if they were reared under relatively benign conditions, gene expression would have its fullest opportunity and relations with respect to heritability would be very high. She studied all identifiable twin pairs in the Philadelphia school system, making careful zygosity determinations and relating twins' achievements in school to their degree of kinship in a standard heritability analysis. She found a heritability coefficient of about .80 for middle-class twins, but heritability coefficients approaching 0 for lower-class twins, particularly black twins. Thus, the same degree of zygosity under these conditions results in a different heritability coefficient as a consequence of the different interaction mixes and contributors to variance. She argues that if you are really interested in the contribution that the genetic differences among individuals make to outcome, you have the responsibility for optimizing the environmental opportunities for their growth because only under optimal conditions will you have the full expression of individual differences in a genetic sense.

On a blackboard, I could lay out a mathematical model with degrees of kinship going down as one column, and systematic variations in environments going across in rows. Each cell would then represent the particular levels product that would attach to populations of given zygosity under given conditions of mix. With this model you can do a very interesting transformation that I have been playing with for the last year or so. Taking the grand mean for the entire matrix, you can subtract the row and column means from each cell and add to it your grand mean, and your residual there is your interaction residual. You can then define which conditions produced the greatest interactions, you can define the quality of interaction, you can make certain theoretical predictions with respect to the model, and so on. It's a fascinating mathematical model and an obvious one to use if you assume a linear system and assume that your task is the partitioning of variance. Then you can explore an appropriate set of graded differences in zygosity and an appropriate set of graded (or scaled) differences in environmental circumstances hypothetically relevant to this issue.

This is the kind of model that we need in all of our work. I haven't used it yet in the nutritional area, but I'm trying to see how it might be used. I would propose it as a model for looking at zygosity relations and outcomes with respect to schizophrenia or any of a variety of other issues. It's a lovely linear model that a child can handle from the point of view of doing an analysis of variance by simple addition, subtraction, and defining an interaction term by arithmetic transformation. You don't need a calculator or a computer, and you can analyze your data in a day. And it is the appropriate model for looking at what we want to look at.

ZUBIN. Some people have tried that, haven't they?

BIRCH. Yes, Fowkes and Jinks in England began a partial attempt in that direction.

ZUBIN. The trouble that they came across, as I am sure you know, is that if you had a measurable quantity, indicating the degree of blood relationship, and if it were linear, you could compute the correlation for closer and closer degrees of relationship. However, when you try to relate the correlation between differences in the environment, or environmental similarities, we don't have any measure for that. Environmental similarity is still not scaled.

BIRCH. Exactly. So what we need to do, and you put your finger on it exactly, is to develop an appropriate scaling method for defining hypothetically different environments, and this we have not yet done.

ZUBIN. These are very exciting models for discussion, and I think what you have done over the course of years is really admirable. Certainly you haven't limited yourself to the physical conditions of known etiology and appreciable ways of measuring the effect of inadequate nutrition. Compared with the problems we have in schizophrenia, this is almost like an open territory — even though, when you have looked at it, it turned out to be far from open territory. Do you ever envisage what to do when you do not know the cause of the condition and you do not have a measure identifying its presence, or any way of seeing how it varies?

BIRCH. When I encounter a condition like that, I pick up a little book by Peter Medawar called *The Art of the Soluble* (1967). In criticizing Koestler, the author, who was speaking about grand breakthroughs in science and attachment to important problems by science, Medawar starts by saying that a working scientist always recognizes that science is the art of the soluble, in the same sense that politics is the art of the possible. Nobody will credit you for valiant work on an insoluble question, so your first task as a scientist is to formulate your problem or subproblem in such a way that it is soluble. We do this in any effective work.

In the area with which we are concerned, there are a family of questions that require more careful resolution and definition if we are to convert concern into practicable scientific inquiry. Concern bears the same relation to science as desire does to demand in economics, where demand is desire backed by the ability to pay. That makes it real. In science, concern not backed by the appropriate formulation and technology is scientific sentimentalism.

Within that framework, what are the particular tasks and problems we have? The first thing, obviously, if we are concerned with a particular outcome, is a set of ground rules for identifying what that outcome condition is. If we are still in the stage of arguing that what you describe as schizophrenia in your studies and what somebody else describes as schizophrenia in his studies are not the same, and you find different findings, this is parallel play. What is required is some uniform definition of the entity, operational definitions that can be effectively applied; in the absence of this, any kind of variations can occur. With respect to consideration of environments, we have to demand far more powerful conceptual and analytic tools than have thus far been forthcoming. The use of Guttman's scaling models, for example, or any of a variety of other models for the scaling of environments is a way in which we can delineate that dimension of the matrix with which we need to be concerned. At present we haven't done it. Certainly, there has been no uniformity in how it is delineated across situations and elsewhere. As a consequence, there can be no comparability among studies, either of effects or of interactions. We can have argument, but we can't have productive controversy. We are at the stage of developing the technologies for studying the problems rather than at the stage of indeed studying the issues.

ZUBIN. If you are in a position where your laboratory and all your ventures are concerned with mental disorders, you can't satisfy yourself with saying, "Well, we aren't ready yet"; you have to do something about it. The solution, I think, lies not in demanding such rigor as you have posed, though that should come eventually; the solution lies in having operational definitions to begin with.

BIRCH. Yes, that's what I said a moment ago.

ZUBIN. And then perhaps setting up "as if" models — that is, venture forth under some daring new concept under the guise of "wouldn't it be funny if this were really the case" — and see where that leads you.

BIRCH. Yes, I think that there is an enormous opportunity in what the physicists call gedank experiments — a kind of brainstorming, the adoption of an as-if attitude.

SCHAIRER. That's called hypothesis, isn't it?

BIRCH. Sometimes. But most hypotheses are the anticipation of a fact rather than the extension of a theory. In other words, most "hypotheses" are really inferences rather than true hypotheses.

RICKS. Knowing of your sequential series of studies, I begin to wonder, What is he going to do next? My guess is to study the intrauterine environment and the nutrition of the mother.

BIRCH. Already did that.

RICKS. You don't have time to tell us about that?

BIRCH. Much of the concern with this area began with the uterus of the mother. A decade ago Marty Gittelman, Margaret Hertzig, and others as well as me began to study the relation of the obstetrical course to intellectual competence in all children in the total population of a city, Aberdeen, Scotland (Birch et al., 1970). Our choice reflected the art of the soluble. In Aberdeen there is a uniform obstetrical service. The obstetrical service is a research unit for the whole community; it's free to the duchess and her cook. There are uniform records for all pregnancies, there is continuous monitoring of the accuracy of information placed in all records by all clinicians working, there is a fulltime data clerk corps that examines all case records and spot-checks physicians' accuracy, and so forth. This has been going on since 1947. It is an obstetrical service which had as its first member an obstetrician with vision, whose first appointment was that of a splendid statistician, whose second appointment was a sociologist, whose third appointment was a splendid epidemiologist, and whose next appointments were obstetricians. He then established a research service. Within this framework, we could look at all pregnancies, all births, and so on. One of the most profitable ways of doing this is to look at the subsequent development of the children about whose circumstances and births we know so much. Again, we were fortunate in that there were available in Aberdeen good medical and educational records for all children attending public schools in the city. And with colleagues in Aberdeen we made detailed clinical studies of appropriately drawn samples of schoolchildren drawn from complete age groups of children.

In our study we compared mentally backward children and children who were backward in learning, with matched controls in the same class at school and with the total population of children of similar age in the city. The numbers were large enough for us to analyze the data by social class of parents; the height, age, reproductive history, and living conditions of the mothers; and the biological and social factors affecting our index cases.

When we looked at the mentally subnormal children in our Aberdeen population we found, as others have, that they could be divided into two broad groups differentiated at about IQ 50 by the severity of their mental handicaps and biological concomitants.

But what of the social conditions in which these children were being reared? The social class, as measured by the occupation of the father, provides a useful index of the familial environment. When we looked at the two sets of retarded youngsters, the severely retarded group and the mildly retarded group, we found that the social class distribution of their families was quite different. Mental subnormality of severe degree is not a respector of social class, and the prevalence rates do not differ by the social class of the parents. But what about relatively moderate and mild subnormality? From the upper to the lower social class, the gradient is like a ski slope. There is a twentyfold increase in the frequency of mild subnormality in the unskilled working class as contrasted with the non-manual working group in the community.

What's this related to obstetrically? Nothing fancy like surgical problems and so on. It's related to how well the baby grows in the uterus. The most striking single finding in this total community study is that whereas 6 per cent of children stratified by appropriate social class designations now in the total population are at low birth weight, 37 per cent of these mild cases are low in birth weight and at low weight for gestational age. So something was wrong with how they grew in the uterus. We looked at their mothers and found that it is not all mothers in the lower social class who are overrepresented in this sample, but it's the stunted mothers. Orr's (1936) dire prediction was being borne out in the study: a mother's being stunted in her childhood is one of the most significant factors influencing her reproductive efficiency, the growth of her offspring, the adequacy of the intrauterine environment, and the size and therefore the risk at which the propositus is.

These kinds of concerns then led a number of us who were working in Aberdeen to move to warmer climates to look at problems of serious malnutrition. Angus Thomson, the epidemiologist in the group, went to the Gambia to look at problems of malnutrition in this community and its interaction with infectious disease, particularly the parasitic disorder known as malaria, which is the major condition in that swamp in Western Africa. I went to Latin America, to Jamaica, and so on. A number of us took on this problem as a consequence of a concern with the very problem that you are posing. I left this out because I had to begin somewhere and I thought I would begin a little earlier.

REFERENCES

Birch, H. G., & Lefford, A. Intersensory development in children. *Monographs of the Society for Research in Child Development*, 1963, 28 (5, Serial No. 89.)

Birch, H. G., Richardson, S. A., Baird, D., Horobin, G., & Illsley, R. *Mental subnormality in the community: A clinical and epidemiologic study*. Baltimore: Williams & Wilkins, 1970.

Birch, H. G., Piñeiro, C., Alcalde, E., Toca, T., & Cravioto, J. Relation of kwashiorkor in early childhood and intelligence at school age. *Pediatric Research*, 1971, 5, 579–585.

Birch, H. G., & Richardson, S. H. The functioning of Jamaica school children severely malnourished during the first two years of life. In *Nutrition, the nervous system and behavior*. Proceedings of the Seminar on Malnutrition in Early Life and Subsequent Mental Development. Mora, Jamaica, Jan. 10–14, 1972. Pan American Health Organization, WHO Scientific Publication No. 251, 1972. Pp. 64–72.

Boas, F. Changes in the bodily form of descendents of immigrants. Immigration Commission Doc. 208, Washington, D.C.: GPO, 1910.

Cabak, V., & Najdanvic, R., Effect of undernutrition in early life on physical and mental development. *Archives of Disease in Childhood*, 1965, 40, 523–534.

Cravioto, J., Birch, H. G., DeLicardie, E. R., Rosales, L., & Vega, L. The ecology of growth and development in a Mexican preindustrial community. Report 1: Method and findings from birth to one month of age. *Monographs of the Society for Research in Child Development*, 1969, 34 (5, Serial No. 129).

Cravioto, J., DeLicardie, E. R., & Birch, H. G. Nutrition, growth and neurointegrative development: An experimental and ecologic study. *Pediatric Monograph Supplement*, 1966, 38, 319.

Davison, A. N., & Dobbing, J. Myelination as a vulnerable period in brain development. *British Medical Bulletin*, 1966, 22, 40–44.

Dobbing, J. The influence of early nutrition on the development and myelination of the brain. *Proceedings of the Royal Society of Medicine*, 1964, 159, 503–509.

Greulich, W. W. Growth of children of the same race under different environmental conditions. *Science*, 1958, 127, 515–516.

Hertzig, M. E., Birch, H. G., Richardson, S. A., & Tizard, J. Intellectual levels of school children severely malnourished during the first two years of life. *Pediatrics*, 1972, 49, 814–824.

Jensen, A. How much can we boost IQ and scholastic achievement? *Harvard Educational Review*, 1969, 39, 1–123.

Keys, A., Brozek, J., Henschel, A., Mickelson, O., & Taylor, H. L. *The biology of human starvation*. Vol. 2. Minneapolis: University of Minnesota Press, 1950.

Lashley, K. S. *Brain mechanisms and intelligence*. Chicago: University of Chicago Press, 1929.

Lesser, G. S., Fifer, G., & Clark, D. H., Mental abilities of children from different social class and cultural groups. *Monographs of the Society for Research in Child Development*, 1965, 30 (4, Serial No. 102).

Medawar, P. *The art of the soluble*. London: Methuen, 1967.

Orr, J. B. *Food, health and income*. London: Macmillan, 1936.

Richardson, S. A., Birch, G. H., Grabie, E., & Yoder, K. The behavior of children in school who were severely malnourished in the first two years of life. *Journal of Health and Social Behavior*, 1972, 13, 276–284.

Richardson, S. A., Birch, H. G., & Hertzig, M. E. School performance of children who were severely malnourished in infancy. *American Journal of Mental Deficiency*, 1973 (in press).

Scarr-Salapatek, S. Race, social class, and IQ. *Science*, 1971, 174, 1285–1295.

Winick, M. Nutrition and cell growth. *Nutrition Review*, 1968, 26, 195–197.

———— & Rosso, P. The effect of severe early malnutrition in cellular growth of human brain. Pediatric Research, 1969, 3, 181–184.

Zamenhof, S., Van Marthens, E., & Margolis, F. L. DNA (cell number) and protein in neonatal brain: Alteration by material dietary protein restriction. *Science*, 1968, 160, 322–323.

DAVID ROSENTHAL *Issues in*
High-Risk Studies of Schizophrenia

In the field of schizophrenia research, a bandwagon movement that would warm a candidate's heart has been gathering increased momentum during the past decade, and at this point we cannot yet tell if the movement has peaked or not. Of course, I am referring to those research projects which have been subsumed under the name "high-risk studies."

The idea of studying people at risk for various disorders is hardly new, and has been used in studies of medical diseases for a long time. Even with respect to mental disorders, the germ of the high-risk idea can be traced at least as far back as Thomas Willis, who in the late seventeenth century stated, "It is a common observation that men, born of parents that are sometimes wont to be mad, will be obnoxious to the same disease." Such a statement cries out for these children of mad parents to be examined, evaluated, and understood.

In the nineteenth century, efforts were made to examine the relatives of people who were thought to have what was called "hereditary taint," with the intention of seeing what the prevalence of such taint would be in the relatives of tainted index cases as compared with the relatives of normal persons. In the twentieth century, investigators invented the term *morbidity risk* for such studies, but the studies became more sophisticated in conception and method. The underlying concept of morbidity risk is statistical, an effort being made to describe the incidence of a given disorder in the relatives of people afflicted with that disorder and the incidence in the population at large or in a selected sample of normal controls. The concept of morbidity risk is still vital to an understanding of the role of heredity in various medical and mental disorders.

Why, then, has the risk concept now taken hold so strongly in schizophrenia research? As I see it, the current trend toward risk research had its beginnings with Barbara Fish (1957) and David Sobel (1961). Fish, who was strongly influenced by the thought and research of Lauretta Bender, tried to identify characteristics that represented early signs of future schizophrenia in neonatal offspring of schizophrenic mothers. She pointed out that research into "the underlying constitutional factors . . . would undoubtedly be advanced if it were possible to detect schizophrenia or its antecedents early in life, and study the developing manifestations by direct observation." She also noted that "it is difficult to prove from the data on adult patients whether the physiological dysfunctions are the cause of schizophrenia or only the end result of many years of severe tension or of conditions secondary to hospitalization."

Clearly, Fish worked under the assumption that schizophrenia was an inherited illness and that manifestations of the genetic defect would already be manifest in affected newborns. She hypothesized that poor integration of neurological development in infancy was the analogue of the manifold integrative disorders found in the later course of schizophrenia. Sobel, who was impressed by Fish's research strategy, but not at all by her theoretical base, examined eight babies, each of which had *both* parents schizophrenic, the mother being a hospitalized patient. Four of the children were reared by their schizophrenic parents, and four were placed in foster homes. Sobel reported that three of the eight babies developed clear-cut signs of emotional disturbance in infancy and that these three babies were reared by their schizophrenic parents, whereas none of the four babies reared by foster parents showed such disturbances. Sobel concluded that it was the severely inappropriate rearing by the schizophrenic parents that led to the emotional disturbances found in the babies. Thus, the stage was set for introducing the heredity-environment issue into high-risk studies of schizophrenia even before the term *high-risk* was introduced into schizophrenia research. Fish pointed out the possibility of early manifestation in hereditary risk, and Sobel's work emphasized the importance of assuring that the loading of hereditary or environmental risk in the child was there, if either was to prove relevant at all.

Still, it is clear that the bandwagon rush to high-risk studies in schizophrenia had its main impetus in the brilliantly conceived study of Sarnoff Mednick and Fini Schulsinger in Denmark (Mednick, 1967; Mednick & Schulsinger, 1968, 1970). There were several reasons for this. First of all Mednick detailed forcefully the disadvantages in trying to learn about the etiology of schizophrenia from a study of schizophrenic patients themselves. He re-emphasized the well-known fact that many of the differences observed between schizophrenics and controls might be reflecting the effects of the schizophrenic illness rather than the causes, and he called special attention to the deleterious psychological and behavioral effects of chronic hospitalization. He elaborated on Fish's point about the advantages of studying individuals in detail before they develop the clinical illness, so that information regarding possible etiology of the disorder would not have to be obtained retrospectively but could be based on information obtained before the illness became manifest. Also, Mednick (1958) had a provocative theory about the etiology of schizophrenia, based on popular learning theory and experimental studies, which seemed to permit confirmation or disconfirmation — a goal that is often difficult to achieve, especially in studies of mental disorders.

Another important factor in their success was Mednick and Schulsinger's evaluation of a large number of subjects at risk. By contrast, Fish and Sobel had been forced to deal with small N's, and Fish, for unfortunate reasons, was unable to accumulate an appropriate control group. Whereas the main data in both the Fish and Sobel studies were based on clinical assessments by the experimenters themselves (years later, when Fish's subjects were age 10 and 18, independent observers confirmed her predictions of schizophrenia; Fish et al., 1965), the Mednick and Schulsinger study invested heavily in objective methods that yielded quantitative data. They obtained 207 index cases who had been born of schizophrenic mothers. They matched the index cases by pairs, so that if one of a pair became schizophrenic, he could be compared with his matched index case. They then selected one control subject for each pair of index subjects, basing the selection on factors that might be implicated in the development of the disorder — age, sex, father's occupational status, rural or urban residence, years of formal education, and institutional-versus family-rearing conditions.

Another reason why they stimulated a bandwagon effect was the simple fact that Mednick and Schulsinger were first to use the term *high-risk* to identify their index subjects. In this way they gave this type of research a name and a sense of identity that facilitated discussion and appreciation of it.

Lastly, the bandwagon effect burgeoned because the Mednick-Schulsinger study turned up so many provocative significant findings that one could almost read them to say "the road to success." Imitation is not only a form of flattery; it suggests that the imitator hopes to derive as much benefit from a given act as the individual who is being imitated. Thus, at least for these reasons, and possibly because researchers in the fifties had not appreciated the strategic implications of the Fish study, Mednick and Schulsinger paved the road along which the bandwagon would roll in the sixties and seventies.

It is worth noting that Mednick's main goal in resorting to the research design he and Schulsinger formulated was no less than the discovery of the cause of schizophrenia. He states, "The 'high-risk sample' method . . . stands out as the research strategy most likely to yield information on the etiology of schizophrenia" (Mednick, 1967, p. 184). This high hope for the method is rather surprising, since most theories of the etiology of schizophrenia are predicated around either a genetic theory with an implied proximal metabolic cause, or a theory of intra-familial behavioral patterns which are thought to be schizophrenogenic. Clearly, however, Mednick never intended to evaluate in any depth either the genetic properties of his sample or the intra-familial climates in which the children were reared.

The term *high-risk* is not to be taken in its literal sense. For example, Mednick-Schulsinger and others usually choose index cases who are the offspring of a schizophrenic parent. The morbidity risk for schizophrenia among such a group of subjects ranges between 7 and 17 per cent, with a median expectancy of about 10 per cent. This means that about 90 per cent of the subjects are not at risk for the clinical illness. Whether this expectancy rate should be thought of as high-risk is a matter of opinion, since if we tried to predict which children would become clinically schizophrenic, knowing nothing else about them, we would be wrong nine times out of ten. If however, one chooses index cases who have both parents schizophrenic, as Erlenmeyer-Kimling has (1968), the morbidity risk runs in the range of 35 to 45 per cent; no one would hesitate to call such index cases high-risk subjects. Reed (1972), of the Dight Institute, which has had over 3,000 genetic counseling cases in the last twenty years, says, "Few people consider a risk of a repetition of a serious defect in their children under about 25 per cent to be serious . . . Risks of under 10 per cent are not considered to be particularly threatening. Risk figures of from 1 to 5 per cent are not of great concern because the usual risk for the whole population of an abnormal child is of about this magnitude" (p. 316). Perhaps the term *elevated risk* would be a more accurate designation of the Mednick-Schulsinger index cases, but the phrase *high-risk* is here to stay.

THE GOALS OF HIGH-RISK RESEARCH

Although Mednick sees the goal of high-risk research as understanding the etiology of schizophrenia, there are actually several important goals of such research. However, in the main, all high-risk studies are essentially prospective-longitudinal studies. The investigators have an end point in mind, the clinical illness itself. Wanting to know something about the background of people who eventually become schizophrenic, the investigator sets out to record what he considers to be the major milestones that the subject traverses along the road toward a schizophrenic outcome. Thus, the method implies that the investigator will have more or less continued contact with the subjects, and that this contact will continue at least until the entire subject sample will have lived through the age of risk for developing the illness. During that time he will administer tests, record observations, obtain reports about the subjects from various sources such as family, school, or clinic — accumulating a mountain of information to be filed, coded, statistically analyzed, and theoretically evaluated.

What the investigator eventually finds and reports will depend in large measure on the kinds of subjects he chooses to study. At the present time, most people are investigating the offspring of a schizophrenic parent because statistical evidence suggests that there will be ten times as many schizophrenics in such a sample as in a sample from the population at large. However, there may be other samples of subjects who may also have an elevated vulnerability for schizophrenia, but who present different prodromal histories and different characteristics of the developing illness. For example, an investigator might choose to do high-risk studies of children who have a broken home, or children who have a domineering mother and a passive father, or children of parents thought to be double-binding or to fragment the child's attention. He could as well begin his study with children who already have some known symptom or feature, such as children who have a reading disability, children who are functioning at a level considerably below their potential, children who are deemed uncontrollable or run away from home, or children who are hyperactive or enuretic, have a low attention span, walk in their sleep, take drugs, are funny-looking, and so on. (Clinical studies of adolescents who are underachieving, or who have run away from home, are being carried out at the National Institute of Mental Health.) Although the yield of subsequent schizophrenia may be lower in such samples as compared with a sample of children who have a schizophrenic parent, the rate of schizophrenia among such samples may eventually turn out to be appreciably higher than the rate in the population at large. Also, quite different experimental and clinical features might be manifested during the maturing years in the different samples of subjects.

Much of the prodromal behavior that Mednick and Schulsinger observe in their subjects, either experimentally or clinically, will reflect either some genetic contribution, some environmental factors associated with having a schizophrenic parent, or perhaps some combination of both. These factors are not easily teased apart. How, then, can the investigators achieve their goal of understanding the etiology of schizophrenia? From Mednick's viewpoint, the problem is not serious because he uses the high-risk method to test a specific theory of the etiology of schizophrenia based on principles of learning, and he makes predictions about what he expects to find in his subjects, according to the theory. If the predictions are borne out, then he can maintain that this evidence supports his theory. If not, then his mission has failed. Thus, from his point of view, the heredity-environment issue has only distal, secondary bearing on the mechanisms, essentially psychological, which he believes lead to clinical schizophrenia.

Does Mednick really find evidence to support his predictions? Yes and no. Mednick's (1958) theory involves the reciprocal augmentation of anxiety and stimulus generalization. The schizophrenic process begins with high anxiety, which is seen as a form of drive. The tendency to high anxiety may be inherited or learned. An important aspect of this high anxiety is that it habituates or extinguishes slowly. When the anxiety is high, stimulus generalization increases so that more stimuli are able to potentiate the slowly habituating anxiety. The increased potentiation in turn leads to increasingly higher anxiety levels, which lead in turn to increased stimulus generalization. This anxiety-generalization spiral culminates eventually in the schizophrenic break. The features of the theory with regard to the schizophrenic illness itself need not concern us here. Since *anxiety* is such a slippery term, Mednick chooses to identify it with responses mediated by the autonomic nervous system, especially electrodermal responses. The theory predicts that the GSR (galvanic skin response) to a loud or stressful stimulus should be greater in the index cases than in the controls. Indeed, this is what he finds. The theory also predicts that the GSR should be overgeneralized in the high-risk subjects, and again, this is what he finds. The theory also predicts that the GSR recovery from stress should be slower in the high-risk subjects than in the controls, but here the finding turns out to be exactly the opposite. Indeed, recovery from stress is considerably *faster* in the high-risk subjects.

Properly enough, Mednick has therefore revised his theory. He now points out why an abnormally fast recovery time is so necessary for the development of schizophrenia, according to his general theoretical paradigm, whereas he had originally pointed out why an abnormally slow recovery time was essential for the development of schizophrenia. A theory that can accommodate two diametrically opposed positions places its advocate in a precarious position with regard to any claim regarding the merits of that theory. Under such circumstances, the claim that the high-risk method, unaccompanied by additional controls, can yield critical information about the etiology of schizophrenia, can be accepted only with considerable reservation. Nevertheless, the modified theory remains viable, and we shall probably hear a lot more about it.

Mednick and Schulsinger are not averse to making inferences about the respective roles of heredity and environment in regard to the mental health of their subjects. In evaluating one body of data, for example, they examined their material in terms of the length of time the child had been separated from its mother during its first five years of life. They found that the high-risk group had markedly poorer mental health than the low-risk group, even when the amount of separation from the mother was equated for both groups. They concluded that the poorer mental health of the high-risk group probably could not be ascribed to separation from their parents, and that it would therefore seem possible to attribute their adjustment difficulties to genetic factors. However, the possibility that environmental factors other than separation might have contributed to the mental health differences in the high- and low-risk groups must be taken into account.

I mention this merely to point up the difficulty in trying to assess etiology from the usual kind of high-risk study. Of course, the possibility always exists that some finding will point toward a variable that seems to play an etiological role. Such a finding was turned up by Mednick and Schulsinger in the form of birth complications. This variable originally had no role in Mednick's theory of schizophrenia, but now Mednick and Schulsinger are doing further research on the potential role of birth complications in the development of schizophrenic disorder. The original finding of an association between perinatal birth complications and illness in their index cases was the kind of chance finding that occurs so often in science, and it was obtained because midwives' reports happened to be available and the investigators took the trouble to study them. If this finding holds up, Mednick and Schulsinger may indeed have brought to our attention a nongenetic but also nonpsychological variable that plays a significant role in determining whether schizophrenic psychopathology becomes manifest or not.

Mednick and Schulsinger have found that separation from the mother in the first five years of life can also make a difference with respect to outcomes in index cases, in that high-risk subjects with greater separation from the mother tended to have poorer mental health than index cases with less separation. Here again, the investigators provide us with a possible etiological factor in schizophrenia, but they recognize that it is difficult to determine whether the children were separated from their mothers because they already had poor mental health and were perhaps too difficult to care for, or whether the poor mental health came about as a result of the separation.

It follows from the above discussion that even though there may be difficulties in drawing hard and fast conclusions about etiology in the usual high-risk study, one clear and significant virtue of this type of research lies in the fact that the investigator may be able to uncover a number of precursors of schizophrenia. Thus, not only can Mednick and Schulsinger point to such precursors as birth complications, early extensive separation from the mother, and reports from teachers about the children's behavior and personality during their school years, but they can also delineate other premorbid variables that characterized the high-risk subjects during the prodromal period, including performance on IQ tests, word association tests, and various aspects of psychophysiological responses in a controlled experimental situation. By delineating a cluster of such aspects of personality functioning, the investigators are able to portray what the prodromal personality is like in schizophrenic disorder. The assessment of the contribution of genes or environments to the various components of the prodromal state is another matter, and perhaps a more difficult one.

I should like to call attention to one more aspect of the Mednick-Schulsinger study, because it seemed to have such great promise which was unfulfilled: that feature of the design in which high-risk subjects were matched in pairs. The intent was to be able to look back retrospectively to see what differences had existed in the two members of a pair when one subject broke down and the other remained healthy. Since they were both high-risk subjects with a schizophrenic mother, it was hoped that any differences found consistently within pairs would provide basic information about the etiological factors leading to illness in the sick subject. Unfortunately, the strategy failed for two reasons, according to the authors. First, the matched index cases who had not broken down were likely candidates for becoming ill, and could hardly be said to have developed more normally. This inference can readily be challenged. Second, the original matching had not included the subjects' psychiatric status at the time of the first examination. For these reasons, the authors abandoned the matched index case idea and turned instead to an analysis of a sick group comprising index cases who had broken down and a well group comprising retrospectively selected index cases whose level of adjustment at the time of the initial assessment was similar to that of the sick group, but who were currently well or even improved over their initial level of adjustment. The revised strategy implies that the initial level of adjustment was an important factor in whether the subjects became sick or not. If this is so, it suggests that the measures taken of the sick group during the initial examinations might not be reflecting etiological factors, but might in fact be measuring the extent to which the disorder had already developed, even if it could not be detected by the clinical interview. This possibility raises some question about the meaningfulness of the retrospective well group–sick group comparison, and arouses increased regrets that the original matching design was abandoned. Comparisons of the sick and well groups might in fact be subject to some of the same criticisms that Mednick had originally made in regard to comparisons of schizophrenic and control subjects.

Also with respect to the sick group–well group comparison, how reliable or meaningful were these ratings of adjustment level? Although Schulsinger, who made the ratings, is a gifted clinician, we have no idea about how difficult it is to make interview-based assessments of adolescents on a five-point scale for "adjustment," a rather loose concept. The judgment was based on "personal and environmental factors," variables which may not be easily weighed, especially when the information about them must be obtained from closemouthed youngsters on the other side of the generation gap.

In fact, when the authors examined the school adjustment of the "sick" and "well" subjects, they found that the "sick" group was indeed more seriously maladjusted in school than the "well" group. Although this finding could be interpreted to mean that the groups were truly matched for adjustment at the time of the interview and that the "sick" group became more maladjusted only in subsequent years, it seems more likely that the "sick" group was always more maladjusted, but that the difference in adjustment between the two groups could not be detected in the interview.

If this inference is correct, then the retrospective matching in regard to "adjustment" was not in order, and we must be prepared to acknowledge that the sick group–well group comparisons are in fact analogous to comparing schizophrenics with normal controls, thus aborting some of the primary aims of the high-risk study. From such comparisons we can learn only what the manifestations of the sickness may be at different ages. Such findings may well have clinical interest, and may be indirectly heuristic as well, but sick-well comparisons by themselves will very likely not tell much about the etiology of schizophrenia.

In my own collaborative studies of schizophrenia, my colleagues and I have also been concerned primarily with the goal of trying to make determinations about the etiology of the disorder. For the most part, we have been trying to elucidate the respective roles of genes and rearing in producing clinical schizophrenia or variant subforms of the disorder.

In our studies in Denmark (Kety et al., 1968; Rosenthal, 1970; Rosenthal et al., 1971), we have used formal adoption to separate the genetic and rearing variables. For example, we selected one group of subjects who had a biological parent who was schizophrenic. A second group of adoptees was selected because neither of their biological parents had had a registered psychiatric illness. A third group of adoptees was selected for study because, although they did not have a biological parent who was schizophrenic, they were given for adoption to a *rearing* parent who had some form of schizophrenic disorder. For additional comparative purposes, we also obtained a group of non-adoptees who had a biological parent who was schizophrenic and who were reared in the parental home for the first fifteen years of life. With these four groups of selected subjects, we are able to make group comparisons regarding a number of characteristics, in the hope of determining whether any of these characteristics are related to the genetic or the rearing factors associated with the clinical illness.

In a study carried out in Israel, we selected a group of index cases who had a schizophrenic parent and a set of matched controls with normal parents. One half of each group was reared in the usual nuclear family, and one half was born and reared in a kibbutz. In the Danish study, we made no effort to control for the manner of rearing, except for the group that we selected because one adopting parent had a form of schizophrenic disorder. However, rearing by parents with such disorders may vary appreciably, and we could not specify the details of such rearing for the entire group of subjects. By contrast, in the Israeli study we are able to specify more precisely the broad differences in the two kinds of rearing environments to which both index cases and controls are subjected. We hope to be able to specify whether certain traits in the subjects reflect the different kinds of rearing, the different kinds of genetic background, or the interactional effects of genes and the two kinds of rearing environments.

By designing studies in these ways, we hope to obtain some leverage on the difficult etiology problem. However, we must recognize that the etiological locus to which we may be able to ascribe different characteristics will be relatively crude — that is, we may not be able to say anything more than the fact that a particular personality trait, or a naturally occurring behavior, or a pattern of performance on a given test, was influenced primarily by heredity or by environment or by their interaction. We did not start out with a relatively well-formulated theory of etiology, on the basis of which we could make specific predictions. In this respect, Mednick's approach to the problem is more advanced than ours, but at this stage of knowledge about the etiology of schizophrenia, both approaches to the problem can make a contribution.

In Denmark, we are pursuing one additional goal of high-risk studies. We hope to be able to specify in our high-risk subjects a number of behavioral-psychological characteristics which can be identified as prodromal or subdromal manifestations of the schizophrenic genotype. The best way to achieve this goal is through comparisons of our index adoptees who had a biological schizophrenic parent with the control adoptees who did not. Both groups were given up for adoption to rearing parents who, we must assume, were selected randomly with respect to our particular goals. Under this assumption, we can infer that differences found between the two groups of adoptees represent the contribution of the independent variable built into the design, namely, having or not having a biological schizophrenic parent. The parental genes, of course, were passed on to the children, but were not accompanied by the behavioral contamination of these biological parents' rearing practices.

We are already able to make a few statements regarding prodromal or subdromal characteristics in carriers of the schizophrenic genotype. For example, we have generated some evidence that whether or not a selected subject emigrated from Denmark depended on whether or not he had a biological parent who was schizophrenic. Although the literature on migration and schizophrenia suggests that schizophrenics emigrate more often than non-schizophrenics, our tentative findings do not point in that direction. In fact, our subjects who did *not* have a biological schizophrenic parent did almost all of the emigrating. By contrast, the subjects who had a biological schizophrenic parent, whether they had been given up for adoption or reared in the parental home, rarely emigrated and, indeed, stayed put. The findings suggest that individuals who have the schizophrenic genotype, whether they are clinically schizophrenic or not, are likely not to be adventurous. They may in fact be manifesting a trait that Shakow (1971) believes to be a fundamental characteristic of schizophrenics, neophobia, which in real life situations may be manifested by an intense reluctance to take on anything new or to experience change. On the other hand, performance on a reaction time task, which has often proved to be an excellent discriminator of schizophrenics and normal controls, turns out to be influenced primarily by non-genetic factors. This is a finding that I had not entirely expected, but it was consistent and clear. Poorer reaction time performance was associated with rearing by schizophrenic parents, not with having the schizophrenic genotype.

In Israel, we carried out a neurological examination on 100 subjects between the ages of eight and fourteen. It was conducted by a child psychiatrist, Dr. Joseph Marcus, who had had special training with this type of examination. For each subject, he obtained a total neuropathology score. In all our studies, both in Denmark and Israel, the examiner had no knowledge of the index or control status of the subject. Dr. Marcus found that the bulk of the variation with respect to neuropathology scores was related to the index or control status of the subjects, and not to their rearing status. The neuropathology scores were significantly higher for the index group than the control group. However, the difference occurred entirely in the younger children. Among those over age eleven, the groups did not differ significantly. These results suggest that the neuropathology findings may reflect an immaturity or disturbance of neurological integration in the index cases, and that the immaturity aspects eventually resolve themselves in most cases with the coming of puberty. This finding lends support to Fish's original hypothesis.

FORMAL CHARACTERISTICS OF HIGH-RISK STUDIES

Age of Subjects. Mednick and Schulsinger chose index cases who were between the ages of ten and eighteen because such subjects were not so young that the investigators would have to wait for many decades to find out which of them would become schizophrenic, and at the same time, the subjects were old enough to be in the age of risk, or close to it, so that it could be safely predicted that a number of them would become schizophrenic before very many years had passed. In fact, the mean age of their sample was 15.1 years, the age which most investigators consider to be the beginning of the risk period. This means that well more than half of the subjects were in their middle to late teens and that some could already be showing early signs of schizophrenic illness. In our Israel study, the subjects were from eight to fourteen years old, and the results of our neurological examination indicated that signs of neurological disorder would be found in younger age groups — from age eight to eleven or even younger.

It may well be that the time to begin a high-risk study is at the very beginning of life. Indeed, a number of investigators have proposed to undertake such studies, and some are already in progress. For example, Garmezy* reports that Sameroff found that offspring of schizophrenic *and* of neurotically depressed mothers tended to have lower birth weights and lower APGAR scores. The greater the psychopathology in these mothers, the fewer spontaneous deliveries and normal fetal EEG's Sameroff found. Garmezy also reports that Schachter found that schizophrenic mothers did not differ from other psychiatric groups in complications of delivery or pregnancy, APGAR scores, abortions, or still births, but did find a higher rate of prematurity. When he exposed the babies to clicking noises at various intensities and intervals, he found the heart rate of the high-risk babies to be more variable and to show a greater rise in level than that of the babies of normal mothers.

Whether these findings have any bearing on a particular high-risk baby's becoming schizophrenic or not is a matter that will have to be resolved after many, many years of waiting and observing. However, such findings do suggest evidence of genetic influences, or the influences of birth and delivery complications, even in the first weeks of life.

Anthony (1968) has dealt with the age problem by stratifying his subjects into three age groups, preschool up to five years, elementary school to eleven years, and high school to seventeen years. In this way,

*These findings were reported by Dr. Norman Garmezy at a Neurosciences Research Program Work Session on Schizophrenia, May 9–11, 1971, and appear in Kety and Matthysse (1972). For more information, see Norman Garmezy, "Children at Risk: The Search for Antecedents of Schizophrenia," *Schizophrenia Bulletin,* in press.

he can directly compare his subjects of different ages, and follow the younger ones as they move into the next stratified age.

Longitudinal Aspects. Once an investigator has made his initial studies of high-risk children, he almost always finds it necessary to continue to study them, to observe their life course and any changes that may occur with respect to the development of psychopathology. Although for some purposes follow-up studies are neither necessary nor compelling, the investigator *must* carry out follow-up studies if he is ever to learn whether the earlier findings had any relation to the etiology of schizophrenic disorder. Thus, he must hope for a long life, a great deal of financial support, and the wisdom to know what kinds of examinations to conduct with his subjects as they progress from one age to another. He must decide how frequently he should try to examine his subjects. He will have to find some way of keeping in touch with the subjects or their parents and of sustaining their interest and cooperation. He must be prepared for the loss of some subjects, and he must be concerned about what effect the subjects' participation in the investigation is having on their own development, and even on their future test performances. The investigator must also consider other ethical matters. For example, if the child is showing signs of decompensating, should the parents be told or not? How will the child interpret his being selected for such a study? What should parents be told when they ask for the results of the examinations? And so on.

The Implicit Model in High-Risk Research. Some investigators hope to circumvent the problems of longitudinal research by carrying out so-called cross-sectional studies. The general scheme supposes that each investigator will examine a high-risk group of a different age. By looking at the findings regarding the various age groups, one could perhaps note the continuities and discontinuities from one age to another, and collate them so as to map out successfully the chronological development of schizophrenic illness. The plan differs from the prospective-longitudinal studies in that in the latter the same group of subjects is examined repeatedly over the years, whereas the cross-sectional studies involve different groups of subjects who, combined, could conceivably yield the same results in the space of a few years if such studies could be coordinated.

Both types of research strategy have strengths and weaknesses, but they both imply the same general model, time-lapse photography. Each examination period in a longitudinal study, or each age group in a series of cross-sectional studies, may be compared with a momentary photograph of a developing process. Many such photographs are taken over a chosen time span. Each yields a picture of the state of the organism at the time. By arranging these pictures chronologically and flipping them successively, we are supposed to obtain a running account, moving picture, or dynamic depiction of the "natural history" of schizophrenia. I do not know if anyone has openly advocated such a viewpoint, but it seems to me to be implicit in the bandwagon rush to high-risk research on schizophrenia. One can use time-lapse photography to see vividly the dramatic ways in which flowers grow, but this procedure alone does not tell us how or why they grow as they do. It is highly probable that the same conclusion can be drawn in regard to the usual high-risk studies of schizophrenia.

Replication, Replication. In the behavioral sciences, it is not often that experiments are carefully replicated. This failure frequently leads to an unruly accumulation of studies in any given area, where the studies co-exist incongruously more often than they build on one another. An investigator who wants to make sense of them collectively often has a difficult time trying to sort out the agreements and disagreements around any given point. When he draws a conclusion, he usually does so with discomforting uncertainty and finds himself forced to leave loose ends dangling.

Now if this is the case in fairly well-controlled experimental studies carried out in a one-shot examination in the laboratory, imagine the difficulties of interpreting numerous findings in the future outpouring of high-risk studies. High-risk investigators use different criteria in selecting their schizophrenic parents or, perhaps as important, their control parents. They prefer to select subjects of different ages for various reasons. Whether they have a theoretical axe to grind or they adopt a more inductive, intuitive, look-and-see approach, their tests, procedures, hypotheses, and independent and dependent variables are going to vary to such an extent that we may never get a true replication of any given point raised by any particular study. Considering the multiplicity, complexity, and duration of any single high-risk project, we should begin to plan even now to assure that at least some replication studies will be carried out as closely as possible.

To illustrate what can happen, let us examine some findings regarding psychophysiological responses of index and control subjects. Mednick and Schulsinger found consistent group differences with regard to the latency of GSR response to a loud auditory stimulus, the latency being shorter for the index cases. However, in my own collaborative studies in Copenhagen, using Mednick and Schulsinger's apparatus and the same auditory stimulus, but employing a slightly different conditioning procedure, we could find no significant differences in GSR response latency between our index and control groups.

On the other hand, Mednick and Schulsinger did not find differences between their groups in regard to GSR baseline levels; but, although we found no *mean* difference between groups either, we did find that our index cases were significantly more *variable* than controls in basal level—a finding consistent with Schachter's finding in regard to heart rate responses to clicks. Interestingly, Schachter's subjects were infants, Mednick-Schulsinger's were pubescent and adolescent, and ours were adults. Why should the infants and adults show such increased variability, but not the adolescents?

Also, why should the latency findings turn out differently in our study and Mednick-Schulsinger's? Is one correct and the other wrong, or are some seemingly minor variations in subject selection or experimental procedure enough to change the direction of the findings? Do the differences really reflect age differences? Or, even more interesting, is it possible that in the Mednick-Schulsinger index subjects, who were reared mainly in the parental home or with relatives, the faster latency reflects one of the effects of such rearing, as compared with our own index cases, who also had a schizophrenic biological parent, but were reared in adoptive homes?

We can easily become intrigued with the many possibilities of interpretation in regard to such differences between projects, but we would be on surer ground if we planned replication studies beforehand and tried to avoid such multiple ambiguities as much as possible. Although I commend to you replication of these complex high-risk studies, I can assure you that at my age I have no intention of being one of the replicators. Not for me the second time around. I am grateful enough just to have survived most of my high-risk period. I hope you survive yours.

NOTE: Commentary on this paper appears on pages 78–85.

REFERENCES

Anthony, E. J. The developmental precursors of adult schizophrenia. In D. Rosenthal & S. S. Kety (Eds.), *The transmission of schizophrenia.* London: Pergamon Press, 1968. Pp. 293–316.

Erlenmeyer-Kimling, L. Studies on the offspring of two schizophrenic parents. In D. Rosenthal & S. S. Kety (Eds.), *The transmission of schizophrenia.* London: Pergamon Press, 1968. Pp. 65–84.

Fish, B. The detection of schizophrenia in infancy. *Journal of Nervous and Mental Disease,* 1957, 125, 1–24.

————, Shapiro, T., Halpern, F., & Wile, R. The prediction of schizophrenia in infancy: III. A ten-year follow-up report of neurological and psychological development. *American Journal of Psychiatry*, 1965, 121, 768–775.

Kety, S. S., & Matthysse, S. Prospects for research on schizophrenia, a report based on an NRP work session. *Neurosciences Research Program Bulletin*, 1972, 10, no. 4.

Kety, S. S., Rosenthal, D., Wender, P. H., & Schulsinger, F. The types and prevalence of mental illness in the biological and adoptive families of adopted schizophrenics. In D. Rosenthal & S. S. Kety (Eds.), *The transmission of schizophrenia*. London: Pergamon Press, 1968. Pp. 345–362.

Mednick, S. A. A learning theory approach to research in schizophrenia. *Psychological Bulletin*, 1958, 55, 315–327.

————. The children of schizophrenics: Serious difficulties in current research methodologies which suggest the use of the "high-risk group" method. In J. Romano (Ed.), *The origins of schizophrenia*. Excerpta Medica Foundation, 1967. Pp. 179–200.

———— & Schulsinger, F. Some premorbid characteristics related to breakdown in children with schizophrenic mothers. In D. Rosenthal & S. S. Kety (Eds.), *The transmission of schizophrenia*. London: Pergamon Press, 1968. Pp. 267–291.

————. Factors related to breakdown in children at high-risk for schizophrenia. In M. Roff & D. F. Ricks (Eds.), *Life history research in psychopathology*. Vol. 1. Minneapolis: University of Minnesota Press, 1970. Pp. 51–93.

Reed, S. C. Genetic counseling in schizophrenia. In A. R. Kaplan (Ed.), *Genetic factors in "schizophrenia."* Springfield, Ill.: Thomas, 1972. Pp. 315–324.

Rosenthal, D. *Genetic theory and abnormal behavior*. New York: McGraw-Hill, 1970.

————, Wender, P. H., Kety, S. S., Welner, J., & Schulsinger, F. The adopted-away offspring of schizophrenics. *American Journal of Psychiatry*, 1971, 128, 307–311.

Shakow, D. Some observations on the psychology (and some fewer, on the biology) of schizophrenia. *Journal of Nervous and Mental Disease*, 1971, 153, 300–316.

Sobel, D. E. Children of schizophrenic patients: Preliminary observations on early development. *American Journal of Psychiatry*, 1961, 118, 512–517.

MARGARET E. HERTZIG] *Neurologic Findings
in Prematurely Born Children at School Age*

THIS PAPER will describe the neurologic status at 5 years of age of a
sample of 68 children who at birth weighed less than 1,750 g. This sample
represents all but 3 of a specially defined series of 71 children selected for
study within two weeks of their birth and followed continuously thereafter.
The initial group of children was composed of a continuous series of socially advantaged cases admitted to two premature centers in New York
City. Only those children who met the following criteria were enrolled:
(a) their birth weights were between 1,000 g (2 lbs 3 oz) and 1,750 g
(3 lbs 14 oz); (b) they had intact families; (c) their social situation was
that of skilled working class or higher; and (d) they derived from pregnancies in which prenatal registration had occurred during the first trimes-
ter, and antenatal care from that time onward had been provided.

Such a sample was selected and followed longitudinally (now into
the tenth year of life) because of the existence of primary questions concerning the relation of prematurity to neuropsychological development.
Almost all studies of the relation of perinatal conditions of risk to defective outcome have been difficult to interpret because of the association of
such risk with social disadvantage. Studies of the contribution made by
prematurity to later neurological, behavioral, or intellectual outcome are
no exception to this general rule. A number of studies provided support
for the view that prematurity has deleterious effects on physical and mental development (Abramowicz & Kass, 1966; Drillien, 1961, 1967; Lillienfeld & Pasamanick, 1954; McDonald, 1967; Pasamanick & Lillienfeld, 1955; Harper & Weiner, 1965). Abramowicz and Kass (1966) have

NOTE: A portion of the present study was carried out during the tenure of a Career
Development Award from NIMH, K01-MH-38832-03, to Dr. Hertzig and received
additional support from the National Institute of Child Health and Human Development, NICHHD 00719, and the Association for the Aid of Crippled Children.

cogently described the problems surrounding the interpretation of the findings of studies of the prognosis of low–birth weight infants with respect to physical well-being and intellectual adequacy — briefly, prematurity, low socioeconomic status, incomplete intellectual development, and poor health are all to be found in the same populations.

This confounding of adverse circumstances has led different workers to assess the contribution made by prematurity to developmental deviations in populations at risk in different and often contradictory ways. For example, Barker (1966) and McKeown (1951) have suggested that low birth weight and defective development are commonly elevated but independently elevated conditions in lower-class groupings. In support of this position, Barker (1966) has suggested that many of the risk conditions for maldevelopment, including low birth weight, derive from a failure to utilize available facilities and services for antenatal care. In his view such a failure occurs largely because expectant mothers in disadvantaged circumstances are intellectually incapable of recognizing the importance to the health and well-being of their prospective offspring of availing themselves of existing opportunities for medical supervision. He has therefore concluded that stupid women have dull offspring on familial grounds, and that these offspring are often of low birth weight because of the mother's incompetent utilization of resources. Richardson (1968) has taken an alternative position, arguing that low birth weight has negative consequences for development because the conditions for postnatal growth in the lower social classes from which the majority of low–birth weight children derive is more influential in its depressing effects upon initially handicapped infants. As a logical extension of this argument, Richardson (1968) has also suggested that the adverse developmental consequences of low birth weight would be markedly reduced or absent in more advantageously situated infants.

None of these points are new. All of them were anticipated by Arthur Benton before the onset of World War II. In his review of the literature at that time, Benton (1940) identified three principal issues which made it difficult to define the relation of prematurity to later development. First, he noted the association between low birth weight and social disadvantage and pointed out the difficulty of separating those features of faulty outcome which were due to low birth weight per se from those which could have derived from more general conditions of disadvantage. Secondly, he indicated that studies of low birth weight had not carefully considered particular ranges of weight, a fact making comparisons across studies impossible. As a third point, he observed that follow-up studies were inconsistent in the developmental stage of the child at the time of follow-up, and since neuro-psychological abnormalities are differentially manifested at different age stages, studies could either be giving undue emphasis to transient delays in development or failing altogether to identify abnormalities potentially present because of the excessive youth of the child. The present study was designed to meet these questions by (a) removing social disadvantage as a condition of risk; (b) considering all children within a given range of birth weight; and (c) following the sample from infancy into the school years.

METHOD

Initially, 71 children (32 boys and 39 girls) who had survived the first two weeks of life were enrolled in the study. These children all weighed between 1,000 and 1,750 g at birth. All, as well, derived from families which were intact, and socially and economically well situated. During the first three months of the study, 3 children were lost to follow-up. Of these 2 died, 1 a crib death at four weeks of age, and 1 as a consequence of congenital heart disease at two months of age. The family of the third child relocated abroad when he was three months old. The remainder of the series, consisting of a total of 68 children, 29 boys and 39 girls, was followed continuously into the fifth year of life.

During the course of the study information has been obtained which describes (a) antecedent conditions of the children and their mothers during pregnancy, birth, and the neonatal period; (b) clinical neurologic status; and (c) behavioral characteristics, at different age-stages of development. The mother's hospital records were systematically reviewed and abstracted to a protocol which provided for notations of mother's age, parity, date of last menstrual period, date of beginning prenatal care, complications of pregnancy, blood type, duration of labor, length of time membranes had been ruptured, complications of labor, type of sedation and anesthesia employed, type of delivery, and presumed reasons for prematurity. The baby's hospital records were similarly reviewed and the following kinds of information abstracted: birth weight, condition at birth, duration of nursery stay, weight at discharge, duration of use of O_2, and complications of nursery course.

First neurologic examinations were scheduled when the child reached a weight of 2,000 g, just before his discharge from the hospital nursery. Subsequent examinations were conducted at 6 months, and at 1, 2, 3, and

5 years of age. The neurologic examinations were complete and age appropriate. In each, the following attributes were described and recorded: developmental level; general behavior and demeanor; degree of cooperation; patterns of speech and language organization; laterality and right-left awareness; intactness of cranial nerves; sensory organization; reflexes; directed and voluntary movement; muscle strength and tone; motor coordination; extinction to double simultaneous tactile stimulation; gait; balance; skill in executing coordinated movement patterns; and adventitious motor movements. Decisions about the clinical neurologic status of the children were made from the entire set of examination protocols by the examiner after an interval of at least 6 months.

A child was judged to be neurologically abnormal if (a) one or more localizing signs of central nervous system abnormality were present or (b) two or more nonlocalizing signs (Paine & Oppé, 1966) of central nervous system CNS dysfunction were found. Localizing signs included such standard findings of CNS damage as abnormalities in reflexes and cranial nerves, lateralized dysfunctions, and the presence of pathologic reflexes. Non-localizing signs of CNS dysfunction included clearly recognizable disturbances of speech, hyperkinesis, failure to maintain balance, disturbances of gait, inadequacies of muscle tone, coordination defects, extinction to criterion in response to double simultaneous stimulation, inability to engage in sequential finger-thumb opposition, graphesthetic disturbances, and excessive degrees of adventitious motor overflow.

The design and scoring of the neurologic examination resulted in three types of findings on the basis of which to classify the children studied: (a) the absence of any abnormal neurologic signs, (b) the presence of localizing signs of CNS damage, and (c) the presence of non-localizing signs of CNS dysfunction. Children with any number of localizing signs of CNS damage as well as children with two or more non-localizing signs were considered to have clinical evidence of CNS damage. However, in the children without any abnormal neurologic signs as well as those with fewer than two non-localizing abnormal signs, the clinical evidence was considered to be insufficient to conclude that the child had a damaged brain (Birch, Richardson, Baird, Horobin, & Illsley, 1970).

The families of the children were visited and interim social, behavioral, and developmental histories were taken every 6 months for the first 2 years of life and annually thereafter. A detailed description of the procedures followed during these contacts has been presented elsewhere (Thomas, Chess, Birch, Hertzig, & Korn, 1963) and can be briefly summarized here. Information was obtained from the parents of each child in the course of a structured interview which covered events in the daily life of the child from the time he got up in the morning until he went to bed at night. Thus, detailed behavioral descriptions of the child's behavior during the routines of sleeping, dressing, feeding, bathing, and playing were obtained. Note was made of the age at which both motor and language developmental milestones were achieved. Changes in familial organization or in the occupational status of the parents were also inquired after, and descriptions of the child's behavioral response to these or other special events were recorded. In addition, full reports of medical and/or psychiatric consultation and treatment have been regularly obtained.

RESULTS

Clinical Neurologic Findings at 5 Years of Age. Table 1 summarizes the neurologic status of the children when examined at a mean age of five years. As may be seen in the table, a total of 30 children (44 per cent) were found to have clinical evidence of neurologic abnormality at this point in time. Half of the abnormal cases (15 children) had localizing neurologic signs, clinically describable as one or another variant of cerebral palsy. The other half was made up of children in whom two or more non-localizing signs of CNS dysfunction were found. The clinical neurologic examination was considered to be within the limits of normal functioning for age in the remaining 38 children. In 29 of these children the clinical examination revealed no evidence of abnormality, and in the remaining 9 only a single deviation from normally expected function was observed.

Table 1. Neurologic Status at 5 Years in 68 Premature Children
with Birth Weights of 1,000–1,750 g

Type of Finding	Boys	Girls	Total
Localizing	7	8	15
Non-localizing	9	6	15
Normal	13	25	38
Total	29	39	68

Of the 30 children with clinical evidence of neurologic impairment at 5 years of age, 16 were boys and 14 were girls. Thus, a somewhat greater percentage of the boys in the study had evidence of neurologic dysfunction (55 per cent) than did the girls (36 per cent). Furthermore, although localizing findings tend to occur with approximately equal frequency in both boys and girls, the proportion of boys among the children with non-localizing findings of CNS dysfunction (60 per cent) is notably greater than girls (40 per cent).

Of the 15 children who had localizing signs of CNS damage, abnormalities involving all four extremities were found in 5 children. Of these, 4 were severely quadriplegic, and 1 had evidence of a less severe degree involvement. In addition, 5 children were paraparetic, 4 children had signs of a left hemiplegia, and 1 child was mildly athetoid.

Two or more non-localizing signs of neurologic dysfunction were found in 15 children. Abnormalities of coordination were noted in 8, of muscle tone in 8, significant speech disturbance in 7, and a disordered gait in 4. Lesser number of children had excessive degrees of adventitious motor overflow, abnormalities in response to double simultaneous stimulation, inability to engage in sequential finger-thumb opposition, graphesthetic disturbances, mild mental retardation, or hyperkinesis.

Thus, the 68 children studied from birth through the fifth year of life can be divided into the following three groups on the basis of their neurologic status at 5 years of age: (a) children with localizing findings of CNS dysfunction, (b) children with non-localizing signs of CNS dysfunction, and (c) children with no clinical evidence of significant neurologic abnormality. These three groups differ as well with respect to their condition at earlier points in time.

The Association between Antecedent Conditions and Neurologic Status at 5 Years of Age. Birth weight in the present study ranged from 1,000 to 1,750 g with a median of 1,445.5 g. Weight at birth tended to bear a significant relationship to neurologic status at 5 years of age. There is a suggestion that those with non-localizing findings of neurologic dysfunction are below the median of the group with localizing findings, but the number of cases is not large enough to establish the significance of this.

There was also a suggestion that gestational age was associated with neurologic status at 5 years of age. The gestational ages of the children as a whole ranged from 26 to 38 weeks, with a median of 32 weeks. Children with non-localizing signs tend to be older than the median gestational age, but the sample is too small for this difference to reach a level of significance.

Thus, children with non-localizing signs of neurologic abnormality as newborns tended to be below the median weight and above the median for gestational age. It therefore appears as if they were less adequately grown for their gestational age — that is, "smaller for date" than other babies in the sample. A systematic examination of the question reveals that this is indeed the case. Internal criteria for the definition of small-for-date babies were established such that a baby was considered to be poorly grown if his birth weight was below the mean weight of all the children in the sample who were of equivalent gestational age. In Table 2 (top), the results of the application of these criteria are presented. As may be seen, nearly 70 per cent of the children with non-localizing signs of CNS dysfunction were considered to be small for date. In contrast, 45 per cent of the children with localizing signs and 35 per cent of the children who were neurologically normal were defined as being small for date. This gradient differs from chance ($p<.10$). When external standards for the definition of poor intrauterine growth, such as those developed by Thompson and Tanner (1970), are used to identify small-for-date babies, this association reaches the 5 per cent level of confidence (Table 2, bottom).

Table 2. The Association between Intrauterine Growth
and Neurologic Status at 5 Years

Criteria	Localizing Findings	Non-localizing Findings	Normal
	Internal Criteria[a,b]		
Small for date	7	11	14
Not small for date	8	4	24
	External Criteria[c,d]		
<5th percentile	7	10	11
≥5th percentile	8	5	27

[a]Internal criteria for small-for-date babies were that birth weight was below the median of all *S*s in the sample of equivalent gestational age.
[b]$\chi^2 = 5.745$, $df = 2$, $p<.10$.
[c]Developed by Thompson and Tanner (1970).
[d]$\chi^2 = 6.55$, $df = 2$, $p<.05$.

A similar trend obtains when the relation of pregnancy complication to neurologic status at 5 years of age is examined. As may be seen from the accompanying tabulation ($\chi_2 = 5.031$, $df = 2$, $p <.10$), approximately half the children in the group with non-localizing findings of CNS dysfunction derived from pregnancies complicated by third-trimester bleeding or pre-eclampsia. In contrast, only 15 to 20 per cent of the children who were either neurologically normal or who had localizing findings of CNS dysfunction were the products of disordered pregnancies. Although this association is significant at only the .10 level of confidence, the finding is of interest because it lends support to the view that a primarily disordered pregnancy might well be an underlying factor contributing to the poor intrauterine growth achievements of children with non-localizing signs of CNS dysfunction.

	Localizing Findings	Non-localizing Findings	Normal
Complications of pregnancy	2	7	8
No complications of pregnancy ..	12	8	31

In contrast with the trend of associations found between antenatal factors and non-localizing signs of CNS dysfunction, postnatal factors appear to be related to the later emergence of localizing signs of neurologic damage. Disturbances of nursery course tended to be most frequent, and conditions were most severe in the children with localizing findings. Respiratory distress, apneic episodes, cyanosis, severe jaundice, or seizures were noted in all but two of these cases, whereas such disturbances were relatively infrequent or less severe in the children with non-localizing signs. As would be expected as a consequence of the greater frequency of occurrence of complications in children with localizing findings, clinical progress in the nursery as measured in terms of the duration of nursery stay and the rate of weight gain was commensurately slower. Length of stay in this sample of children ranged from 16 to 86 days, with a median of 41 days. Twice as many of the children with localizing findings remained in the nursery for longer than the median number of days; among the children with non-localizing findings or no significant findings of CNS dysfunction, approximately equal numbers were above and below the median. Weight gain per day was determined by dividing the difference between discharge weight and birth weight by the number of days in the nursery, and was found to range from 12.75 to 68.12 with a median of 20.01 g. A greater proportion of children with localizing findings were below the median for weight gain on a daily basis than was the case in either of the other two groups.

The group of children with localizing findings of CNS dysfunction were also distinguishable from those with non-localizing signs by virtue of the nature of the course of their illnesses over time. The group of children with localizing findings were characterized by enormous consistency. With one exception, all of the children identified as having localizing findings by 2 years of age had them at 5 years. In contrast, the course of the children with non-localizing findings was quite different: of the 15 children having two or more non-localizing findings at 5 years of age, only 4 had been identified by 3 years.

DISCUSSION

The data of the present study suggest that even in the absence of social disadvantage, birth weight of less than 1,750 g is associated with a high frequency of neurologic abnormality. Almost one fourth of the children followed were found to have symptoms characteristic of cerebral palsy in clinical neurologic examinations conducted at 5 years of age, and an equivalent number were found to have clear, though non-localizing signs of CNS dysfunction. Only slightly more than 50 per cent of the children were found to be without frank evidence of neurologic abnormality.

These findings suggest, therefore, that the neurologic impairment consequences of prematurity are not uniform, with respect either to severity or to kind. Even within the relatively narrow range of birth weight which provided the basis for the selection of the subjects of the present study, two distinguishable types of neurologic dysfunction are suggested. These two types of CNS disorder, one with localizing and the other with non-localizing signs of dysfunction, were found to be differently associated with antecedent conditions of risk during the prenatal and neonatal period. The greatest condition of risk, most particularly with respect to the development of non-localizing signs, attached to being small for date. The prevalence of this risk condition was not elevated, however, in children with localizing signs of CNS damage. Moreover, children with non-localizing signs of CNS dysfunction were far more likely to have derived from pregnancies complicated by pre-eclampsia or third-trimester bleeding than were children with localizing disorders. In contrast, such complications of nursery course as respiratory distress, apneic episodes, cyanosis, severe jaundice, or seizures were more frequent and more severe in children with localizing disorders. Children with localizing findings also gained weight more slowly and tended to remain in the hospital for a longer period than the other children.

These differences in the pattern of association between the two types of CNS dysfunction identified clinically at 5 years of age and antecedent conditions of risk suggest that different mechanisms may be operative in the two instances. It appears that whereas non-localizing signs may well be the consequence of general developmental debility associated with complications of pregnancy and failure to grow at expected rates, localizing signs are more directly associated with the detrimental effects of such postnatal conditions as respiratory distress, apneic episodes, jaundice, or seizures on a developing and growing nervous system. A high frequency of occurrence of such conditions during the first days and weeks of life in premature infants, particularly those of very low birth weight, is well known and has been attributed to the immaturity of biologic mechanisms underlying these functions. The continued development of sophisticated techniques of management and treatment have resulted in the steady improvement in survival rates for low–birth weight infants during the past quarter century (Silverman, 1961). The relative immunity of the small-for-date babies in the present study to postnatal complications may be accountable in terms of their relative maturity and resulting increased ability to withstand the demands of extrauterine existence despite their low weight. Then, too, the different developmental course of these clinically disparate types of CNS abnormalities supports the view that they are etiologically distinct disorders. The typical picture observed in children with localizing findings was one of early identification of disorder and a stable clinical course. In contrast, non-localizing findings, which in fact represent developmentally emerging abnormalities, did not become clinically apparent until much later in the course of the life of the child. Over 70 per cent of the children with non-localizing findings of CNS dysfunction did not come to clinical notice as impaired until 5 years of age, despite the fact that they were the subjects of regular and systematic examination.

It is of interest to compare these findings with those of other follow-up investigations of low–birth weight children. The rate of dysfunction in the present sample does not differ strikingly from the rates reported by Drillien (1961, 1967) and McDonald (1967), both of whom conducted their follow-up investigations of low–birth weight children during the early school years. This close correspondence is maintained despite the fact that the subjects of the present study constitute a socially advantaged group, whereas Drillien's and McDonald's inquiries into the consequences for development of prematurity were heavily weighted for social disadvantage. The findings of the present study suggest that even when social contributions to dysfunction are eliminated, low birth weight per se results in an elevation of risk for neurologic maldevelopment. Furthermore, the similarity in rates of impairment in studies whose subjects derived from disadvantaged as opposed to advantaged backgrounds suggests that within this weight range, the frequency of neurologic impairment in prematurely born children is probably independent of social class.

NOTE: Commentary on this paper appears on pages 78–85.

REFERENCES

Abramowicz, M., & Kass, E. H. Pathogenesis and prognosis of prematurity, *New England Journal of Medicine*, 1966, 275, 878–885, 938–943, 1001–1007, 1053–1059.

Barker, D. J. P. Low intelligence and obstetrical complications, *British Journal of Preventive and Social Medicine*, 1966, 29, 15–21.

Benton, A. L. Mental development of prematurely born children. *American Journal of Orthopsychiatry*, 1940, 10, 719–746.

Birch, H. G., Richardson, S. A., Baird, D., Horobin, G., & Illsley, R. *Mental subnormality in the community. A clinical and epidemiologic study*. Baltimore: Williams & Wilkins, 1970.

Drillien, C. M. The incidence of mental and physical handicaps in school-age children of very low birthweight. *Pediatrics*, 1961, 27, 452, 464.

————. The incidence of mental and physical handicaps in school-age children of very low birthweight. *Pediatrics*, 1967, 39, 238–247.

Harper, P. A., & Wiener, G. Sequelae of low birthweight, *Annual Review of Medicine*, 1965, 16, 405–420.

Lillienfeld, A. M., & Pasamanick, B. Association of material and fetal factors with the development of epilepsy. 1. Abnormalities in prenatal and paranatal periods. *Journal of the American Medical Association*, 1954, 105, 719–724.

McDonald, A. *Children of very low birthweight*. Spastics Society Medical Education and Information Unit Research Monograph No. 1. London: Heinemann, 1967.

McKeown, T., & Gibson, J. R. Observations on all births (23,790) in Birmingham, 1947. IV. Premature birth. *British Medical Journal*, 1951, 2, 513–517.

Paine, R., & Oppé, T. *Neurologic examination of children*. London: Spastics Society Medical Education and Information Unit, 1966.

Pasamanick, B., & Lillienfeld, A. M. Association of maternal and fetal factors with development of mental deficiency, 1. Abnormalities in the prenatal periods. *Journal of the American Medical Association*, 1955, 159, 155–160.

Richardson, S. A. The influence of social-environmental and nutritional factors in mental ability. In N. S. Scrimshaw & J. E. Gordon (Eds.), *Malnutrition, learning and behavior*. Cambridge, Mass.: MIT Press, 1968.

Silverman, W. A. *Dunham's premature infants*. 3rd ed. New York: Paul B. Hoeber, 1961.

Thomas, A. T., Birch, H. G., Chess, S., Hertzig, M. E., & Korn, S. *Behavioral individuality in early childhood*. New York: New York University Press, 1963.

ALEXANDER THOMAS
STELLA CHESS
JANET SILLEN
OLGA MENDEZ | *Cross-Cultural Study
of Behavior in Children
with Special Vulnerabilities to Stress*

DURING the course of several ongoing studies, we have had the opportunity to compare the behavior patterns of Puerto Rican working-class children and non–Puerto Rican middle-class children. The studies yielded clinical samples of youngsters with behavior problems reflecting the impact of special environmental stresses and cultural values.

This paper will report on several significant differences between the two groups with regard to the severity of behavior disorders, the type of systems, and the age of onset. We shall consider various reasons for these differences in light of the characteristic patterns of family relationships, child-care practices, and home and community environments. Such a cross-cultural study may help clarify the role of specific environmental influences in the ontogenesis of behavior disorders and the factors involved in symptom choice.

Sample. The first clinical sample consists of 31 children from Puerto Rican working-class (PRWC) families. The clinical cases are drawn from studies of 95 preschool children and 155 of their school-age siblings. The second clinical sample comprises 42 children of middle- and upper–middle-class background drawn from a group of 136 youngsters whose behavioral patterns have been investigated in the New York Longitudinal Study (Thomas et al., 1968). The backgrounds of the two groups present a sharp contrast — economically, socially, and culturally — yet certain variables affecting behavioral development are comparable.

NOTE: This study was supported in part by grants from the NIMH (MH-3614) and the NYC Health Research Council (U-1618).

The total sample of 250 PRWC children derives from 72 predominantly Spanish-speaking, working-class families. Some 2 per cent of the fathers are skilled workers, 37 per cent are semiskilled, and 60 per cent unskilled; one is a lawyer.* Over 92 per cent of the mothers are full-time homemakers. The fathers attended school for a mean duration of 8 years 1 month, and the mothers for 8 years 8 months. Of the fathers 95 per cent and of the mothers 88 per cent were born in Puerto Rico; the remainder were born in New York City of Puerto Rican parentage. All of the families had lived in the continental United States for at least ten years. During the period of interviewing, the vast majority lived in low-income public housing projects in that part of Manhattan commonly called Spanish Harlem or East Harlem.

The group of 95 preschool PRWC children was drawn consecutively from new infants registered at two municipal baby health stations in Spanish Harlem. The behavioral development of these youngsters has been followed longitudinally from early infancy through age 5. The group of 155 school-age children consists of their siblings, ranging in age from 6 to 18 years.

The 136 middle- and upper–middle-class children in the New York Longitudinal Study were all residents of New York City or its suburbs when enrolled in the study. Almost all the parents were born in the United States. The families are predominantly Jewish (78 per cent), with some Protestant (15 per cent) and Catholic (7 per cent) families. Of the mothers 40 per cent and of the fathers 60 per cent have both college and postgraduate degrees, and only 8 per cent of the fathers and 9 per cent of the mothers had no college education at all. Of the fathers, 75 per cent are professionals or business executives, 20 per cent are small businessmen, and 5 per cent are highly skilled artisans. By the time the children reached 3 years of age, 18 per cent of the mothers had returned to full-time and 25 per cent to part-time employment, usually in a professional occupation.

Despite these striking differences between the two groups, there were some important similarities. Both samples showed a relatively high degree of family stability. Although the frequency of disruption by divorce, separation, or parental death was somewhat higher in the PRWC group, this difference was not statistically significant. The majority of the children

---

*The child of this professional family did not become a behavior problem. The 31 clinical cases in the Puerto Rican sample came entirely from working-class families.

lived in two-parent homes in which geographical and economic stability (albeit at different levels) prevailed. In addition, there were no significant differences in the number of prenatal and perinatal complications in the middle class and preschool PRWC children, though no accurate data on this issue are available for the older PRWC children (the siblings). It is therefore likely that such complications did not significantly determine differences in the incidence of behavior disorders in the two groups.

Methods. During the longitudinal study of the preschool PRWC children, periodic interviews were held with the parents, usually the mothers. The protocols were those used in the New York Longitudinal Study (Thomas et al., 1963; 1968). They provided details of each child's behavioral development. The parental interviews and routine psychological testing of the children were conducted by Spanish-speaking staff members of Puerto Rican origin. In cases where a child showed troublesome behavior which could not be handled by changes in parental management, the child was referred to a Spanish-speaking psychiatrist for evaluation.

Although the school-age siblings were not followed longitudinally, behavior problems in this group were identified through the use of a Symptom Inventory devised for this study and by a follow-up psychiatric evaluation.

Because of their long-term association, the staff interviewers became closely acquainted with these PRWC families, their child-care approaches, the neighborhood environment, and special stresses in the family. In addition, special interviews were held with parents to determine their aspirations for the children's education. We obtained further data about parental functioning in the course of the psychiatric work-up when a behavior problem arose. The psychiatrist's subsequent meeting with the parents to review his findings and recommendations usually yielded additional information on parental attitudes and practices.

Methods of data collection and of behavior problem identification in the middle-class sample paralleled those used with the Puerto Rican group and have been described in detail elsewhere (Thomas et al., 1968).

Because the data on the middle-class sample extended only to the age of 9 years, when the present comparison was made, the data for the PRWC sample tabulated below considers only children up to this age. Therefore, although a total of 31 PRWC children were diagnosed as having a behavior problem, only the 15 who were younger than 9 years at the time of diagnosis are compared with the middle-class sample of 42 children, all of whom were 9 or under. It should be noted, however, that the total sample in each group is used for culling descriptions of family practices and attitudes.

FINDINGS

Age at Diagnosis of Behavior Disorder. A greater percentage of the middle-class children were diagnosed as having behavior problems by the age of 9 years (42 out of 136, or 31 per cent) as compared with the PRWC sample (15 out of 143,* or 10 per cent) (Table 1). Of the 42 middle-class cases, 17 (40 per cent) came to attention before 5 years of age, whereas only 4 (27 per cent) of the 15 PRWC cases came to attention in this early age period.

Table 1. Age at Diagnosis

Age in Years and Months	Males Middle Class	Males PRWC	Females Middle Class	Females PRWC	Total Middle Class	Total PRWC
2–2.11			1		1	
3–3.11	4	1	3	1	7	2
4–4.11	5	2	4		9	2
5–5.11	7	1	3		10	1
6–6.11	3	4	2		5	4
7–7.11	5	3	1	1	6	4
8–8.11	2	2	2		4	2

The middle-class parents were child-problem oriented, and even slight behavioral disturbances in their children were reported promptly to the interviewers for review by the staff psychiatrists. As a group, these parents were well aware of currently influential theories of child psychiatry and psychology, which place great stress on the child's development in the first 5 years of life as being crucial to his later psychological functioning. Therefore, these parents were especially concerned about evidence of a behavior problem that appeared in their children at a young age.

The PRWC parents were also concerned about the well-being of their offspring, but they were not preoccupied with the psychological significance of a behavioral deviation in their young children unless it was fairly severe. Rather than viewing mild disturbances with alarm as a portent of future difficulties, as did the middle-class parents, their attitude was typically expressed by the remark, "He's a baby — he'll outgrow it."

Of the PRWC children, 4 developed behavior disorders before the

*143 is the total number of PRWC children age 9 or younger.

age of 5. In all cases the difficulties were rather severe — 3 of the youngsters were mentally retarded. The combination of disturbed behavior and retardation resulted in serious management difficulties; the children had not developed the capacity for self-care, had speech problems, and were easily frustrated. One also showed "bizarre" behavior. The mother of this child had sought psychiatric advice in a city hospital clinic before evaluation by the project psychiatrist. The other PRWC children presenting symptoms before the age of 5 also were very difficult to handle. They were aggressive with siblings and peers, and presented disciplinary problems at home and in kindergarten.

It is possible that the earlier presentation of symptoms in the middle-class group also stemmed from the greater demands for task performance made upon them both at home and in school. Their parents emphasized the early accomplishment of self-care activities, particularly feeding and dressing. They also encouraged their children to master the use of toys and stressed the educational value of play. In addition, many adaptations to new situations and new people were required of the preschool middle-class children because their involvement in nursery school and kindergarten brought them into contact with unfamiliar experiences. Of the entire middle-class sample of 136 children, 89 per cent attended nursery school; 10 per cent began schooling with kindergarten; and only one child did not start until the first grade. It is true that the demands to adapt to these new social relations and play work patterns were met easily by most of the children. However, these demands were quite stressful to some who had the temperamental characteristics of slow adaptability to new people or situations (Thomas et al., 1968).

In contrast, the demands on the PRWC children in the first 5 years of life and their extrafamilial experiences with new people and new situations were much more limited (Hertzig et al., 1968). They were not expected to feed or dress themselves ("If I do it for him I get done faster"), and there was little insistence that the children follow through on verbal task directions. Most of the PRWC parents regarded toys as amusements: educational toys were not purchased, and the children usually amused themselves with household objects in a self-determined manner. None of the children in the group from which the clinical sample was derived went to nursery school; only 26 per cent attended kindergarten; and only two children in the clinical sample were in kindergarten at the time of psychiatric evaluation.

Almost all of the social experiences and relationships of this group were intrafamilial, consisting of visits exchanged with close relatives. There was also considerable visiting back and forth with other families in the same apartment house. The preschool children were essentially house-bound. The mothers as a group did not give a high priority to systematic exposure of their children to social experiences with other children and therefore did not plan regular daily excursions to outdoor play facilities. They were also fearful of permitting their children to go to playgrounds unescorted or to play unsupervised with other children in the neighborhood because of concern for their safety. Periodic trips to the beach and playground were often the only outdoor excursions.

Differences in Presenting Symptoms. As indicated above, a significantly larger number of the middle-class sample came to attention for behavior problems (42 out of 136) than did the PRWC children (15 out of 143).* However, the symptoms of the 15 PWRC clinical cases were much more severe than those of the middle-class cases. The PRWC parents did not actively complain about their children's difficulties or seek help until the symptoms became severe enough to create marked problems for the child or serious difficulties in management for the parents. This did not reflect family disorganization or indifference to the welfare of their children on the parents' part. The mothers were actively concerned about their children, cooperated actively with our research staff in the interviews and psychometric testing, were responsive to the suggestion that they consult the research staff psychiatrist, and were communicative and cooperative in the clinical workup. In addition to the lesser tendency to view mild disturbances with alarm as a portent of future difficulties compared with the middle-class parents, the PRWC parents were pessimistic regarding the possibility of getting effective help for a child's problem from the school or municipal hospital clinic. This pessimism, unfortunately, had all too much of a basis in reality in the Harlem community. As a result, they sought help generally only when they began to feel that the child's problems were becoming dangerously unmanageable.

As Table 2 indicates, from infancy through 9 years both samples present the largest number of symptoms in the areas of discipline, mood, and social relationships. These three symptoms appear as a constellation more

---

*This difference is still apparent even if the comparison is extended to include the older age periods. In the age period beyond 9 years, the same trend appears as in the under-9-year group — namely, that a greater proportion of PRWC children who develop behavior problems present at an older age group as compared with the middle-class group. Our comparison of the over-9-year group is incomplete because of the relatively younger age of the middle-class sample.

Table 2. Presenting Symptoms in Children to Age 9 Years

Symptom Area	Children Aged 0–4.11		Children Aged 5–8.11		Total	
	Middle Class[a]	PRWC[b]	Middle Class[c]	PRWC[d]	Middle Class	PRWC
Learning	1	1	4	13	5	14
Mood	4	7	7	11	11	18
Social relationships	4	10	8	18	12	28
Discipline	4	5	9	12	13	17
Sleep	1	8	5	3	6	11
Speech	3	6	1	4	4	10
Feeding		1	5	1	5	2
Elimination	3	2	3	1	6	3
Motor activity	2	5	6		8	5
Somatic	1	3	1	3	2	6
Self-inflicted injuries	2		5		7	
Habits	1	3	3	2	4	5
Excessive fears	2	1	3	4	5	5
Others	1	2	7	4	8	6

[a] $N = 4.$ [b] $N = 17.$
[c] $N = 11.$ [d] $N = 25.$

frequently among the PRWC children, with 11 of the 15 youngsters displaying all three. Complaints about excessive motor activity were reported by the parents of 53 per cent of the PRWC children but only 12 per cent of the middle-class group. In addition, all the PRWC children who were reported to be excessively active also showed the three-symptom constellation described above.

It is pertinent to examine some of the symptom areas where differences between the groups, both in terms of the child's behavior and the parents' handling, are especially clear. These areas include sleep and feeding, motor activity, discipline, learning, and self-inflicted injuries.

a. Sleep and Feeding Problems. Judging from interview and observation data, child-care practices were much less structured and demanding in the preschool years in the PRWC than in the middle-class families. The young PRWC child, in the course of daily functioning, had few rules and regulations imposed on him. The time for sleeping, for example, was elastic and could begin at midnight and end late the next morning, even at noon.

When the PRWC children approached school age, however, the situation usually changed dramatically. As they began school (and first grade was typically their first exposure to formal education), they had to go to sleep and get up promptly at regular hours, eat without dawdling, dress quickly, and arrive at school on time — all functions that they had not previously been required to perform.

Almost half of the PRWC clinical sample that came to notice between the ages of 5 and 9 presented sleep problems, whereas only one child under 5 had a sleep difficulty. In most instances, the parents complained of a child's unwillingness to adhere to a regular bedtime, with accompanying temper tantrums. Some of the children's sleep problems also took a more vigorous form, such as nightmares, frightening dreams, sleepwalking, and inability to sleep alone or without a light.

These problems may be attributed to the sudden new demand on the children for sleep regularity combined with the stresses that resulted if the child resisted learning this new behavioral pattern. The parents presenting these complaints indicated that they exerted great pressure on the children for full compliance with their new rules. The psychiatric reports show that the child's resistance to this pressure frequently created disciplinary problems, with the parents forming an image of the youngster as a bad boy or bad girl who was being deliberately disobedient or disrespectful. Thus, in view of all the new stresses that emerge at school age plus the central demand for regularity at bedtime, it is not surprising that sleep difficulties were frequent and sometimes severe.

The development of sleep problems at the time of school entry may also be related to the new stresses and demands posed by the school situation for these children. The school day in effect begins when the child retires the night before. Going to sleep is the act which precedes arising and preparing to face the school day. If school represents a stress, whether in terms of the demands for learning, apprehension over the teacher's discipline, or discomfort owing to movement restraint, the anticipatory apprehension may show itself as difficulty in falling asleep or interruption of sleep on the night preceding a school day.

In contrast, complaints about sleep problems in the middle-class group were more numerous in the preschool period and declined sharply after the children began school. In general, this reflects a difference in child-care practices and the fact that for these middle-class parents the ease with which a preschool child approached bedtime was crucial. As a group, these parents were not tolerant of deviant behavior in this area. A child who intruded repeatedly on his parents' evenings instead of going to bed quickly and quietly, or who awakened his parents during the night, inconvenienced them and even impaired their functioning. Many of these parents also believed that a child's sleep irregularity, even if not in itself inconvenient to them, might reflect a psychological problem that was not to be treated lightly. The middle-class parents were therefore likely to make an issue of the child's bedtime and sleep behavior. These differences in handling are reflected in the fact that 8 middle-class children (47 per cent of the clinical sample) had sleep difficulties at this young age.

Basically, however, the middle-class parents' complaints about a preschooler's sleep pattern did not necessarily indicate the onset of a fixed long-term behavior disorder so much as they reflected the parents' focus on training the child. Thus, by the time these youngsters reached the age of 5, bedtime regularity had usually been achieved and sleep schedules ceased to be a source of problems.

Neither group of parents reported feeding as a problem area. Although irregularity of feeding was described by many of the middle-class parents, it rarely became the basis of a specific complaint. The irregularity was generally noted and then dismissed by the parent as not important because the child's health did not suffer. If the child picked and chose what he ate, the parents were generally unconcerned because "it is so easy and inexpensive" to prepare something the youngster likes especially. In the PRWC families food was prepared for the entire family. Refusals by the child to eat were treated very casually.

b. Motor Activity. In the PRWC clinical sample, there was a strikingly high incidence of parental complaints about excessive and uncontrollable motor activity: 53 per cent of this group under 9 years of age presented such symptoms, whereas only one middle-class child displayed hyperactivity (and this was a brain-damaged youngster). This difference is significant ($p < .001$).

We suspect that some, if not most, of the "hyperactivity" complained about in the PRWC children was due to the circumstances of their environment. The families usually had several children and lived in small apartments in which even the normal fooling around and active play of a youngster greatly impinged on others and could appear to the family as excessive motility. Furthermore, those children who temperamentally had a high activity level were even more likely than others to be cooped up at home for fear that if they ran around in the streets they would be in special danger of accidents.

In addition, the PRWC families were very conscious and concerned over the real dangers of street life in East Harlem. For a child to go down to the street or even to a playground meant all kinds of dangers — aggressive gangs, bad companions, traffic accidents. Even the use of recreational centers carried the risks to be met on the street coming and going. These parents did not have the opportunities available to middle-class families to chauffeur their child to and from safe playgrounds and school or Saturday recreational groups. The solution easily available to the PRWC parents was to keep their children under supervision at home at all times. It was assumed that the child could and should learn to restrain his motor activity.

It is altogether possible that if these families lived in an environment with more space for physical activities and fewer hazards, the number of complaints about hyperactivity would be greatly diminished. In fact, one child who had been described by his teachers as "uncontrollably active" and by his parents as a "whirling dervish" became much more manageable when the family moved to a private house with a small yard.

In most cases, however, the parents could offer few opportunities for active play to their children. Furthermore, they frequently interpreted the youngster's lack of compliance to their demands for restraint as deliberate disobedience. As a result, many of the parents who reported excessive activity in their children stated that they employed restrictive and sometimes punitive practices to control them. (One mother said that she forced her child to stay on his knees whenever his jumping and moving about the apartment became excessive; other mothers indicated that they spanked their offspring with a belt when their physical activity exceeded the limits of their tolerance.) If a child is scolded or punished for infractions of rules he is unable to follow, he may in turn decide that there is no point in trying to please his mother and may, in fact, become even deliberately disobedient. It is interesting that all of the Puerto Rican children reported to be too active by their parents were also said to be disciplinary problems.

In the middle-class group, no child was brought to notice with the specific complaint of excessive motor activity except for the one child with brain damage. (The other four children had other types of motor problems.) The middle-class parents had the financial resources to provide ample living and play space for their children, indoors and out. It was possible, therefore, for highly active children to engage in motor activities without endangering themselves or encroaching on the needs of other family members. As a result, there was little or no conflict between the needs of the parents for quiet and the needs of the children for motoric release.

It seems very possible, then, that the different incidence of complaints about excessive activity in the two clinical groups can, in great part, be attributed to environmental conditions rather than intrinsic psychological differences among the children. Certainly, it is highly questionable to label the high activity levels of the PRWC sample as "hyperactivity due to minimal brain damage" thus adding to the loose use of the term in the psychiatric literature. In these samples there is no significant difference in the incidence of neurological disorders to account for the high motility of the PRWC youngsters. It is likely that this high motility did not represent pathological hyperactivity as such but, rather, the normal temperamental characteristic of high activity level which became exacerbated and the basis for a behavior problem development because of environmental constraints (Thomas et al., 1968).

Discipline. The incidence of disciplinary problems is more than two times higher in the PRWC than in the middle-class sample (significant, $p<.01$). In addition, the PRWC children more frequently displayed symptoms of negative mood, poor social relations, and excessive motor activity, all of which appear related to parental complaints about discipline.

The majority (over 75 per cent) of the PRWC parents in our entire study said that children should implicitly obey their parents. Strict obedience to parental directives was a common demand. The comments of one parent illustrate this attitude, "I think children should always obey their parents. Of course, if they accidentally spill water on the bathroom floor, I don't spank them. But I don't let them get away with anything. Whenever they do anything wrong, I spank them. I always punish them when they disobey us, when they say bad words or when they fight with each other. They respect us." When queried about her demands for obedience of her younger children, the same mother stated, "Usually I reprimand the younger ones once or twice. If they do not obey, then I spank them. If I tell them to stop fighting and they continue, I get out a slipper or a strap. With the older ones I do the same. Last Thursday, I told the three boys that I didn't want them to go down to play. They waited 'til I went to my room and then went down without my permission. I called to them through the window. When they came up, I spanked them all with a strap."

This demand that a child "do as he is told" may be related to significant situational variables. For example, lateness in arriving home from school clearly aroused parental concern over trouble the child might have got into; failure to comply with parental directives, answering back, or use of bad language often symbolized to the parents the child's potential lack of control over dangerous environmental factors. As long as the child obeyed and was a good boy or a good girl, anxiety over the effects of ghetto living could be held in abeyance.

For the PRWC parents, a child's defiance or even questioning of their demands also represented a direct challenge to their authority, was interpreted as lack of respect, and conjured up all the possibilities of serious delinquency and trouble with the authorities. Confrontations and stress over even small disciplinary issues were therefore frequent in these families living in the ghetto.

Most of our middle-class parents, though by no means all, by contrast, tolerated a great deal of questioning and challenging of disciplinary rules by their children. Such challenges did not carry the same dangerous antisocial implications they did to ghetto families. Some middle-class parents even expressed satisfaction that their children were learning how to "stand up for themselves."

Because only four of the PRWC children in the clinical sample were followed longitudinally from early infancy on (the remainder were part of the sibling study), we cannot trace the development of these child-care practices from infancy to the point of psychiatric evaluation. It is therefore difficult to know whether the restrictive or punitive handling gave rise to the negative mood and disciplinary problems that were reported or, conversely, grew out of the parents' frustration and inability to cope with a child manifesting "difficult" temperamental characteristics from the beginning (Thomas et al., 1968).

The middle-class parents used different management techniques to deal with their disobedient children. The denial of privileges was the most frequently used disciplinary measure. Verbal criticism and nagging, often in an intense and rejecting manner, was also a common approach.

d. Learning. As can be seen from Table 2, learning problems were more common in the school-age middle-class children than in their PRWC peers. This may appear to be surprising finding in that none of the middle-class youngsters in the clinical sample had a below normal IQ (in fact, over half scored in the superior or very superior range), whereas approximately three quarters of the PRWC children in the clinical sample did have a below-normal IQ. One might have expected, therefore, to find learning problems much more frequently in this group. Two factors may help to explain this apparent paradox.

In their life situation, these PRWC families necessarily gave priority to problems other than learning. As one mother said of her son, "He gets only C's, but he passes. The important thing is that he behaves well and he is a good boy." Although the parents would have liked their children to do well in school, their actual expectations were tempered by an objective view of the limited opportunities for a meaningful education open to the children. Their attitude is, in fact, an adaptive environmental response. Thus, even in the case of the retarded children, academic issues were not usually the focus of the parents' complaint. How such a child performed in school was certainly of interest to them, but any signs of behavior that might get him into trouble (usually with the law) were of paramount concern.

Similarly, from what we know about the schools of East Harlem, it is likely that the teachers had minimal expectations for these children and that they were often indifferent if a child's academic progress was below average. Thus, even though about two thirds of the youngsters scored below their school grade norm in achievement tests, a finding in line with the situation defined and described by many others studying ghetto children (Clark, 1965), no one thought to make an issue of their obvious learning problems. At worst, the schools emphasized only their custodial role, and, at best, seemed to settle for whatever limited learning they expected from these "disadvantaged" children.

In sum, then, the paucity of learning problems reported in the PRWC sample testifies not to their absence but to their acceptance by both parents and teachers as a fact of life.

In turn, the presence of learning problems among the middle-class children does not necessarily reflect true academic failure but rather the parents' overriding concern with scholastic success. Interviews with the middle-class parents revealed that they exerted considerable pressure on their children for superior cognitive performance. A child's academic achievement, for this group of families, took precedence over all other problems. This priority reflects an adaptation to an environment quite different from that of the PRWC parents. Having achieved what they considered to be a superior professional, economic, and social status, the parents were keenly aware of the competitive necessity for excellent performance in order to maintain this status. This necessity is communicated to the children, so that even in the preschool period emphasis is placed on cognitive performance and participation in a wide variety of cultural activities. When the middle-class child begins school, the parents are always checking on his performance. Their relationships with school personnel are such that difficulties in the child's performance are promptly brought to their attention. And, if the child fails to assume an adequate academic role, as this is understood by the parents, they are quick to report learning problems. Thus, the discrepancy in the reported prevalence of learning problems may reflect a difference in priorities that masks the true incidence of these symptoms in the two groups studied.

In general, the middle-class parents assumed a direct continuity between early childhood behavior and later functioning, and the PRWC parents tended to take each succeeding stage as a separate issue. The middle-class parents focused particularly on ease of socialization and early experience with educational tasks as essential building blocks toward later success. For some youngsters this emphasis appeared to be consonant with the children's capacities, but in others the demands were premature or inappropriate and produced excessive stress, with anxiety or defensive protective mechanisms such as avoidance of academic tasks. Such anxiety or defensive responses were usually apprehended by the parents or teacher and deemed to be a sign of maladaptation.

In contrast, the PRWC parents as a group assumed that the children ought to be able to handle new developmental tasks when they arose. Learning was considered to be the responsibility of the school, and it was expected that the child would be capable of handling the social and educational demands of first grade when he arrived at the proper age. Prior exposure to educational tasks, such as learning the alphabet, was not traditionally seen as preparation for school, nor was there a deliberate training of the child to carry to completion a task that had been begun, as is characteristic of the education-oriented middle-class family. Thus, by contrast with the middle-class families, it is unlikely that the PRWC children would have been pressured to master social and learning tasks if they were not developmentally ready for such mastery.

e. Self-Inflicted Injuries. Seven PRWC children in the clinical sample under 9 years of age were reported by their parents to have inflicted injuries on themselves. These resulted from banging their heads and bodies against walls, and sustaining burns and razor cuts. Several of these children threatened to commit suicide when they were disciplined or frustrated. No self-inflicted injuries were reported among the middle-class children in the clinical sample.

Although the reasons for this difference in the incidence of self-inflicted injuries are not clear, we may speculate on its possible relationship to the handling of disciplinary restrictions in the two groups. In the middle-class families the children were usually permitted and even encouraged to voice their objections to restrictive rules and to discuss them freely with the parents. This was not true in the PRWC families, and the resulting suppressed and repressed aggression may then have been turned inward against the self.

DISCUSSION

In these two samples of children presenting behavior disorders before the age of 9, we found certain specific differences in age of onset and the types of symptoms. These differences can be explained in terms of variations in the environmental influences, demands, and stresses. Although these correlations are necessarily impressionistic and qualitative because of the small size of the sample, there appears to be a striking relationship between symptoms and specific environmental influences.

The study emphasizes the need for understanding a child's social and cultural background if one is to evaluate what constitutes excessive stress. This is of special concern because systematic criteria of normal behavioral development have been established primarily for white, native-born, middle-class children. The uncritical application of these middle-class norms to lower-class children of varying ethnic background has often resulted in faulty diagnosis and treatment (Chess et al., 1953). In evaluating personality, a psychiatrist must recognize that the same overt behavior patterns may have different meanings in individuals from different socioeconomic and cultural backgrounds. The incidence and types of presenting symptoms may reflect parental expectations as much as they do problems of functioning intrinsic to the child (Thomas et al., 1968). These expectations, in turn, cannot be understood apart from their social and cultural matrix.

NOTE: Commentary on this paper appears on pages 78–85.

REFERENCES

Chess, S., Clark, K. B., & Thomas, A. The importance of cultural evaluation in psychiatric diagnosis and treatment. *Psychiatric Quarterly*, 1953, 27, 102–114.

Clark, K. B. *Dark ghetto.* New York: Harper, 1965.

Hertzig, M. E., Birch, H. G., Thomas, A., & Mendez, O. A. Class and ethnic differences in the responsiveness of preschool children to cognitive demands. *Monographs of the Society for Research in Child Development*, 1968, 33 (1, serial no. 117).

Thomas, A., Chess, S., Birch, H. G., Hertzig, M. E., & Korn, S. *Behavioral individuality in early childhood.* New York: New York University Press, 1963.

Thomas, A., Chess, S., & Birch, H. G. *Temperament and behavior disorders in children.* New York: New York University Press, 1968.

MARK A. STEWART
HELEN PALKES
RAY MILLER
CAROL YOUNG
ZELA WELNER] *Intellectual Ability and School Achievement of Hyperactive Children, Their Classmates, and Their Siblings*

THE FIRST systematic description of the pattern of behavior which we now call hyperactivity, was published by Still in 1902; a number of the children whom he described had lesions of the brain. Twenty years later, many children who recovered from the acute form of encephalitis lethargica developed personality changes which would now be diagnosed as severe hyperactivity (Ebaugh, 1923; Leahy & Sand, 1921). More recently, Ingram (1956), Laufer and Denhoff (1957), and Clements and Peters (1962) published detailed descriptions of hyperactive behavior in children who had actual or presumed brain damage. Since the early reports on this behavioral syndrome linked it with lesions in the patients' brains, it is hardly surprising that the hyperactive child syndrome has become synonymous in the minds of many clinicians, teachers, and parents with brain damage, or the attenuated version of this concept, minimal brain dysfunction.

Confusion between *brain damage* and *hyperactivity* persists, in spite of demonstrations that the relationship between the two entities is complex. Paine, Werry, and Quay (1968) found a disturbing lack of correlations between historical, neurological, and psychological findings on a group of children who had been diagnosed as having minimal cerebral dysfunction. Rutter, Graham, and Yule (1970a), in an epidemiologic study of neuropsychiatric problems in children, showed that there are several

NOTE: The research reported in this paper was supported in part by the U.S. PHS Grants MH-05804 and MH-13002.

patterns of behavior associated with brain damage or dysfunction, and no one-to-one relationship between brain dysfunction and hyperactivity.

One unfortunate result of this confusion has been a difficulty in answering the question whether hyperactivity is commonly associated with specific problems in learning. In their classic description of the hyperkinetic behavior syndrome in children, Laufer and Denhoff (1957) reported that most of their patients were of normal intelligence, but that they frequently had "specific learning difficulties, usually in arithmetic but frequently in reading" and "disturbances in tasks involving visuo-motor function." Clements and Peters (1962) reported similar observations. There seems to have been an element of circularity in the reasoning of these and later reports. The perceptual problems and other handicaps in learning were taken as signs of neurologic disturbances and this premise then led to the conclusion that the whole pattern of behavior was a result of brain dysfunction. This influential idea, and the widespread assumption that specific reading disability and other learning handicaps were also part of a single syndrome of minimal brain dysfunction, have made it hard to disentangle the relationships between the behavior pattern of hyperactivity and specific learning disabilities. Other investigators, such as Chess (1960), Werry, Weiss, and Douglass (1964), and Stewart et al. (1966), have used a purely behavioral definition of the hyperactive child syndrome and made no assumptions about the etiology of the disorder. With this definition they have found that only a small proportion (less than 15 per cent) of the children studied had a definite history of brain damage, and that hyperactive children did not have histories of difficult delivery and similar events more often than control children (Minde, Webb, & Sykes, 1968; Stewart et al., 1966).

A behavioral definition of hyperactivity allows such simple questions as, Are hyperactive children handicapped by specific learning difficulties, such as reading disability? Do they tend to have perceptual blocks, or visuomotor defects? On the average, do they have the same intellectual ability as their classmates? How does their school achievement compare with that of their classmates? The three studies described here give beginning answers to these questions. Final answers will be important in a practical sense as well as being interesting theoretically for what they may tell us about the nature of hyperactivity as a behavioral problem. Most hyperactive children are brought to physicians, psychologists, or other professional people, primarily because of poor school performance. This is not to say that parents do not have troubles with hyperactive children at home, but they are usually most concerned about what is happening at school. The teachers of hyperactive children are, similarly, more concerned about the child's apparent underachieving rather than about difficulties in controlling his behavior. These observations make it important to discover whether hyperactive children are truly performing below their potential, whether they are learning at a slower rate than they should, and whether the difficulties that they have with schoolwork stem from impulsiveness and distractibility, or from specific cognitive problems.

First Study
(Helen Palkes and Mark Stewart)

The subjects were 32 consecutive new patients attending the St. Louis Children's Hospital Psychiatry Clinic who fitted the following criteria: the subjects' parents reported that they persistently suffered from overactivity, distractibility, impulsiveness, and excitability, and their teachers also reported overactivity and distractibility; they were attending regular public schools; and they were free from any continuing neurologic disorder, such as epilepsy, or special sensory handicap. The subjects were all boys, white, and mostly from middle-class families.

For controls 34 subjects were obtained from a St. Louis suburban public school which served a neighborhood of professional, managerial, and white-collar families. They were matched by the school secretary as closely as possible with the hyperactive child group on the variables of sex, age, grade, race, and socioeconomic class. Children who were known to have behavior problems in school, from records or current teacher reports, were not included in the control group, nor were children who had skipped or repeated grades or been in special classes. All of the control children and three quarters of the children in the hyperactive child group attended the same public school; the concentration of patient subjects in one school was due to a close working relationship between the school social worker and the investigators. Several of the remaining 8 hyperactive children attended comparable suburban schools, so that the two groups were quite well matched on educational opportunity.

Each subject was given the following battery of psychological tests: Wechsler Intelligence Scale for Children (wisc); Bender Gestalt Test for Young Children; Jastak Wide Range Achievement Test; Gray Oral Reading Test; Goodenough-Harris Drawing Test; Hidden Figures Test; and Peabody Picture Vocabulary Test.

The patients were tested in the Psychology Laboratory of St. Louis

Children's Hospital, and generally took four hours for each subject. Control subjects were tested at the school that the children attended. The senior author, or one of two psychometricians under her supervision, gave the tests and followed the standard procedures described in the respective test manuals. At times when children were inattentive, questions were repeated so that they were not penalized for failing to respond.

For each of the WISC IQ scores (see accompanying tabulation), the mean of the control group was significantly higher than that for the hyperactive group ($p<.01$) The t test modified for unequal variances was used for these comparisons, since the hyperactive group showed more variation than the control group on the WISC Performance IQ ($p<.01$) and on the WISC Full-Scale IQ ($p<.05$).

	Verbal	Performance	Full Scale
Mean			
Control	109.0	111.6	111.3
Patient	101.0	99.8	100.3
SD			
Control	11.95	8.40	9.91
Patient	14.69	13.82	13.73

The significant data for performance of the two groups on the WISC subtests are presented in Table 1. The control group had higher scores on all of the subtests, but since the scores represent nonindependent values, the probability levels had to be adjusted by the use of Bonferoni's t. Using this statistic for comparison, the control group's performance was better than the hyperactive group's on the Similarities ($p<.01$), the Picture Completion ($p<.01$), and the Mazes ($p<.05$) subtests.

To compare the scores of the two groups on the Wide Range Achievement and Gray Oral Reading Tests, the group means were adjusted for WISC Full-Scale IQ and grade level. The adjusted means were higher for the control group, but the differences were not significant.

Table 1. WISC Subtest Scores

	Mean		SD		P—	Adjusted P—
	Control	Patient	Control	Patient		
Similarities	13.41	10.71	2.95	3.20	<.001	<.01
Digit Span	9.82	8.53	2.56	2.65	<.05	n.s.
Picture Completion	12.14	9.34	3.11	3.16	<.005	<.01
Picture Arrangement	11.61	10.09	2.37	2.97	<.05	n.s.
Block Design	12.35	10.46	2.71	3.12	<.05	n.s.
Object Assembly	12.44	10.96	2.61	2.95	<.05	n.s.
Mazes	10.08	8.56	1.83	2.21	<.005	<.05

When the mean scores on the Bender-Gestalt Test, Developmental Score, and Hidden Figures Test were adjusted for WISC Full-Scale IQ, neither test distinguished between the two groups significantly: Developmental Score [Koppitz Scoring] (3.5 vs. 3.1; $F = -0.27$; n.s.); Hidden Figures Test (30.7 vs. 26.1; $F = 1.49$; n.s.).

The findings in this preliminary study of cognitive function in a group of behaviorally defined hyperactive children were these: The hyperactive children performed significantly less well on tests of intelligence than did their controls and did less well on tests of school achievement and perceptual-motor performance. However, the latter two differences disappeared when the variable of intelligence was controlled. The most obvious explanation for the deficit in measured intelligence would be that we simply demonstrated the hyperactive child's impulsivity and distractibility. Weighing against this explanation are the care we took to allow for such handicaps, and the common clinical observation that hyperactive children are on their best behavior in a strange situation with one other person.

This study suggested that hyperactive children are at a disadvantage in school because of intellectual handicaps as well as behavior problems. However, a major reservation about the findings stems from the fact that our subjects were patients, and the possibility that intellectual handicap was one of the factors that had determined their being referred to a psychiatric clinic. Our findings also suggested that hyperactive children actually learn skills in school at a rate normal for their measured intellectual ability. Presumably, the widely held idea that they are underachievers is related to the gap between their potential and that of their classmates, as well as to their difficulties in concentrating and finishing assignments. Teachers may also overestimate the intelligence of hyperactive children because of their apparent curiosity, alertness, and energy, and therefore expect too high a standard of work from them.

Second Study
(Ray Miller)

While H. P. and M. S. were doing the work that has just been described, R. M. was screening a large grade school population in order to determine the prevalence of hyperactivity in a suburban school district serving middle-class families. Later we were able to collaborate in comparing the scores on intelligence tests of the hyperactive children picked up in his screening with the scores of their classmates, and thus to find whether the differences we had observed between hyperactive children and their classmates also distinguished non-patient hyperactive children from their classmates.

The procedure involved in the screening was as follows: R.M. gave a standard presentation to the teachers at four elementary schools. He asked the teachers to name any children in their class who showed restlessness, lack of attention, inability to sit still, distractability, low tolerance of frustration, and who were hard to manage. He then interviewed each of the teachers in a standard way about the children named. The essential part of the interview consisted of a review of twenty-eight specific items of behavior such as "never seems to be still for a moment," "finishes classroom assignments," and "is easily upset by changes in things around him." Children were diagnosed as hyperactive if the teachers reported them to be overactive and distractible, and to have any five other symptoms from this list of twenty-eight items. In the third, fourth, fifth, and sixth grades, 849 children were screened in this way, 41 boys being diagnosed as hyperactive (9.3 per cent) and 6 girls (1.5 per cent). These figures are quite similar to those reported by Werner et al. (1968) in their epidemiologic study of children on the Island of Kauai. Scores on Lorge-Thorndike group intelligence tests were available for 22 hyperactive boys; these are compared with the scores of classmates in the accompanying tabulation. The differences between the hyperactive children ($N = 22$) and their classmates ($N = 296$) are in the same direction as those found in our first study and somewhat greater. We do not know how many of these children were patients. Teachers may have been more likely to nominate children whom they knew were patients, but it is also possible that hyperactive children who were being treated with drugs might have been doing so well in the classroom that they were not named by their teachers. This study suggests that the IQ deficit is not simply due to selection as a patient.

	Hyperactive Boys	*Normal Boys*
Verbal		
Mean............	94.0*	104.3*
SD.............	14.2*	16.3*
Nonverbal		
Mean..........	95.1**	110.2**
SD.............	15.7**	16.6**
Full scale		
Mean..........	94.9**	107.3**
SD............	14.1**	15.3**

*$p<.01$.
**$p<.001$.

Third Study
(Mark Stewart, Helen Palkes,
Carol Young, and Zela Welner)

We next compared the intellectual ability, school achievement, life history, and self-esteem of hyperactive children with those of their siblings, and did a parallel study of control children and their siblings. Here we present only the data on intelligence.

Using a standard interviewing technique, we interviewed the mothers of 45 hyperactive children (all boys and white) who were attending the Psychiatry Clinic of St. Louis Children's Hospital, or who were private patients of M. S., in order to get systematic data on the current behavior, school performance, and development of all their children. We also interviewed the hyperactive children themselves and their siblings between the ages of six and sixteen, and tested the patients and their siblings with the same battery of psychological tests we had used in the first study. For this study children were called hyperactive only if their mothers reported a long history of overactivity, short attention span, impulsive behavior, and emotional lability. As in the earlier study, these children had to be living with their natural families, attending school, and free from neurologic disease (cerebral palsy and epilepsy, for example) or special sensory handicap.

We asked the parents of all the boys in the fifth and sixth grades of two elementary schools in the Webster Groves School District for permission to interview the mother and to interview and test the boy and his siblings between the ages of six and sixteen. The only qualification that a subject had to have was that he had one or more siblings between these ages. Of the parents, 44 sets out of 74 agreed to the interviewing and testing. The socioeconomic levels of the families served by the two schools roughly matched those of our patients' families.

Of the original hyperactive children 10 had one or more siblings who also was diagnosed as hyperactive on the information given by the mother; these children and their siblings were dropped from the statistical comparisons shown here. Also, 9 control families were dropped from the main statistical analyses because they contained one or more hyperactive children. The hyperactive children picked up in these families did provide data for some other interesting comparisons.

As shown in Table 2 there were no differences in WISC scores between the hyperactive patients and their siblings, and only slight differences between index control children and their siblings. There were signifi-

Table 2. WISC Scores of Hyperactive and Normal Children
and Their Siblings

Children	Verbal	Performance	Full Scale
Hyperactive			
Ss ($N = 35$) 103.01		106.3	105.1
Siblings ($N = 49$) 106.6		106.8	107.5
Normal			
Ss ($N = 35$) 112.9		116.1*	115.9*
Siblings ($N = 64$) 109.7		112.3*	111.9*

*$p<.05$.

cant differences between the average level of intelligence of the hyperactive patients and that of the index control children, and between those of their respective siblings, but these differences have no particular meaning for the study. There were significant differences between the control children who were diagnosed as hyperactive and the index control children, which were meaningful since the children in the two groups were classmates or schoolmates (see accompanying tabulation).

The lack of difference between the scores of hyperactive children and those of their siblings argues against the possibility that the lower scores of hyperactive children are due to their behavior in the testing situation, since there is no obvious reason why the healthy siblings of the hyperactive children would be at a similar disadvantage. However, it is possible that the siblings also tend to be impulsive and distractible, though not qualifying for the label *hyperactive*. The data we collected in the interviews may answer this question after we have analyzed them. The finding that siblings share the intellectual deficit of hyperactive children also works against the idea that the apparent deficit is a result of parents' and teachers' being more likely to describe a dull child as hyperactive.

The lower IQ's of the hyperactive children who were found in the control population (see tabulation) serve to confirm the findings of our second study. These children were diagnosed as hyperactive from information given by the mother rather than by the teacher, but the differences between their measured intelligence and that of their classmates were the same. This study also shows that there was a greater difference between

	Verbal	Performance	Full Scale
Hyperactive controls ($N = 9$) ...	102.8*	101.1**	102.2**
Normal controls ($N = 35$)	112.9*	116.1**	115.9**

*$p<.05$.   **$p<.01$.

the Performance IQ's of hyperactive children and their classmates than there was between the Verbal IQ's of the two groups. This relationship can be seen in the data from all four sets of comparisons between hyperactive children and control children.

Discussion

The deficit in measured intelligence that we have found in hyperactive children has been noted by other investigators. Minde et al. (1971) found a mean difference in IQ of eleven points between a group of 37 hyperactive children and controls who were their classmates. Quitkin and Klein (1969) found a seven-point difference between young adult psychiatric patients who were diagnosed retrospectively as hyperactive and a control group of young patients who did not have a history of childhood disorder. The latter report suggests that the intellectual deficit of hyperactive children may be stable over time, but we make this comment hesitantly because Quitkin and Klein's population is a special one.

Rutter has reported that psychiatric disorder in children is associated with lower intelligence in the general population (Rutter, Tizard, & Whitmore, 1970b) and in neuro-epileptic children (Rutter et al., 1970a). These reports raise the question whether our findings reflect a specific association between lower IQ and hyperactivity, or are part of a nonspecific association between lower IQ and psychiatric disorder in children. Since the hyperactive child syndrome, as we have defined it, may well be the commonest psychiatric disorder among children in general and among those with brain dysfunction, it is possible that the association reported by Rutter and his colleagues may be largely due to a specific association between hyperactivity and lower intelligence. Actually Rutter et al. (1970b) found that among boys with psychiatric disorder, only those diagnosed as antisocial had a significantly lower IQ than that of the controls, (the difference was about eleven points). It is difficult for us to tell where the children that we diagnosed as hyperactive would fit into the diagnostic scheme used by Rutter and his colleagues, who define hyperkinetic syndrome differently. It seems quite likely that our patient population would correspond to their group of "conduct or antisocial disorder" rather than "neurotic disorder" and "mixed conduct and neurotic disorder," but there is probably some overlap with the latter two categories.

Our findings could be explained as a function of hyperactive children's impulsivity and distractibility, rather than a lack of intellectual ability, in spite of the arguments that we have raised to the contrary.

Garner, Percy, and Lawson (1971) found that intellectual impulsivity was negatively related to scores on the WISC among boys and girls. Other evidence that seems to support this explanation indirectly is the improvement in WISC scores of hyperactive children brought about by treatment with amphetamines (Conners, 1972; Conrad et al. 1971). It seems reasonable to assume that the effects of drugs on measured intelligence are mediated through effects on concentration and impulsivity. We do not know, however, whether normal children's scores might not be affected in the same way by stimulant drugs and, therefore, prefer not to attach too much weight to these observations.

The findings can also be explained by an opposite relationship between the abnormal behavior and the lower IQ. It is possible that children with lower intelligence develop behavior problems because they need to express resentment over, or compensate for, their failures in school. This explanation is favored by Rutter and his colleagues, but it cannot be applied readily to hyperactive children since the majority of them have been noted by their parents to have unusual behavior from an early age, and nearly all of them have caused problems before they entered school (Mendelson, Johnson, Stewart, 1971; Stewart et al., 1966; Stewart, Thach, & Freidin, 1970).

Another possibility is that dull children are more likely to be labeled by parents and teachers as hyperactive. Such a bias in selection seems quite probable, but our finding that the apparently healthy siblings of the hyperactive children share their intellectual deficit argues against this explanation. This particular observation needs to be confirmed, but it suggests an independent variable operating in families that determines both lower intelligence and hyperactivity. We have already found evidence that hyperactivity may pass from one generation to another (Morrison & Stewart, 1971), and we have data on families of adopted hyperactive children which suggest that this transmission is genetic rather than social (Morrison & Stewart, in press). We think it likely that the deficit in intellectual ability of hyperactive children and their siblings is a sign of an inherited defect.

Whether the intellectual deficit we have found is a sign of a primary lack of intellectual ability or the result of impulsivity and lack of concentration, there is a functional deficit in intelligence which has important practical implications for parents and teachers of hyperactive children. In order to accept the hyperactive child or pupil, and to have positive regard for him, parents and teachers need to form realistic expectations about his performance in school. These expectations can best be based on a full battery of psychological tests. Expectations that are rationally based are likely to be met by the average hyperactive child according to our data, so that parents and teachers should be able to avoid the sense of frustration they usually feel with such children. An important step in this direction, especially for teachers, is to make a clear distinction between the performance of assigned work and the process of learning. Hyperactive children do less assigned work than their classmates, and the quality of their work is less satisfactory, but they appear to learn the required skills at the same rate as classmates of equal intelligence. We believe that the improved understanding and acceptance of a hyperactive child's performance in school which can follow from this research should help to sustain his self-esteem.

COMMENTARY

CHESS. We shall discuss the first four papers together, since they are interrelated.

WIRT. Rosenthal's paper seems to me to be an excellent discussion of the problems of research in high-risk populations, not just in schizophrenia. The other papers, I think, show some of the kinds of difficulties researchers have in choosing what factors to study and what will be essential, what relevant, and how these are to be measured. We get stuck with the results of such decisions many years later. The problem of replication remains in all longitudinal research because we always see ways in which we could improve what we did or what somebody else did; thus, nothing ever gets replicated precisely.

ROFF. Dr. Thomas, do you have any comparison of the mental health level of adults in the same two ethnic-class groups, even though such information was not longitudinally obtained and did not deal with the same persons at all? In other words, is it possible to get any reasonably accurate descriptions of the current mental health pictures in adults of the two groups?

THOMAS. This is an important issue, and it would indeed be interesting if we could compare the differences in the children in our two populations with differences in adults of similarly contrasting ethnic-class backgrounds. Unfortunately, to our knowledge there are no definitive studies or satisfactory data on this issue. There are comparative data on schooling, income level, crime, and so on, but not on mental health status. Several limited studies have been reported, but their findings are at best suggestive.

WATT. I have received correspondence from Dr. A. Hoffer saying that he has observed in the children of schizophrenic parents an unusual number of hyperactive children. Dr. Stewart, do you have any information about the prevalence of hyperactive children among schizophrenics or their offspring?

STEWART. I can't answer your question directly, but in our family study we have found no relation. Parents and adult relatives of hyperactive children tend to show alcoholism and sometimes sociopathy and hysteria. That observation definitely needs to be confirmed. Perhaps there is some excess of bipolar affective disorder. We had only a small group of Ss, some 50 hyperactive children and 50 controls. But though we found these other things, rather to our surprise, we found no schizophrenics.

CHESS. In the identification of hyperactivity, it is rather difficult to separate out how frequently, how fast, and how goal directed the hyperactivity is. It is clearly recognized that a child is being hyperactive when his behavior is also disorganized, whereas a child who moves at high speed, but who functions in an organized and purposeful manner, may not be getting in your way. It is certainly true that schizophrenic children's behavior is disorganized. In my clinical experience, there is also a proportion of children referred to as hyperactive who, on close examination, are not in fact hyperactive in the sense of how fast and how often.

ROSENTHAL. I would like to call your attention to the book by Paul Wender on minimal brain dysfunction. Wender, my long-time research colleague, has made this one of his major interests. We don't have any hard data at this point, but Wender believes that minimal brain dysfunction is genetic, and he also believes that at least one subgroup among hyperactive kids probably will turn out to be schizophrenic when they grow up. In a study now under way, Wender is also looking at the relatives of these hyperactive kids.

ZUBIN. Did you correct for regression effect when comparing your hyperactive children and their siblings?

STEWART. That is the kind of question I can't answer. There were various interaction effects looked for, and none found.

BIRCH. I think there are at least three or four features of these four papers that cannot be permitted to stand without challenge. In the first place, there has been a very loose discussion of *genetic*. Everything is genetic, everything. Benson Ginsberg some years ago remarked that everything is genetic, but nothing is determined. What we are concerned with is the interaction between particular familial antecedents and the circumstances in which certain frequencies of phenotypical manifestations occur. None of the data presented gives us a sufficient basis for considering these two contributors to variance and their interaction in the development of any phenotype, whether this is discussed in connection with schizophrenia or with hyperkinesis. I could develop many other fancy theories to account for any of the interactions presented. For example, I could take a position that children of lower IQ more frequently have difficulties in middle-class schools than do other children, and that this then reactively produces conduct and behavior disorders that are classified as hyperkinetic. I see no control for this in any of Stewart's studies.

STEWART. How about their siblings?

BIRCH. Their siblings are also lower IQ. And there is a 33 per cent risk rate for hyperkinesis in lower IQ children. OK? Thus, 33 per cent of the children in a sibship who are duller than the community in which they live exhibit hyperkinesis. This is what your data show, and nothing more. They show that the sibs don't differ from the hyperkinetic kids — both are duller than the other children in the community with whom they are matched. One could advance this hypothesis. Or, if one has a little more imagination, one could advance another hypothesis, that the mothers of these sibships are ineffective reproducers. Look at Rutter's data, look at our data in Aberdeen, look at data anywhere, and you will find that the frequency with which behavior disturbances occur are related systematically to the birth weight of the children and the frequency with which mothers have had disturbances of pregnancy, and that these often run in families. In other words, the sibs whose mothers are poor reproducers also are poor reproducers. I would like to know your data with respect to the reproductive course of children in all of these sibships and so on before I accept, even for an instant, any of your very, very bold generalizations with respect to a genetic effect.

Other questions have occurred to me. For example, Rosenthal's statement about the lack of finding of neurologic abnormalities in individuals above preadolescence is in contradiction to the findings of Hertzig and myself with respect to adolescent schizophrenics, in whom one finds an excessive frequency of neurologic abnormalities. I would suggest that this is probably a function of the ceiling effect of the neurologic examination performed. Pediatric neurological examinations become undiscriminating after preadolescence, and one has to use a more refined and more developed examination. I don't think that Rosenthal would necessarily disagree on that.

Thomas gave us beautiful vignettes. He argues that certain of the sleep disturbances are the developmental consequence of sleep being the initiation of the school period, that going to sleep the night before is in fact the beginning of the school day. Implicit in his statement and almost explicit at one point was the implication that sleep difficulties, nightmares, disturbances, etc., should be more frequent on Sunday through Thursday nights than on Friday and Saturday nights. I should like to know whether he has analyzed his data from this point of view and whether he plans to do so. I think these are fascinating questions, but I think that we stay too much on the surface of the phenomena with which we are concerned, and haven't boldly explored alternatives and pointed to new oportunities for study.

THOMAS. Knowing that Birch would come up with a stimulating discussion, I was careful to say that he was taking no responsibility for this aspect of the study. What he says is absolutely true, and it illustrates one of the problems in a longitudinal study — that when you start to analyze the data in applying certain relationships, you realize there are all kinds of questions that you should have asked and all kinds of data that you should have gotten that you didn't at the time. The reason for my emphasis on this being impressionistic is that we don't have these data. What could be done — and it doesn't require the same sample, obviously — is to study a group of children of this background with sleep problems.

ROSENTHAL. As long as we're responding, certainly the last point Dr. Birch made in reference to our Israeli study is correct. In the fall of 1972 we shall start re-examining our Israeli *S*s, and we shall include another neurological examination. I'm not sure what form it will take, but we'll have a chance to see if there are additional kinds of neurological disturbance in this population. This is something that can be tested empirically.

You do raise a special kind of problem when you say that everything is genetic. Not everything really is genetic — except in the sense that we have to have genes to be alive, to move, to talk, to see, and to write. Let's assume that the organism is here. What we are really trying to do in studying mental illness is to see whether specific kinds of genetic mechanisms play a role in the disorder — whether, for example, we can identify either a single gene or a certain genotype pattern that will be specific to schizophrenic disorders. When we start working on the affective disorders, we'll have the same kind of plan in mind. There is a very good chance that we'll be able to point to genetic mechanisms at work.

The interaction between genes and environment has been of concern to us from the very beginning, but it's not easy to isolate. For example, our Israeli study is designed for teasing out gene-rearing interactions, and some interesting findings do emerge. But the relatively small number might be expected just by chance alone. I still believe in gene-environment interactions, and I'm still looking for them. We may not have detected them in Israel, but we know they have to exist.

ZUBIN. I was very taken with Rosenthal's findings that in the light of his new studies, reaction time is related more to the home environment than it is to the genetic component. Now, this raises a whole series of questions. Is it only the autonomic system that seems to be the differential between the high risk for schizophrenia group and the normal controls? Our own work leads me to conclude (although I would like to know whether Rosenthal would agree, or would like to carry out some of these studies on his population) that the central nervous system, aside from the autonomic system, is also involved. For example, even in reaction time, in his own laboratory and in ours, we have been able to show that although the schizophrenic himself is rather slow (as would be indicated by the fact that the people brought up in schizophrenic families would be slow in reaction time), when we compare in succession the response to sound coming after light as compared with the response to sound coming after sound, there is a much longer retardation in the schizophrenic when you switch modalities on him. It seems to me that that could not be explained by slowness owing to family upbringing.

One might try to explain the retardation in reaction time by postulating that the uncertainty regarding the next stimulus is the disturbing factor — that is, that if the patient expects a light and receives instead a sound, reaction time is increased owing to the unfulfilled expectancy or set, and that the training in schizophrenic families makes them most vulnerable to disappointments. In order to examine this question, all uncertainty was removed by telling the patient what the next stimulus would be and placing his finger on the key for the particular modality that was next in the sequence. The elimination of this uncertainty reduced but did not eliminate the differential retardation between normals and patients. There seems to be a central nervous system difference in the processing of successive stimuli in patients compared with normals which is hardly explicable on the basis of family upbringing.

Another difference between schizophrenics and normals in the processing of information is the finding that critical duration following the **Bunson Roscoe Law** or Bloch's Law is shorter in schizophrenics suffering from thought disorder than in other types of schizophrenics and in depressives and normals. In this experiment, reaction time was again used as the response to brief stimuli. It was noted that for normals full integration of the delivered energy held true despite differences in its packaging (short duration of very intense stimuli versus long duration of less intense stimuli) as measured by the constancy of the reaction time response. This full integration held for as long as 13 msec of stimulation for the particular energy system used in our laboratory. For schizophrenics, full integration continued only up to 4 msec of stimulation, the reaction time rising when the same energy was delivered over a period of 6 msec (including a 2-msec interval of darkness) rather than in 4 msec. Here again, it is difficult to attribute such findings to family upbringing. It seems as if the energy cup for the schizophrenic fills up at 4 msec, and energy delivered beyond that interval spills over and does not affect the response. All attempts thus far to get normals to alter their response at 4 msec has failed.

The other point that I wanted to make is perhaps a little more urgent. That is, why, when we have rather systematic structured interviews for assessing the presence of schizophrenia in adults (we haven't got them for children yet), do we still depend on case histories and discursive descriptive approaches? In the studies that are going on in Denmark and also in this country, why don't you utilize more systematic structured interviews that are reliable and have shown themselves to differentiate between affective and schizophrenic disorders? At the present time, I'm not too sure that the mere fact that the patients are in hospitals labeled as schizophrenic guarantees that they are characterized by a schizophrenic syndrome. We find that 60 per cent of the people suffering from morbid depression in this country are called schizophrenic by some state hospital psychiatrists. I don't mean to say that Rosenthal's diagnoses of schizophrenia are suspect, but why use labels based merely on consensus when reliable profiles across dimensions of behavior are available?

The last thing that I wanted to say refers to the genetic versus environmental argument. I believe that there are no genetic diseases nor environmental diseases. We call a disease genetic because we don't yet know the genotypes required for it. And I can at least conceive of a genotype that can survive in any of the worst niches you place it in; by the same token, there may be a niche that will crumple the best genotype you can think of.

ROSENTHAL. Well, which point to address first? No genetic diseases, no environmental diseases. You're absolutely right that when we use the term *genetic disease*, it's almost always shorthand to imply that some kind of genotype is involved in the disease, that it has a certain specificity. And of course, there always has to be environment.

It would be nice to use a Spitzer interview, and in a way I wish we had. It certainly would have made my life easier. There were various reasons why we could not use this kind of interview in Denmark, although by now we may have convinced our Danish colleagues that it is perfectly all right to use a structured interview. If we ever replicate the study, perhaps we shall use one. However, there are advantages in an open-ended interview, lasting from three to five hours, where the psychiatrist examines all aspects of the individual's personality, whether they are nicely reliable or not, and does not restrict himself to some items. We have a wealth of material that we never would have obtained if we had stuck to a structured interview. Compromise may be the best answer to this problem, but you can only examine a patient for so long, and a three- to five-hour interview is exhausting. Several aspects of our open-ended interviews, can be analyzed quite fruitfully, and we are doing this.

Now the reaction times. Can reaction times be influenced by a family? I really doubt it. I have clear evidence that the subjects in hospitals who were reared by a schizophrenic parent (either a biological schizophrenic parent or a parent to whom he was given up for adoption) had poorer reaction time than did the subjects who were selected because they did not have a schizophrenic parent. You can't discard these findings simply because you believe that they are impossible. What about these phenomena that you mentioned, the shifts in modality? And even the shifts with respect to reaction time performance? I am now convinced that reaction time probably has nothing to do with upbringing in any direct sense, and I am equally convinced that it has nothing to do with genes in any direct sense. And I am pretty well convinced that it has to do with the clinical illness itself. This is simply one kind of phenomenon, one manifestation, of what it means to be clinically schizophrenic.

ZUBIN. Why do you say that it is not genetic?

ROSENTHAL. We have not completed analysis of the reaction times. But into this huge reaction time study, we have built characteristics that are based on differences between clinical schizophrenics and normal controls, especially with respect to the variations in preparatory intervals. What I have reported is an overall finding with respect to the performance on all aspects of the reaction time experiment. We have performed experiments under regular and irregular conditions — where the preparatory interval is shorter and longer, and variations of that sort. We shall analyze that data to see whether the patterns in clinical schizophrenics follow the patterns that in our subjects, who are not clinically schizophrenic, but who are related or not related to a schizophrenic. My guess is that we won't get the same kinds of patterns in our subjects and in clinical schizophrenics, but I'll let you know as soon as we get the data analyzed.

RIEDER. Dr. Stewart, your study that revealed no difference between hyperactive children and their sibs excluded those families where there was not more than one hyperactive child. Assuming that there may be multiple etiologies for hyperactivity, if you take out that group which has more than one hyperactive child, then you may be selecting against genetic loading. You have a group of families, and a group of children, in which a greater number of the children would be hyperactive on the basis of another cause. If there is a predominance of other causes, such as "learned" hyperactivity, that may explain why you don't see something underlying the hyperactivity, such as an intellectual defect. It's difficult to make a genetic hypothesis after you have selected out the families that are presumably genetically loaded for this.

STEWART. I didn't formulate any genetic hypothesis. It is just a simple description.

RIEDER. Dr. Thomas, I wanted to ask you about the PRWC hyperactive offspring. You seemed to indicate that there was sort of a "closed room" syndrome that produced hyperactivity. I was wondering whether these *S*s were typically hyperactive in the sense that Stewart outlined, having defects in impulsivity and concentration, and whether they responded to Dexedrine. Secondly, I wonder whether this group of PRWC hyperactive offspring were actually the ones who were the most cooped up.

THOMAS. Well, this relates to a general question of activity as a temperamental characteristic, in which there is a normal range of activity level as a temperamental characteristic of a child, from a low to a medium to a high level. There are high active children who are normal, basically — they are not hyperactive in a pathological sense — and who are found also in our middle-class population and other studies. The question of how much freedom of motor activity the children have can make a great difference as to whether his high activity level remains as a normal characteristic of the child — in some cases the parents may not like this level, and in other cases they may delight in it, depending on the parents. But it doesn't become the basis of a behavior problem. Compare that with an environmental situation in which the child does not have the same free play for expression of his motor activity, and in which then there is a pathological development, with a combination of what appears to be hyperactivity and also the development of other problems with it — disciplinary problems, negativism, and so on. In other words, one always has to look at the child's characteristics in interaction with what the environment is. A particular activity level in the middle-class children may not lead to the development of behavioral problems because of the freedom of interaction with the environmental possibilities. In the PRWC children the outcome may be different because of the restrictions on them. These are not children who fall in the pathological hyperactive syndrome, whether one relates this to brain damage or other causes, and that was my point about not using the term *hyperactivity*, owing to minimal brain damage, loosely to characterize all of these children. Given a different environment, some PRWC children who now appear hyperactive might be within the normal range, though highly active, whereas there are others who would be hyperactive in the pathological sense (though we would want more specific clinical criteria before making this diagnosis).

REFERENCES

Chess, S. Diagnosis and treatment of the hyperactive child. *New York State Journal of Medicine*, 1960, 60, 2379.

Clements, S. D., & Peters, J. E. Minimal brain dysfunctions in the school-age child. *Archives of General Psychiatry*, 1962, 6, 185.

Conners, C. K. Psychological effects of stimulant drugs in children with minimal brain dysfunction. *Pediatrics*, 1972, 49, 5.

Conrad, W. G., Dworking, E. S., Shai, A., & Tobiessen, J. E. Effects of amphetamine therapy and prescriptive tutoring on the behavior and achievement of lower class hyperactive children. *Journal of Learning Disabilities*, 1971, 4, 9.

Ebaugh, F. G. Neuropsychiatric sequelae of acute epidemic encephalitis in children. *American Journal of Diseases of Children*, 1923, 25, 89.

Garner, J., Percy, L. M., & Lawson, T. Sex differences in behavioral impulsivity, intellectual impulsivity, and attainment in young children. *Journal of Child Psychology and Psychiatry*, 1971, 12, 261.

Ingram, T. T. S. A characteristic form of overactive behavior in brain damaged children. *Journal of Mental Science*, 1956, 102, 550.

Laufer, M. W., & Denhoff, E. Hyperkinetic behavior syndrome in children. *Journal of Pediatrics*, 1957, 50, 463.

Leahy, S. R., & Sands, I. J. Mental disorders in children following epidemic encephalitis. *Journal of the American Medical Association*, 1921, 76, 373.

Mendelson, W., Johnson, N., & Stewart, M. A. Hyperactive children as teenagers: A follow-up study. *Journal of Nervous and Mental Disease*, 1971, 153, 273.

Minde, K., Lewin, D., Weiss, G., Lavigueur, Douglas V., & Sykes, E. The hyperactive child in elementary school: A 5 year, controlled, follow-up. *Exceptional Child*, 1971, 38, 215.

Minde, K., Webb, G., & Sykes, D. Studies on the hyperactive child VI — Prenatal and paranatal factors associated with hyperactivity. *Developmental Medicine and Child Neurology*, 1968, 10, 355.

Morrison, J. R., & Stewart, M. A. A family study of the hyperactive child syndrome. *Biological Psychiatry*, 1971, 3, 189.

————. The psychiatric status of the legal families of adopted hyperactive children. *Archives of General Psychiatry*, in press.

Paine, R. S., Werry, J. S., & Quay, H. C. A study of "minimal cerebral dysfunction." *Developmental Medicine and Child Neurology*, 1968, 10, 505.

Quitkin, F., & Klein, D. F. Two behavioral syndromes in young adults related to possible minimal brain dysfunction. *Journal of Psychiatric Research*, 1969, 7, 131.

Rutter, M., Graham, P., & Yule, W. *A neuropsychiatric study in childhood.* Philadelphia: Lippincott, 1970. (a)

Rutter, M., Tizard, J., & Whitmore, K. *Education, health and behaviour.* London: Longman, 1970. (b)

Stewart, M. A., Pitts, F. N., Jr., Craig, A. G., & Dieruf, W. The hyperactive child syndrome. *American Journal of Orthopsychiatry*, 1966, 36, 5.

Stewart, M. A., Thach, B. T., & Freidin, M. R. Accidental poisoning and the hyperactive child syndrome. *Diseases of the Nervous System*, 1970, 31, 403.

Still, G. F. Some abnormal psychical conditions in children. *Lancet*, 1902, i, 1077.

Werner, E., Bierman, J. M., French, F. E., Simonian, K., Connor, A., Smith, R. S., & Campbell, M. Reproductive and environmental casualties: A report of the 10-year follow-up of the children of the Kauai pregnancy study. *Pediatrics*, 1968, 42, 112.

Werry, J. S., Weiss, G., & Douglas, V. Studies on the hyperactive child I: Some preliminary findings. *Canadian Psychiatric Association Journal*, 1964, 9, 120.

JON E. ROLF
NORMAN GARMEZY ⟧ *The School Performance*
of Children Vulnerable to Behavior Pathology

THIS PAPER concerns the relationship of biographical and academic performance data contained in grade school records to the development of psychopathology. The aim of this prospective research project has been to avoid the difficulties of retrospective error and uncontrolled pharmacological or psychological therapies inherent in the study of mentally ill adults and to concentrate on different target groups of elementary school children who are considered to be vulnerable to psychopathology in adulthood.

There are two concepts of major importance to our ongoing research: *vulnerability* to psychopathology and *competence*. Garmezy (1969; in press) has discussed the utility of these concepts for research with children. Vulnerability determined the types of children who were chosen, while competence provided a means of selecting the forms of behaviors that would be useful in differentiating, within the vulnerable groups, children who are apparently healthy from others who show evidence of maladjustment.

Vulnerability to adult psychopathology can be a function of genetic high risk (the biological mothers of one of our target groups have had a history of schizophrenic pathology); a function of deviant parental models (another target group have mothers who have received no psychotic psychiatric diagnoses in the course of hospitalization or outpatient treatment); a function of learned externalizing, antisocial, or internalizing

NOTE: Grateful acknowledgment must be made for the generous advice and assistance of Beverly Kaemmer, Ceci Littwin, and Judith Parizer. This research was in part supported by grants from U.S. PHS–NIMH (NH-06170) and from the Supreme Council 33, A. A. Scottish Rite, Northern Masonic Jurisdiction (N. Garmezy, principal investigator).

neurotic childhood habits (two of our target groups have been seen in child guidance clinics for diagnosis and treatment); or as a function of some organic deficits described elsewhere in this volume. But whether one espouses a genetic high-risk or a social learning theoretical model to explain the etiology of a particular behavior disorder, there should be ready agreement regarding our target children's manifest vulnerability as measured by their lack of social and academic competence. In the initial study (Rolf, 1972) which led to the present investigation, it was discovered that among the first four of these target groups the trend of the rankings based upon *peer-rated* social competence* measures indicated that for both sexes externalizing children were lowest, followed in order of ascending competence by the children with schizophrenic mothers, the internalizing children, and the children whose mothers' symptomatology was nonpsychotic and essentially of an internalizing nature. This order also obtained for the girls when the *teacher-rated* competence† scores were considered. For the boys teachers rated externalizers lowest, internalizers next lowest, but generally did not discriminate to a significant extent between male target groups with mentally ill mothers and their control groups. Thus, peers and teachers held striking differences of opinion in regard to the competence of sons of schizophrenic mothers. Peers had rated their social competence as significantly lower than their respective matched and random control groups in 75 per cent of the comparisons and nearly as low in overall competence as the externalizers. In marked contrast, the teachers never judged the sons of the schizophrenic mother group on the teacher's rating scale as significantly less competent than their control groups. In addition, they tended to rate these children highest in overall competence of the four target groups (excluding, of course, the control groups, who were always judged more competent).

What could account for these discrepancies between peer- and teacher-rated competence of target groups who had mentally disturbed mothers? Were teachers less perceptive or less willing to report signs of behavior pathology? One step toward answering this question would be to look at report card grades to see if this standard type of teacher's rating would better differentiate between these same four target groups of chil-

---

*The primary social competence rating device was a modification of E. M. Bower's "The Class Play," where each child plays the role of the director and casts his classmates into seventeen positive and negative roles.

†The teacher-rated competence measure consisted of a rating scale containing 26 bipolar items and 3 five-point scales of overall adjustment. These clustered items were derived from Norman Watt's clustering of J. Conger's and W. Miller's rating scales.

dren and their respective control groups. A second step would be to examine a different kind of teacher-recorded data, the biographical information on their students' families, information which perhaps could influence the teacher's perception or judgments. The cumulative records contain information on the socioeconomic and marital status of the parents, the child's sibling status, his changes in residence, as well as his attendance records for up to six years. Would there be important differences between a target group and its control group or among the four target groups on these variables? A third step would be to analyze the teacher's year-end descriptive comments about each pupil. These brief paragraphs are also recorded on the cumulative records, and Watt's (e.g., Watt et al., 1970; and see Watt, pp. 194–211) work with similar material (based on children who later developed schizophrenia in adulthood) suggests that teachers may make predictively useful ratings in this context. This paper will present our findings regarding the utility of the first two of these steps — namely, the teacher-rated academic performance data and the teacher-recorded biographical data — in discriminating between vulnerable children and their controls.

Method

Subjects. Two target groups of children were considered to be vulnerable because of their mothers' psychiatric disorders. One of these two groups contained 14 boys and 17 girls whose mothers had been diagnosed as schizophrenic, and the other contained 13 boys and 13 girls whose mothers had exhibited primarily neurotic depressive symptoms. The remaining two target groups did not, as far as was known from their own clinical records, have a parent who had been formally diagnosed as mentally ill. Instead, these children had been referred for psychological evaluation or treatment either for disturbing externalizing behavior (19 boys and 17 girls) or internalizing symptomatology (16 boys and 11 girls).

There were several reasons for using Achenbach's (1966) internalizing-externalizing dichotomy for categorizing symptoms in the present study: (a) it provided a useful means for grouping most functional childhood behavior disorders; (b) it also could be used to characterize certain types of symptomatic behaviors often viewed as potential precursors of schizophrenia (e.g., antisocial behavior as suggested by Robins [1966] and Roff [1963] and "avoidance orientation" as reported by Higgins [1966]); and (c) the inclusion of internalizing and externalizing children of both sexes permitted a comparison of their psychosocial competence levels with those of the children with psychologically disturbed mothers. In this way, one would be able to rank the four target groups of vulnerable children from best to worst on the basis of their respective performances on the various criterion measures of competence.

Control children were selected from the target child's own classroom. One child — the matched control — was matched on the following demographic variables: sex, age, grade, social class, intactness of the home, previous standard achievement test scores, and IQ score (if the latter was available). The random control child was of the same sex and grade as the target child but otherwise was chosen randomly from among the children in the class who were not manifesting problems. Children with physical handicaps or with behavior disorders known to school officials were not eligible to become random controls.

The target plus his two controls formed a classroom triad. The total number of Ss in the triad groups was 356 (targets $=$ 120, matched controls $=$ 120, random controls $=$ 116), and they were located in 113 classrooms in 30 elementary schools in a midwestern city. Ss in this study had an average age of ten years, had attained an average fourth-grade level in school, and were largely from blue-collar families. A more detailed description of these and other demographic variables will be presented below.

Procedure. The procedure for locating the mentally ill mothers,* identifying their school-aged children and tracing them to their respective

*The mothers themselves were identified by screening all female psychiatric admissions to the three major public psychiatric facilities of a midwestern city in "Lakeland County" for the period January 1, 1967, to May 1969. Women were placed into schizophrenic and nonpsychotic groups on the basis of diagnoses and other information contained in their hospital records. (The authors have confidence in the validity of this grouping procedure, but validity checks are under way which employ independent, experienced judges.) Women were automatically excluded from the study if they were: nonwhite; not born United States citizens; exceeded the age range of 18 to 50 years; gave evidence of being mentally defective as measured by standardized intelligence tests; or had been given a primary diagnosis suggesting an organic brain syndrome. Of 260 "Lakeland County" women with a current diagnosis of schizophrenia, 162 were excluded for the following reasons: 65 had no children, 12 had left the county, 25 were separated from their children (with the children no longer residents of the county or state), 11 had given up their children through adoption, 1 mother had her only child incarcerated; for 27 mothers the children were older than school age, and for 20 mothers they were younger. Of the 98 schizophrenic mothers who were not eliminated from the study by the exclusion criteria, 65 were in our city target area, but only 21 mothers had children in elementary school. Of the potentially available children of urban schizophrenic mothers, only 70 were locatable in the city schools. (Of those who could not be located, 26 were in private

schools, enlisting the cooperation of the principals and teachers — all without betraying any confidentiality or jeopardizing the child's status in the classroom — has been reported (Rolf, 1972). Only procedures pertaining to the collection of academic achievement data will be reported here.

The peer- and teacher-rating materials were distributed to the classroom teachers and collected a week later in a two-month period preceding the ending of school. Shortly thereafter, during the end of May and throughout June, one of the authors and an associate returned to the central office of each school to photocopy the cumulative record file materials for the triad children. Each cumulative record file contained the following information: parents' names, addresses, occupations, marital status, the child's sibs and his ordinal position, attendance records, course grades and yearly teacher's comments for grades one through six, all standard achievement and intelligence test scores, health records and some physical fitness scores, and notes about a child's special abilities or handicaps. At the time of photocopying, all names and other specific identification were obliterated, and a subject code number was substituted to assure confidentiality.

Results and Discussion

THE ACADEMIC PERFORMANCE VARIABLES

There were five standard coursework areas and one physical health area recorded on the cumulative records: Social Studies, Science, Reading, Math, Language, and Health. A trichotomous rating system was used in which 1 = above average, 2 = average, and 3 = below average performance for each of these areas. A series of 2×3 chi-square analyses was computed to determine whether the triad groups differed in frequency of above average, average, and below average grades. Since the matched controls were, in part, selected for the similarity of their achievement test scores to those of their respective targets, one would expect to find fewer significant differences between targets versus matched controls than between targets versus random controls.

schools or unidentified foster homes; for 43 we lacked sufficient information to attempt to locate them; and 64 were definitely lost to the study — i.e., no longer in school, too young or too old, left the city, or were institutionalized.) Thus, 31 of the potentially available 70 children of schizophrenic mothers were located in the city's elementary schools.

For the internalizing (depression, anxiety reaction, phobic reaction) mother group, 47 met the criteria of the study with a total of 100 potentially available children. Of these 100, 26 were located in the city's elementary schools.

For the current year's grades, the target groups always received lower average grades than their controls. The differences were statistically significant only in the following areas: The sons of schizophrenic mothers were poorer than their random controls in Social Studies ($p<.05$) and Science ($p<.025$); the daughters of schizophrenic mothers were poorer than both their matched and random controls in GPA ($p<.05$).* For the internalizing mother group, sons were poorer than their random controls in Social Studies ($p<.05$); the daughters were poorer than both their matched ($p<.025$) and random ($p<.05$) control groups in Reading and their matched controls in Language ($p<.05$). Among the externalizers, boys were significantly poorer than their matched controls in Social Studies ($p<.025$) and Language ($p<.05$), and with the exception of Health, both male and female externalizers were significantly poorer than their random controls in all coursework areas including their overall GPA ($p<.05$ to $p<.001$). For the internalizers, males were poorer than both their matched and random controls in Reading, Math, and Language and GPA ($p<.05$ to $p<.001$) but poorer than their random controls only in Social Studies ($p<.025$) and Science ($p<.05$); in contrast, the female internalizers were poorer than their matched controls only in Math ($p<.05$).

There were no significant differences in GPA among the male target groups. Among the female target groups, there was an overall significant difference in the pattern of GPA's ($\chi^2 = 17.20$, 6 df, $p<.01$). The performance of the daughters of schizophrenic mothers was the poorest (50 per cent below average), the externalizers performed less poorly (0 above average and 37 per cent below average), the daughters of internalizing mothers are best described as average (79 per cent), and the internalizers performed either very well (40 per cent above average) or very inadequately (40 per cent below average). However, during the previous year both the sons and the daughters of schizophrenic mothers performed significantly more poorly than their respective controls in many subject areas. The children of internalizing mothers also received significantly lower grades than their controls during this year. It is probable that this poorer performance by the children occurred during their mothers' psychological breakdowns, for it was during this previous academic year that

*A child's GPA was computed by adding his six grades and dividing by six. Chi-square comparisons of GPA were made by ranking a group's GPA's as 1 = above average (GPA's of 1.0–1.4 or 4 of 6 areas with above average grades), 2 = average (GPA's of 1.5–2.4), and 3 = below average (GPA's of 2.5–3.0 or 4 of 6 areas with below average grades).

most of the disturbed mothers were hospitalized or received outpatient psychiatric treatment. Table 1 summarizes the significant probability values obtained from the chi-square analyses.

Table 1. Summary of Chi-Square Probability Values for Comparisons of Grades from Current Academic Year

Groups	Social Studies	Science	Reading	Math	Language	Health	GPA
*S*s with schizophrenic mothers							
Male T[a] vs. MC[a]			<.10	<.10			
Male T vs. RC[a]	<.05	<.025	<.10	<.10			<.10
Female T vs. MC							<.05
Female T vs. RC		<.10	<.10	<.10			<.05
*S*s with internalizing mothers							
Male T vs. RC	<.05			<.10			<.10
Female T vs. MC			<.025	<.10	<.05	<.10	<.10
Female T vs. RC		<.10	<.05	<.10			<.10
Externalizers							
Male T vs. MC	<.025			<.10	<.05		<.01
Male T vs. RC	<.01	<.025	<.05	<.01	<.05		<.001
Female T vs. MC ...	<.01	<.01	<.01	<.025	<.01		<.01
Female T vs. RC	<.01	<.01	<.01	<.01	<.001	<.025	<.001
Internalizers							
Male T vs. MC	<.10	<.10	<.01	<.05	<.01		<.05
Male T vs. RC	<.025	<.05	<.01	<.025	<.001		<.025
Female T vs. MC			<.10	<.05	<.10		<.10

[a]T = target; MC = matched control; RC = random control.

Among the externalizers, both the girls and the boys achieved at approximately the same poor level in relation to their respective control groups as they did in the current academic year. For the internalizers, especially the females, the previous year seemed to have been a more trying one. Figure 1 illustrates the relative GPA distributions for the male and the female target groups. Whereas there had been significant differences between certain target and control groups, there were no significant differences in GPA between target groups of the same sex.

Four conclusions can be drawn from these data based on academic performance. All target groups were clearly differentiated from their respective controls by their poorer academic grades, while for both the previous year (except for one instance involving math) and the current year's grades, there were no significant differences between matched and random control groups. Second, the children of schizophrenic and depressive mothers did particularly poorly during the previous year — a time corresponding in a number of cases to their mothers' hospitalizations or out-

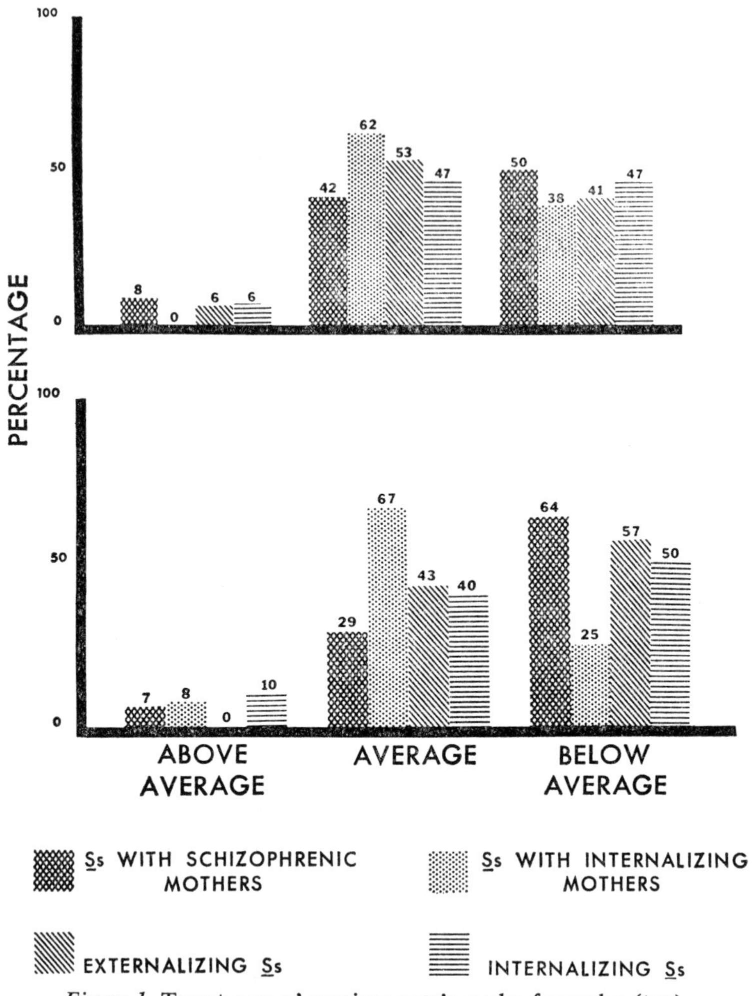

Figure 1. Target groups' previous year's grades for males (top)
and females (bottom).

patient treatments. Third, for all male and female target groups, the previous year, for whatever reasons, seemed to be a rather unhealthy one (from the standpoint of school performance) in comparison with their respective controls. It is possible that in some cases poor physical or emotional health in that year handicapped children during the following, current* school year even though there were very few significant differences in health manifested within the triads at that time. Fourth, during

**Current year* refers to the 1968–1969 academic year, when the peer and teacher ratings were made and the cumulative records were photocopied.

the previous year the children of psychologically disturbed mothers changed residence significantly more often than either their matched or random controls or the externalizing and internalizing target groups. Thus, it may be that poor grades reflect the effects of maternal breakdown and certain other demographic variables as well.

THE DEMOGRAPHIC VARIABLES

Many students of psychopathology, the authors included, give considerable weight to sociocultural variables in the etiology of behavior disorders in children. It would be foolish to study and compare target groups of "vulnerable" children without thorough attention to their social origins, their family's living conditions, their residential mobility patterns, and the like. One must control for these experiential factors, but how? It wasn't practical to be too selective in matching target children on the basis of their home environments — the number of grade school children of schizophrenic mothers is too small to permit the investigator to exclude Ss on the basis of atypical social class status or a history of a twice-broken home. However, one can be confident of at least a modicum of control if one chooses to select within the same classroom a control child for each target child, matched on the important variables of sex, grade, SES, family intactness, and intellectual aptitude. Such a control group matched to samples of four deviant, pathological populations is probably not representative of a "normal" population of grade school children. Therefore, the decision was made to use both randomly selected classmate controls and matched controls to provide a more balanced picture of the effects of these demographic variables on our dependent variables.

There were not many differences in age, grade, and SES level among target groups and their respective controls or even among all target groups of both sexes. However, there were a few differences. The mean parental occupational index score for the internalizing boys indicated a significantly higher SES level than for the internalizing girls and the sons of schizophrenic mothers. In addition, in three instances random control groups came from significantly higher SES families than their respective target groups. Therefore, in these four cases any observed differences in these groups for peer- or teacher-rated social or academic competence as well as grades could be partly a function of social class–related modes of conduct and acculturated levels of academic motivation. However, the data do not permit simple interpretation. For example, the sons of schizophrenic mothers are rated lower than are their controls in competence by peers, higher in competence by teachers, and tend to get better grades than the internalizing boys who are drawn from a higher SES group.

Family Intactness. It has been argued by some investigators (e.g., Wahl, 1956) that one variable which may increase differences in premorbid vulnerability between schizophrenic and non-schizophrenic control groups is family intactness. As reviewed by Garmezy and Streitman (in press), 44.6 per cent was the average rate of broken homes in ten studies reporting on the intactness of the consanguineous families of schizophrenic adults. Among the target groups of children whose mothers were schizophrenic in the present study, the incidence of broken homes was somewhat higher (sons 79 per cent, daughters 53 per cent); but these rates were virtually the same for the target groups of children with internalizing mothers (sons 77 per cent, daughters 54 per cent). However, there were no significant differences in family intactness among the *female target* groups, and among the male target groups, only the internalizing boys came from significantly more intact homes than the sons of schizophrenic mothers or sons of nonpsychotic, internalizing mothers. Turning to the target versus control group comparisons, the incidence of broken homes was higher than the respective control for all but two of the eight target groups even though efforts were made to match on this variable. In six instances (7.5 per cent of the chi-square comparisons) there were significant variations in family intactness: the random control group of the sons of schizophrenic mothers and the daughters of internalizing mothers as well as the matched control group of the externalizing girls had significantly fewer broken homes than their respective target groups.

Given differences in family intactness, is there a simple relationship across all target groups between this independent variable and the dependent variables of peer- and teacher-rated competence or grades? The answer appears to be no, for the following reasons: (a) While both the target and matched control groups have significantly more broken homes than their random control group, only the target versus random control group comparison on the dependent variables produced significant results, whereas a similar matched control versus random control group comparison did not. (b) There are instances in which significant differences occurred only between the target and matched control groups having very similar patterns of broken homes but not between the target and its random control group despite the latter having many fewer broken homes: (c) Although more of the male externalizers came from intact homes than did the sons of psychiatrically disturbed mothers, they were consistently judged to be less competent by teachers and peers. (d) Although there were relatively few broken homes (19 per cent) among male internalizers, this group was rated the second lowest in overall competence, exceeded only by the externalizers.

In summary, any presumed causative effect of marital disintegration on our dependent variables could not be supported across all groups. It remains possible that family intactness could have more discrete interactions with specific independent variables. Indeed, in the case of children with mentally disturbed mothers, the broken home may be but another symptom of maternal personality disturbance, with the impact on the child of the divorce or separation per se secondary to the more significant history of the child's association with a disturbed mother.

Family Mobility. Family mobility probably interacts with the SES and broken home variables. One would expect such an interaction to occur under a variety of circumstances: a working-class, divorced mother is hospitalized for a long period of time; an emotionally disturbed mother is forced to move because of friction with neighbors and landlords; a working mother accepts a series of temporary jobs, or necessity forces her to return to the protection and care of her parents. Table 2 presents the average number of moves for each triad group for the current and previous years. In the families of the two groups with disturbed mothers, there is a pattern of higher mobility rates in the previous year and reduced rates in the current year; the exception appears as a significant sex difference in the current year ($p<.04$) with the sons of internalizing, psychotic mothers maintaining a higher rate of mobility from the previous year than their female counterparts.

In summing up the evidence on family mobility, the children of disturbed mothers changed residences during the previous year significantly more often than their respective controls ($p<.002$). Further, there was a significant difference among all the target groups in the average number of changes in residence during that previous year ($p<.003$) but not during the current year. It is interesting to speculate about the cause of a family move — is it related to a mother's hospitalization, to marital discord, or to an effort to find a more tolerant teacher and school for a disruptive child or to be near other support figures during a period of familial stress? Some of these questions might be answered by studying a mother's hospital records or comparing hospitalization dates with address changes on the child's cumulative record. A more efficient method would be to interview the parents about past moves and to continue to monitor

Table 2. Mean Number of Residential Moves for Current and Previous Years

Moves	Current Year			Previous Year		
	T[a]	MC[a]	RC[a]	T	MC	RC
*S*s with schizophrenic mothers						
Male means	.43	.29	.07	.92[b]	.25	.08
Male *N*'s	14	14	14	12	12	12
Female means	.38	.29	.33	1.00[b]	.14	.17
Female *N*'s	16	17	15	14	14	14
*S*s with internalizing mothers						
Male means	.62[c]	.29	.36	.50[b]	.29	.00
Male *N*'s	13	14	14	14	14	13
Female means	.14	.29	.07	.54[b]	.23	.08
Female *N*'s	14	14	14	13	13	13
Externalizers						
Male means	.41	.28	.12	.18	.21	.18
Male *N*'s	17	18	17	17	19	17
Female means	.56[b]	.06	.12	.38	.07	.20
Female *N*'s	16	17	17	13	14	15
Internalizers						
Male means	.27	.31	.25	.27	.20	.27
Male *N*'s	15	16	16	15	15	15
Female means	.36	.27	.18	.20	.20	.10
Female *N*'s	11	11	11	10	10	10

[a]T = target *S*s; MC = matched controls; RC = random controls.

[b]Significantly more moves ($p < .002$) for the target group than for its respective controls.

[c]Significantly more family moves by sons than by daughters of internalizing mothers.

the adaptation of children over time in a manner similar to that employed by Anthony (1970) in his study of children at risk.

Attendance Data. One would expect the frequencies of tardiness and absences to be related to family disintegration, to heightened mobility, and to the target status of children. All target groups tend to be tardy more often than their respective controls, but in only three instances are these differences statistically significant (children of schizophrenic mothers and externalizers in the previous year and internalizers in the current year). This does not hold true for the pattern of absences, since in nine cases control groups were, on the average, more frequently absent than their respective target groups. However, in only two instances were there statistical and apparently meaningful differences; children of schizophrenic mothers were absent more often than their controls ($p < .05$) in the previous year (sons with 11 and daughters with 18 days absent versus their respective matched controls' 9 and 6 days absent), as were the internalizers ($p < .05$) during the current year (boys with 10 days and girls with 13 days absent versus their respective matched control groups' 5 and 6 days absent).

Useful attendance data were not obtained for a number of Ss, especially for the current year. This loss was due to the very high mobility of some Ss during the academic year, which made it difficult for the teacher to collate the attendance records from several schools. In spite of the incomplete nature of the data, two tentative inferences from attendance records are possible. First, for the current year, the target groups, with the exception of the internalizers, were not tardy or absent significantly more often than their controls. (It would be interesting to check the internalizers' clinic records to ascertain whether these children tended to feign physical illness or to exhibit other school phobic types of symptoms in an effort to avoid school.) Second, the children with emotionally disturbed mothers were tardy or absent significantly more often during the two previous years, perhaps as a function of their mothers' breakdowns. This latter point can be verified only by a closer examination of the mothers' psychiatric records in relationship to their children's cumulative record data.

SOME DATA COMPARISONS WITH OTHER STUDIES

Several studies have employed public school records as a means of describing the childhood personality attributes, intellectual achievements, and social experiences of psychologically or socially deviant adults. Most of these studies share the advantage of having available both the known pathological adult status and the historical premorbid data which had been collected during childhood. Illustrative of this group are the studies of intellectual competence at school age of pathologically disturbed adults (e.g., Lane & Albee, 1966, 1970), the follow-up studies of deviant children grown up (e.g., Robins, 1966), the adolescent adaptation of children with a high risk for schizophrenia (e.g., Mednick & Schulsinger, 1968, 1970), and the numerous studies in the education literature which focus on the prediction from school-related problems of personality maladjustment (e.g., Conger & Miller, 1966). In brief, as a group, pathological adults generally have been described as having shown the following school behavior in childhood: their tested intelligence was lower than their classmates' and perhaps lower than that of their healthy siblings evaluated at the same age; they were poor utilizers of their intellectual ability and may even have shown a declining achievement pattern through the grades; and they also had poorer relationships with their peers (Roff, 1963, 1970).

If one limits the discussion to reports identifying potential precursors of schizophrenia, the design of most earlier studies is not directly comparable with the present study. Data comparison is difficult because most previous studies have focused on the records of older children and have used different types of control groups. For example, Bower (1969) reported lower IQ's, lower GPA's and a lower rate of graduation for preschizophrenic high school students. The present study has found some evidence that the GPA's of the children (especially daughters) of schizophrenic mothers were significantly lower than some of their control groups, most markedly during the year before the collection of the records. However, this was also the case for the children of the nonpsychotic mothers and for the externalizing and the internalizing children.

Several investigators have noted declining IQ or achievement scores in their prepsychotic samples (e.g., Bower and his co-workers, Lane and her co-workers, and Rosenthal in his biography of the Genain quadruplets). There are probably too few prepsychotic children in the present study, and those there are may be too young to manifest definite trends of declining achievement in elementary school. What can be said is that both groups with psychologically disturbed mothers have had difficult academic years, especially during a time of probable family disruption and mobility. However, performance during the current year generally improved rather than worsened.

It seems reasonable to expect that differences in family mobility would produce differences in the number of subjects available to retrospective and prospective studies. Although the present study was successful in pursuing and locating subjects who were highly mobile within a large midwestern city (though some may yet leave the state), some potential subjects were not studied because they had moved into the suburban school systems or to another community. A number of earlier retrospective reports on the premorbid school adjustment of schizophrenic adults have had relatively nonmobile subjects. This appears to have been true of the Watt "Maybury" study (Watt et al., 1970; and see Watt, pp. 194–211). In that study, the probands were selected by checking old high school enrollment lists against names drawn from the Massachusetts Mental Health Registry; controls were selected from classmates without a discoverable history of mental illness. Pre-schizophrenics who changed schools frequently or who were hospitalized in another state or in a private facility were probably lost to the study.

Aside from these differences in subject selection, there are several reasons why Watt et al.'s study is an important one to compare with the present study, even though their subjects were older. In terms of social adjustment, if not academic performance, Watt et al. characterized the teachers' comments on the "Maybury" cumulative school records as indicating more general disagreeableness for the male but not the female pre-schizophrenics. In the present study the teachers' annual comments have not yet been analyzed, but a teacher's rating scale based on Watt's own cluster analysis was employed. On this measure, both the sons and daughters of schizophrenic mothers were rated as generally more socially disagreeable than the children of internalizing nonpsychotic mothers or their normal controls; but the group differences were not statistically significant. The peer ratings identified the sons but not the daughters of schizophrenic mothers as more disagreeable than both their controls and the children of the internalizing, neurotic mother group. The lack of statistical significance in the teachers' ratings should not be surprising since epidemiological data indicate that only 10 to 14 per cent of children born to schizophrenic mothers will themselves become schizophrenic. In contrast with Watt's retrospective study, we could not preselect this highly deviant subset of children. In fact, there were some children of schizophrenic mothers who had to be excluded from our sample because their psychological disturbances had required that they be institutionalized and removed from the public schools.

Beisser et al. (1967) also did not select an already schizophrenic sample to study retrospectively but, instead, they reported on teachers' ratings of elementary and junior high school children with schizophrenic, neurotic, and normal mothers. Their inclusion of another disturbed mother group led them to conclude, rather conservatively, that while the children with schizophrenic mothers were rated as substantially more deviant than the control children with psychiatrically "well" mothers, they were not rated by teachers as significantly more deviant than the children of neurotic mothers. Aside from some minor discrepancies in sex differences (sons versus daughters), the teachers' ratings in the present study are essentially similar.

The inclusion of a target group of children born to mothers with marked internalizing symptoms presented us with other interesting results when compared with earlier reports of temperamental differences among pre-schizophrenic and other children. For example, Higgins (1966) described his mother-reared group as withdrawn and socially unresponsive and his reared-apart group as irritable and emotionally labile. Similarly,

Mednick and Schulsinger (1968) reported that teachers and psychiatrists described the high-risk children as deviating from their low-risk controls by being either much more passive and nervous or more aggressive and disruptive in school. In the present study, teachers rate the following percentages of target groups as withdrawn, shy, and generally socially introverted: 37 per cent of the sons and 53 per cent of the daughters of schizophrenic mothers; 46 per cent of the sons and 62 per cent of the daughters of internalizing mothers; 26 per cent of the male and 38 per cent of the female matched controls. Thus, both target groups with disturbed mothers were definitely less socially assertive than the combined matched control children, but for both sexes a larger percentage of children with internalizing nonpsychotic mothers appeared to be more socially disengaged than were the children of schizophrenic mothers. The differences in the findings on the social withdrawal variable between the present study and the Danish studies may result from differences in the Ss' ages, in the number of target groups studied, or in the cultural milieu. In addition, the present strategy of having a teacher rate three pupils in the context of a normative study of "school achievement and adaptation" without labeling the target child may have elicited less rating of pathology than Mednick and Schulsinger's procedure of identifying one pupil as being of particular interest to a psychological research institute.

In contrast with the data on shyness, there is stronger confirmation in the present study for the findings of these Danish studies and of Roff (1963) that some children of schizophrenic mothers are very aggressive and disruptive in school. Similarly, Beisser et al. (1967) has indicated that children with schizophrenic mothers were reported by teachers to behave in more aggressive, antisocial ways than the two groups of children with depressive or normal mothers. The results of the present sample also indicated that the sons and especially the daughters of schizophrenic mothers display more antagonistic behavior than the sons and daughters of nonpsychotic mothers or their combined same-sex matched controls (Rolf, 1972). These findings are consistent with the retrospective studies of pre-schizophrenic children by Nameche and Ricks (1966) and Robins (1966). In the latter study, 74 per cent of the clinic children who later became schizophrenic had been referred for antisocial behavior. Thus, antisocial or externalizing behavior may prove to be one of the more powerful discriminators between high-risk children with schizophrenic mothers and vulnerable children whose mothers generally suffer from neurotic, internalizing symptoms.

SOME CONCLUSIONS

The decision to pursue four target groups of vulnerable children and two different groups of control children has provided us with useful baseline information for a prospective study of developmental psychology. The inclusion of both a matched and a randomly selected control group has yielded information regarding the relationship of such independent variables as intactness of the home and social class membership to our initial dependent variables. Tables 3 and 4 summarize most of the variables which have been analyzed to date, and these tables can serve as a point of reference for the following tentative conclusions:

a. Matching control children to four groups of vulnerable target children tends to produce a group of controls who are tardy and absent more often, who achieve poorer grades, and who are rated more negatively by peers and teachers than their randomly selected classmates.

b. Family mobility appears to be a very important variable which must be controlled when studying academic achievement and social adaptation among grade school children.

c. All target groups have achieved significantly lower grades than controls, especially their randomly selected controls, at some time in grade school. For the children with psychologically disturbed mothers, poorest school performance may coincide with maternal breakdown.

d. Peers, teachers, and school records with biographical contents provide supplementary information regarding competence. One source of data is not sufficient.

e. When compared with children of internalizing neurotic mothers, the children of schizophrenic mothers share some similar problems (e.g., social withdrawal, family mobility), differ in degree with respect to more severe problems (e.g., lower GPA, lower peer status), and exhibit different varieties of behavior disorders (e.g., unsocialized aggressiveness for both sexes and more negative teachers' ratings for the girls).

f. The inclusion of internalizing and externalizing target groups has permitted observations which suggest that children of schizophrenic mothers more closely resemble children who externalize their distress in antisocial ways.

g. Children of nonpsychotic, depressive mothers manifested some behavior disturbances and some difficulties in school, but of all the target groups, they most closely resembled the control children.

h. Simplistic interpretations of the influences of lower SES, broken homes, and family mobility on children's adaptation in school are contra-

Table 3. Summary of Significant Differences (x) among All Subject Groups[a]

	Males		Females	
Item	T vs. MC	T vs. RC	T vs. MC	T vs. MC
Ss with Schizophrenic Mothers				
Peer ratings				
Positive roles		x		
Negative roles	x	x		
Teachers' ratings				
Emotionally stable				x
Emotional adjustment			x	x
Intellectual potential			x	x
GPA				
Current year			x	x
Previous year		x	x[b]	x
SES, by parental occupation		x		
Broken homes		x		
Ss with Internalizing Mothers				
Peer ratings, positive roles			x	
GPA, previous year		x	x	
SES, by parental occupation				x
Broken homes		x		x
Externalizers				
Peer ratings				
Positive roles	x	x	x	x
Negative roles	x	x	x	x
Externalizers				
Teachers' ratings				
Emotional stability	x	x	x	x
Socially agreeable	x	x	x	x
Emotional adjustment	x	x	x	x
Social adjustment	x	x	x	x
Intellectual potential	x			
Positive social extroversion	x	x		x
Positive academic behavior	x	x	x	x
GPA				
Current year	x	x	x	x
Previous year	x	x	x	x
Broken homes			x	
Internalizers				
Peer ratings				
Positive roles	x	x	x	
Negative roles	x	x		
Teachers' ratings				
Emotional stability	x	x	x	x
Socially agreeable	x	x		
Emotional adjustment	x	x		
Social adjustment	x	x		
Intellectual potential	x	x		
Positive social extroversion	x	x		
Positive academic behavior		x		
GPA				
Current year	x	x	x	
Previous year	x	x	x	x
SES, by parental occupation				x

[a]T = target; MC = matched control; RC = random control.
[b]$p < .06$.

Table 4. Summary of Significant Differences[a] (x) in Moves, Tardiness, and Absences among All Subject Groups

Item	Ss with Schizophrenic Mothers	Ss with Internalizing Mothers	Externalizers	Internalizers
Moves				
Current year			x[a]	
Previous year	x	x		
Tardiness				
Current year				x
Previous year	x		x	
Absences				
Current year				x
Previous year	x	x		

[a]Significant two-way ANOVA F ratio.

dicted by the observation that the internalizing boys demonstrated very poor social and academic competence, even though this target group contained families which were more frequently intact, drawn from a higher SES, and manifested lower family mobility relative to the other target groups.

There are some obvious limitations to the present study. First, there are the shortcomings that inhere in the cumulative record itself. The contents of such records tend to be sparse. For example, parents' occupations on which social class judgments are often based provide no adequate description of job activities or job level. Teachers' commentaries are often minimal and may be influenced by prior judgments that are part of the child's record. Social promotions reduce the discriminability of grades (although they do make obtained differences even more significant). Further, interpretations of such data often require extended inference. Finally, a growing (and rightful) concern with the invasion of privacy has alerted school authorities to the potential consequences of premature and inadequate judgments about children. Thus, one can foresee even greater restrictions on both what will be recorded on cumulative records and how these evaluations will be used by researchers. Given these many faults, what does the cumulative record have to offer? Its importance lies in the fact that it provides one external criterion of economic (i.e., early work) competence — and thus provides measures which warrant correlation with other data related to the psychological and biological adaptation of the child at risk.

The more specific limitations of the current study include the size of the N's in each group. These are small when sex and target status are taken into account. Certain inescapable biases in selection (with the exception of male externalizers) suggest that each target group cannot be considered a random sample of its population of vulnerable children. Furthermore, the selection of young disturbed mothers leaves undetermined the question of what their ultimate diagnostic label may be; nor would it be safe to assume the reliability of their current diagnosis. Similarly, any of the children of the various target groups may, in terms of an ultimate criterion, have a favorable outcome, suffer a schizophrenic or spectrum disorder, or attain other forms of adult adjustment or maladjustment. Such diversity of outcome precludes a too-ready acceptance regarding precursory signs of schizophrenia. Perhaps the more important question revolves around the issue of which of these target children will overcome his or her vulnerability and why? Other investigators have described some children of schizophrenic mothers as model students who achieve superior grades, still others are said to show a creative bent. Will it be these talented children who survive, or will it be the less exceptional individual who makes a steady, if less dramatic, climb to maturity and adult competence? Time joined by further studies of children at risk will provide the answer to that provocative question.

REFERENCES

Achenbach, T. M. The classification of children's psychiatric symptoms: A factor-analytic study. *Psychological Monographs,* 1966, 80, (7, whole no. 615).

Anthony, E. J. The impact of mental and physical illness on family life. *American Journal of Psychiatry,* 1970, 127, 138–146.

Anthony, E. J. Primary prevention with school children. In H. H. Barten & L. Bellak (Eds.), *Progress in community mental health.* Vol. 2. New York: Grune & Stratton, 1972. Pp. 131–158.

Beisser, A., Glasser, N., & Grant, M. Psychosocial adjustment in children of schizophrenic mothers. *Journal of Nervous and Mental Disease,* 1967, 145 (6), 429–440.

Bower, E. M. *Early identification of emotionally handicapped children in school.* 2nd ed. Springfield, Ill.: Thomas, 1969.

Conger, J. J., & Miller, W. C. *Personality, social class, and delinquency.* New York: Wiley, 1966.

Garmezy, N. Vulnerable adolescents: Implications derived from an internalizing-externalizing dimension. In J. Zubin & A. Freedman (Eds.), *Psychopathology of adolescence.* New York: Grune & Stratton, 1969.

————. Children at risk: The search for the antecedents to schizophrenia. Part I (in collaboration with S. Streitman). Conceptual models and research methods. Part II. Review and critique of ongoing programs. *Schizophrenia Bulletin,* in press. (a)

————. Competence and adaptation in adult schizophrenic patients and children at risk. In S. R. Dean (Ed.), *Prize lectures in schizophrenia: The first ten Dean awards.* New York: MSS Information Corporation, in press. (b)

Heston, L. L. Psychiatric disorders in foster home reared children of schizophrenic mothers. *British Journal of Psychiatry,* 1966, 112 (2), 819–825.

Higgins, J. Effects of child rearing by schizophrenic mothers. *Journal of Psychiatric Research*, 1966, 4, 153–167.

Lane, E. A., & Albee, G. W. Early childhood intellectual differences between schizophrenic adults and their siblings. *Journal of Abnormal and Social Psychology*, 1964, 68, 193–195.

————. Intellectual antecedents of schizophrenia. In M. Roff & D. F. Ricks (Eds.), *Life history research in psychopathology*. Vol. 1. Minneapolis: University of Minnesota Press, 1970. Pp. 189–207.

Mednick, S. A., & McNeil, T. F. Current methodology in research on the etiology of schizophrenia: Serious difficulties which suggest the use of the high risk group method. *Psychological Bulletin*, 1968, 70, 681–693.

————. Some premorbid characteristics related to breakdown in children with schizophrenic mothers. In D. Rosenthal & S. Kety (Eds.), *The transmission of schizophrenia*. Oxford: Pergamon Press, 1968. Pp. 267–291.

————. Factors related to breakdown in children at high risk for schizophrenia. In M. Roff & D. F. Ricks (Eds.), *Life history research in psychopathology*. Vol 1. Minneapolis: University of Minnesota Press, 1970. Pp. 51–93.

Nameche, G. F., & Ricks, D. F. Life patterns of children who became adult schizophrenics. Paper presented at the meeting of the American Orthopsychiatry Association, San Francisco, April 16, 1966.

Robins, L. N. *Deviant children grown up*. Baltimore: Williams & Wilkins, 1966.

Roff, M. Childhood social interactions and young adult psychoses. *Journal of Clinical Psychology*, 1963, 19, 152–157.

————. Some life history factors in relation to various types of adult maladjustment. In M. Roff & D. F. Ricks (Eds.), *Life history research in psychopathology*. Vol 1. Minneapolis: University of Minnesota Press, 1970. Pp. 265–287.

Rolf, J. E. The academic and social competence of school children vulnerable to behavior pathology. Ph.D. thesis, University of Minnesota, 1969.

————. The social and academic competence of children vulnerable to schizophrenia and other behavior disorders. *Journal of Abnormal Psychology*, 1972, 80, 225–243.

Siegel, S. *Nonparametric statistics for the behavioral sciences*. New York: McGraw-Hill, 1956.

Wahl, C. W. Some antecedent factors in the family histories of 568 male schizophrenics of the United States Navy. *American Journal of Psychiatry*, 1956, 113, 201–210.

Watt, N. F., Stolorow, R. D., Lubensky, A. W., & McClelland, D. C. School adjustment and social behavior of children hospitalized for schizophrenia as adults. *American Journal of Orthopsychiatry*, 1970, 40 (4), 637–657.

JEAN PIERRE JORDAAN
DONALD E. SUPER

The Prediction of Early Adult Vocational Behavior

IT IS EASY, when deeply involved in a specialty, to fail to take note of relevant work that is being done with somewhat different terminology in another branch of a discipline. Thus, a decade ago a group of distinguished psychologists published a volume entitled *The Study of Lives* (White, 1963) with no reference to *work, occupation, vocation,* or *career*: it is as though men and women did not work, as though work plays no part in their lives. And yet White (1952) himself, in one of his works, drew heavily on work histories for the understanding of personality development, and Roe (1956) and many others (Osipow, 1968; Super, 1957; Vroom, 1964) have documented the psychological importance of work and occupation in theory and in research. It is the purpose of this chapter, first, briefly to relate some of the theoretical and empirical work of vocational psychologists to some kindred work of personality theorists, then to describe in greater detail some of the work of one longitudinal study of career development and of vocational maturity, and finally, to point up some of the implications of this work for understanding personality development in adolescence and young adulthood.

Vocational Psychology. In the year 2000 anyone reviewing the development of vocational psychology during the past hundred years is likely to identify the 1950's as a turning point in the history of this specialty. It was in these years that there was a significant shift away from the study of occupations to the study of careers, and a corresponding shift from the essentially static concept of vocational choice to the more dynamic concept of vocational development. As Super (1968, 1970) has pointed out, an approach which is limited to predicting future vocational status (e.g., occupational level at age 25) from present status (e.g., high school test scores) and which does not inquire into prior and subsequent developments, can throw only limited light on the process of choice and adjustment. What is needed is a developmental approach which focuses on the evolution of vocationally significant traits and behaviors and on the manner in which successive decisions are approached, clarified, revised, and implemented. The focus should thus be on vocational histories rather than on status at a single point in time and on career criteria rather than occupational criteria, and the approach needs to be longitudinal rather than cross-sectional.

Although there may be differences of opinion about the directions in which vocational development proceeds, there is general agreement on at least four points. First, development is multi- rather than uni-dimensional; second, individuals differ in their rate of development; third, some developments are more characteristic of certain life stages than others; fourth, these developments are predictive of later occupational behavior and outcomes.

The Process of Career Development. The constructs of life stages, of developmental tasks, and of maturity have played a major role in vocational or career development theory, as in Piagetian and in Freudian theory. Super (1942) made early applications of these concepts to vocational choice and adjustment. After World War II, Ginzberg and associates (1951), Havighurst (1953), Super and associates (1951, 1953, 1957a, 1957b, 1963), and Tiedeman and O'Hara (1963) directed the attention of counseling psychologists to the possible contributions of a developmental approach to occupational choice and adjustment.

Processes of special interest have been those of continuity and discontinuity, life stages, exploratory behavior, adjustment (a *retrospective* and contemporaneous construct), maturity (a contemporaneous and *prospective* construct), and future orientation. Elder (1968, pp. 240–249) wrote, "Movement from . . . high school to either college or occupational roles represents potentially critical points in the life course for growth or regression. The psychological continuity or discontinuity across these transitions depends on the nature of the change in the environment and on the characteristics of the adolescent, both social and psychological." Havighurst's (1953) stressing of the importance of coping with the developmental tasks of one life stage as a prerequisite for coping with those of the next stage deals with the same issues: adjustment is an outcome of the coping behavior which constitutes maturity. One important kind of coping behavior is future-oriented exploration based on hypothesis formulation and testing, dealt with in differing ways by Berlyne (1960), Piaget (Flavell, 1963), and Jordaan (1963). And future orientation is, as M. B. Smith (1966) found in Peace Corps trainees, an important factor in career as well as in personality development.

Among theorists, Ginzberg (1951), Super (1957, 1963), and Tiedeman and O'Hara (1963) have been the most explicit in describing the order in which certain developments in careers might occur. Among researchers, Super and his associates (Jordaan & Heyde, in preparation; Super, Kowalski, & Gotkin, 1967) and Gribbons and Lohnes (1968, 1969) have conducted long-term studies on the nature and significance of these developments. This paper focuses on the first of these studies, the Career Pattern Study at Teachers College, Columbia University.

CONCEPTUAL FRAMEWORK: LIFE STAGES, DEVELOPMENTAL
TASKS, AND VOCATIONAL MATURITY

Life Stages and Tasks. Vocational development is conceived of as a process which begins in childhood and continues up to and beyond retirement. It encompasses five stages: Growth, Exploration, Establishment, Maintenance, and Decline. The Career Pattern Study subjects were first studied at age 14 or 15 and most recently at age 25. Consequently, the emphasis to date has been on the second and third of these stages, Exploration and Establishment. In 1973 the subjects were approximately 36 years old, at which time they were hypothesized to be in the advancement substage of the Establishment stage.

The task to be accomplished in each stage or substage (Table 1) is called a vocational developmental task. Thus the tasks of the Exploratory stage are to crystallize, specify, and implement a vocational preference, and the task of the early Establishment stage is to settle down and secure a place in the chosen occupation.

Having identified what they believe to be the vocational developmental tasks of each stage and substage, Super and his associates (1957, 1960, 1963, 1967) have outlined the attitudes and behaviors which facilitate or exemplify the accomplishment of those tasks. Thus, for example, the behaviors and attitudes which are involved in specifying a vocational preference are thought to be:

1. Awareness of the need to specify a vocational preference
2. Use of resources in specification
3. Awareness of factors to consider
4. Awareness of contingencies which may affect goals
5. Differentiation of interests and values

6. Awareness of present-future relationships
7. Consistency of vocational preferences
8. Possession of information concerning the preferred occupation
9. Planning for the preferred occupation
10. Wisdom of the vocational preference
11. Confidence in the preference.

Vocational Maturity. If, as has been hypothesized, vocational development is systematic rather than unsystematic and proceeds in certain identifiable directions, it should be possible to assess not only how much of the road the individual has covered, but also how fast he is traveling in comparison with others who are embarked on the same journey. Super has suggested (1957) that rate and progress along this road might be an indication of an individual's vocational maturity.

There are two ways of assessing a person's vocational maturity. One is to compare where he is in his development with where a person of his age might be expected to be (VM_1). The other is to compare his performance with that of others who are in the same stage as he (VM_2). Thus, a man in his thirties who is moving from one occupation to another instead of settling down as most men his age have done might be described as vocationally immature (VM_1). He is still in the Exploratory stage, whereas most 30-year-olds are already in the Establishment stage. A 16-year-old who is in the tentative substage and who has made much greater progress in crystallizing a vocational preference than other boys his age would be judged more mature than they (VM_2). In the one instance, the question is, Are the tasks the individual is addressing himself to those which are usual for persons his age? In the other it is, How well is he coping with these tasks in comparison with others in his life stage?

The Career Pattern Study

The Career Pattern Study is a 21-year longitudinal study of some 280 eighth- and ninth-graders from Middletown, New York, initiated in 1951.

The subjects have been studied at several points in time: when they were in the eighth or ninth grade (age 14 or 15), at age 18, at age 21, again at age 25, and most recently at age 36. The primary sources of data have been: at ages 14, 15, and 18, questionnaires, tests, and interviews; at age 21, a questionnaire; at ages 25 and 36, questionnaires and tests followed by an interview. The procedures and findings through age 25 have been described by Super et al. (1957), Super and Overstreet (1960),

Table 1. Vocational Life Stages

Stage	Period	Vocational Developmental Task	Explanation
Growth stage	Childhood and early adolescence	Forming a picture of the kind of person one is. Developing an orientation to the world of work and an understanding of the meaning of work	Through role-playing (often as a result of identification with admired adults and peers) and participation in school, leisure, and other activities, the individual learns what he can do well, what he likes, how he differs from other people, and incorporates this knowledge into his picture of himself.
Exploratory stage Tentative substage ...	Early and middle adolescence	Crystallizing a vocational preference	Possibly appropriate *fields* and *levels* of work are identified (partial specification).
Transition substage ...	Late adolescence and early adulthood	Specifying a vocational preference	Transition from school to work or from school to further education and training. Generalized choice is converted into a specific choice.
Trial (little commitment) substage	Early adulthood	Implementing a vocational preference	A seemingly appropriate occupation having been located or prepared for, a beginning job in it is found and tried out as a life work. Commitment to the occupation is still provisional, and may be strengthened or weakened by experiences encountered on the job or in training. If weakened, the individual may change his goals and repeat the process of crystallizing, specifying, and implementing a vocational preference.

Table 1.—*Continued*

Stage	Period	Vocational Developmental Task	Explanation
Establishment stage Trial (with commitment) and stabilization substage	Early adulthood to about age 30	Settling down, securing a permanent place in the chosen occupation[a]	Having acquired the necessary skills, training, or work experience, the individual commits himself to the occupation and seeks to establish a place for himself in it. Thereafter, changes which occur are changes of position, job, or employer, not changes of occupation.
Advancement substage	30's to mid-40's	Consolidation and advancement	The individual consolidates and improves his status in the occupation by acquiring seniority, developing a clientele, demonstrating superior performance, improving his qualifications, etc.
Maintenance stage	Mid-40's to retirement	Preservation of achieved status and gains	The individual is less concerned with registering new gains than with maintaining present status in the face of competition from younger, more enterprising co-workers who are in the advancement substage.
Decline stage	Age 65 on	Deceleration, disengagement, retirement	The individual faces the problems of actual or impending retirement, and must plan and find other sources of satisfaction (a part-time job, volunteer work, leisure activities, etc.) to replace those lost through retirement.

[a]There are individuals who for psychological, personal, or economic reasons do not achieve stable jobs or do so only intermittently. In their case what gets stabilized is an unstable career pattern. For such individuals the vocational developmental risk is to recognize, and plan for the inevitability of instability (Super, 1963).

113

Super, Kowalski, and Gotkin (1967), and Jordaan and Heyde (in preparation).

The ninth-grade group (consisting of 142 subjects) was used in some instances to test and in others to generate hypotheses. The eighth-grade group was used to replicate findings obtained with the ninth-grade group.

Data from the original ninth-grade group have since 1960 been subjected to more refined study using factor analysis and stepwise multiple regression analysis. Since these methods have not yet been applied to the original eighth-grade group, this report is limited to the original ninth-grade group and to the years between age 18 (when those who had not dropped out of school were high school seniors) and age 25 (when most had finished their studies and were at work).

Data were obtained from 88 per cent of the surviving ninth-graders at age 21, and from 94 per cent at age 25. However, complete data for *all* four time periods (ages 15, 18, 21, and 25) were available for only 93 of the 140 surviving ninth-graders. It is this group of 93, which has been shown not to differ significantly from the remainder of the ninth-grade sample with respect to such important variables as IQ and socioeconomic status, which is considered in this paper.

TYPES OF MEASURES

The measures were of four types: (a) *Conventional* predictor measures of personal characteristics, background, and achievement, such as grades, socioeconomic status, high school curriculum, and level of aspiration; (b) *novel vocational maturity* predictor measures, some based solely on interview data (e.g., specificity of planning), others on a combination of interview and test data (e.g., agreement between the subject's intellectual ability and the intellectual requirements of the occupation he thought he might enter); (c) *conventional* criterion measures of adult vocational behavior focusing on *occupation*, such as self-estimated occupational success; and (d) *novel* criterion measures of *career*, such as floundering-stabilizing and equity change.

Vocational Maturity Measures. There were 62 hypothetical measures of vocational maturity, designed to tap ten different aspects or dimensions of adolescent vocational development:

> Crystallization of Interests
> Appropriateness or Wisdom of Preference
> Work Experience
> Occupational Information (including Awareness of
>   Significant Aspects of Occupations)

Extensiveness and Quality of Sources of Information
Acceptance of Responsibility for Choice
  and Decision-making Planning
Awareness of Contingency Factors
Weighing of Alternatives
Implementation

Some of the foregoing were represented by only one measure, others by several measures. Grouping of the measures as described above was done initially on an a priori basis. Subsequently, a factor analysis was performed in order to determine whether the measures did in fact cluster in the expected manner.

A principal components analysis with varimax rotation yielded 19 factors in both grades 9 and 12, a larger number than called for by the investigators' a priori grouping of the measures.

A comparison of ninth- and twelfth-grade factors revealed similarities as well as differences. Six of the factors had similar structures at both age levels (the same measures loading .65 or above), seven had somewhat similar structures (some of the same measures loading .65 or above), and the remainder had no clearly identifiable counterpart.

The *factors* extracted in the twelfth grade and the factor scores based on them were defined as follows:

Occupational Information: Preparation (Content)
Occupational Information: Material Conditions
  of Work
Specification of Vocational Preference
Crystallization of Interests
Work Experience: Independence
Accessibility of Vocational Preferences
Occupational Information: Advancement and Transfer
Commitment to Vocational Preferences
Weighing of Alternatives
Occupational Information: Supply and Demand
Implementation: Work Experience
Agreement: Ability and Vocational Preferences
Occupational Information: Preparation (Cost)
Work Experience: Size of Establishment
Acceptance of Responsibility for Implementing
  Career Decisions
Occupational Information: Psychological
  Requirements
Occupational Information: Hours of Work
Implementation: Activities
Occupational Information: Entry Opportunities

Measures of Adult Vocational Behavior. There were 33 criterion or outcome variables. Time and space do not permit a discussion of all of them. An analysis of the intercorrelations of these measures shows that they fall into six logically meaningful clusters rather than into the hypothesized occupational-career dichotomy (Super, Kowalski, & Gotkin, 1967):

1. *Career satisfaction criteria* (largely novel), including self-estimates of career establishment*, career success, career satisfaction*, occupational satisfaction*, and utilization of assets.
2. *Self-improvement criteria* (largely novel), including objective measures of educational level attained*, improvement in educational status after high school*, realism of reasons for changing positions*, and occupational level attained.
3. *Job getting and holding criteria* (conventional), consisting of number of times unemployed* and number of months unemployed*.
4. *Economic self-sufficiency criteria* (conventional), consisting of an objective measure of self-support after leaving high school* and of a self-estimate of occupational success.
5. *Early establishment criteria* (largely novel), a cluster of three measures assessing improvement of socioeconomic status by age 25, attainment of the occupational goal set at age 25*, and (negatively weighted) number of position changes since leaving high school*.
6. *Occupational satisfaction criteria* (mixed conventional and novel), among which are included self-estimates of opportunity for self-expression, occupational satisfaction*, position satisfaction, and utilization of assets, together with objective measures of occupational level attained by age 25 and of stabilizing versus floundering behavior at the same age*.

*Only those variables for which there were complete data for all the subjects ($N = 93$) are included in the analyses which follow. They are indicated here by an asterisk.

The criteria are of several types. Some are static (e.g., Level of Occupation), others are developmental or progress measures (e.g., Change in Equity); some are objective (e.g., Number of Moves), others are subjective (e.g., Self-reported Occupational Satisfaction); some are self-estimates (e.g., Self-estimated Career Success), others are judges' ratings or categorizations (e.g., Realism of Reasons for Moves). The progress or change measures are best viewed as *career* variables. They contribute information which *occupational* variables (which evaluate status at a given point in time) cannot provide. Super, Kowalski, and Gotkin (1967) point out, "static criteria of career success such as salary or occupational level attained . . . cannot accurately describe the vocational progress of young men who may still be in training or in the initial stages of getting established." Their search for more suitable criteria led to two sets of measures: seven career development scales which assess progress or improvement over time, and four measures designed to assess the subjects' coping behavior.

116

The Career Development Scales assess: Improvement in Equity (carry-over and improvement of experience, pay rate, training, and benefits), Realism of Reasons for Moves (remedying or lessening of dissatisfying aspects of previous jobs), Goal Attainment, Improvement in Educational Qualifications, Improvement in Socioeconomic Status, Improvement in Fit between Job and Measured Abilities, Improvement in Fit between Job and Measured Interests. Progress scores can be examined individually, but they can also be summed, after being converted into standard scores, to yield a global or composite measure of career progress.

Coping Behaviors refer to the way the subject deals with the developmental tasks of the exploratory and establishment stage. These are specifying and implementing a vocational preference, committing oneself to a particular type of work, and making a place for oneself in it.

Super, Kowalski, and Gotkin (1967) identified five types of coping behaviors: floundering, stagnation, trial, instrumentation, and establishment. *Floundering* is defined as illogical, poorly conceived, or random changes of position; *stagnation* as remaining in a position after the point of diminishing returns has been reached; *trial* as purposeful exploration; *instrumentation* as behavior which moves the subject closer to his goal; and *establishment* as settling down and making a place for oneself in the chosen occupation.

Trial, instrumentation, and establishment are positive behaviors, floundering and stagnation negative behaviors. Classification of the subject's behavior can be based on what *he* says about a given job or training move (internal frame of reference) or on *judges'* evaluations (external frame of reference). The subject's or judges' evaluation may be based on psychological criteria (interests, abilities, values, etc.) or on socioeconomic criteria (earnings, status, level of responsibility, etc.). The subject's job and training moves since leaving high school can thus be viewed from four different frames of reference: Internal Psychological, External Psychological, Internal Socioeconomic, and External Socioeconomic.

THE SUBJECTS AT TWENTY-FIVE

By age 25 (Super, Kowalski, & Gotkin, 1967) four fifths of the 250 subjects contacted in 1962–1963 were in possession of a high school diploma or its equivalent. One fourth had completed two years of post–high school education, and approximately one fifth a bachelor's degree.

The average subject had changed positions six times. Half of the training or job moves made in the seven-year period could be characterized as floundering (random or aimless movement). A third of the subjects evidenced considerable floundering, half little floundering, and about one sixth equal proportions of stabilizing and floundering behavior. By age 25, however, most of the subjects, including about half of those whose modal behavior had been negative, appeared to be settling down and getting established.

Few of the subjects (about one in four) entered one of the occupations which they were considering when they were in the twelfth grade: Some 5 per cent were in professional or managerial positions and 25 per cent in semiprofessional and lower managerial positions. About 30 per cent were in skilled occupations, another 30 per cent in semiskilled occupations, and 10 per cent in unskilled occupations. The great majority of the subjects felt they were doing as well as, or better than, others of the same age in the same field. Most (about 80 per cent) said they were satisfied with their present occupation, but many (about half) were not sure they would or wanted to continue in it.

FINDINGS

Previous analyses of the prediction data were based on standard correlation procedures which have two defects: first, they examine the predictors one at a time, and second, they do not take into account the fact that some of the predictors (e.g., school achievement and intelligence) are not independent of one another.

The present analysis attempts to overcome these defects by using stepwise multiple regression procedures. From the list of predictors the computer selects the variable which correlates most highly with a given criterion. It then identifies the predictor which correlates most highly with that criterion when its relationship to the first predictor has been partialled out. Each successive variable is selected on the basis of the contribution it makes when its relationship to the previously entered variables have been partialled out. Analysis stops when the *F* level or tolerance is insufficient for further computation. In analyzing the results particular attention is paid to variables which increase the MRSQ by 1 per cent or more.

The foregoing procedures were applied first to the 15 conventional measures (IQ, Curriculum, Parental Occupational Level, etc.), then to the 19 specially devised vocational maturity measures, and then to all 34 predictor variables. Thus, the utility of the two types of measures can be compared, and the combination of measures yielding the best predictions can be identified.

There are three questions which are of special concern in any predictive study: How good are the predictions? Which criteria can be predicted best? Which are the best predictors?

PREDICTIVE VALIDITY OF THE TWO TYPES OF MEASURES

Tables not reproduced here but obtainable on request from the authors indicate the following:

1. *Career Satisfaction* criteria are predicted reasonably well by both types of measures. For the conventional measures the r's range from .47 to .56 with a median of .51, and for the vocational maturity measures from .51 to .62 with a median of .60.

The vocational maturity measures are clearly superior to the conventional measures in predicting Career Establishment, both in terms of the number of measures needed to achieve an r of a given size and of the final r. Only four vocational maturity measures (Occupational Information: Supply and Demand; Preparation Required; Hours of Work; and negatively weighted Implementation of Preference through Activities), are needed to achieve an r of .50, and the addition of four other variables (Agreement between Ability and Preference; Accessibility of Vocational Preference; Work Experience: Independence; and negatively weighted Size of Establishment) raises the r to .60. Six conventional measures (Grades, Extent of After School Employment, Curriculum, Parental Occupational Level, Extent of Participation in After School Avocational Activities, and Extent of Summer Employment) are needed to achieve an r of .50, and the addition of further variables raises the r only to .51.

The Occupational Satisfaction criterion in this cluster is predicted equally well by both types of measures. In either instance only three measures (Occupational Information: Preparation Required; Supply and Demand; and Hours of Work in the case of the vocational maturity measures, and Grades, Curriculum, and Extent of After School Employment in the case of the conventional measures), are needed to achieve an r of .50. The final r employing eight measures is about the same in both instances, .60 and .56.

The findings with respect to Career Satisfaction follow the same general pattern. The number of measures needed to achieve an r of .40 is about the same, four in the case of the vocational maturity measures (Occupational Information: Hours of Work and Preparation Required; Work Experience: Independence; and Agreement between Ability and Preference) and three (Grades, Extent of After School Employment, and Parental Occupational Level) in the case of the conventional measures. Additional variables, six in the one case, five in the other, result in roughly similar final r's of .51 and .47.

2. *Self-Improvement* criteria are the most predictable of all the criteria. For the conventional measures the r's range from .60 to .75 with a median of .62, and for the vocational maturity measures from .55 to .72 with a median of .59. However, here the conventional measures outperform the vocational maturity measures, for only two conventional measures (Grades and Level of Aspiration) are needed to achieve an r of .70 with Educational Level at age 25, and only one (Grades) to achieve an r of .50 with Educational Improvement and Realism of Moves. The numbers of vocational

119

maturity measures needed to achieve *r*'s of this size are, on the other hand, 7, 4, and 4 respectively.

3. *Job Getting and Holding* is less well predicted by both types of measures. For the conventional measures the *r*'s are .41 and .39 and for the vocational maturity measures .32 and .34. In some instances 5 and in others 6 variables are needed to achieve these modest *r*'s.

4. *Early Establishment* is predicted fairly well by the vocational maturity measures (*r* = .51 and .52) and less well by the conventional measures (*r* = .35 and .30), the number of measures needed to achieve these *r*'s ranging from 5 to 7.

5. *Economic Self-Sufficiency* as judged by Months of Self-Support is predicted somewhat better by the conventional measures (*r* = .37) than by the vocational maturity measures (*r* = .33), but the size of the correlations is unimpressive considering the number of variables (7 and 6 respectively) needed to achieve these *r*'s.

6. *Occupational Satisfaction* criteria, a cluster of five, are best predicted by vocational maturity but reasonably well by both types of measures. For the conventional measures the *r*'s range from .43 to .56 with a median of .50, and for the vocational maturity measures from .52 to .62 with a median of .58. Although the number needed to achieve an *r* of .40 is about the same in both instances (typically three), generally fewer vocational maturity measures than conventional measures are required to achieve an *r* of .50, and in several instances *r*'s in the 50's and .60's can be attained only with the former.

Summarizing the relative utility of conventional measures of adolescent status and behavior as compared with novel measures of vocational maturity in predicting adult career behaviors, the conventional measures are superior to the novel with three types of criteria, inferior with three, and equally good with two. Vocational maturity in adolescence thus appears in this analysis to be a useful construct.

The accompanying tabulation furnishes data on the predictability of career movement. The criterion in this instance is a composite measure of career progress since leaving high school. It considers improvement in equity (carry-over and improvement of experience, pay rate, training, and benefits), realism of reasons for changing positions (remedying or lessening of dissatisfying aspects of previous jobs), goal attainment, improvement in educational qualifications, improvement in socioeconomic status, and improvement in fit between the requirements of the job and the individual's measured interests and abilities. The tabulation shows that career progress defined in this fashion is predicted about equally well by both types of measures but more economically by standard measures than by the special vocational maturity measures.

Only three standard measures (Grades, Participation in Avocational Activities, and negatively weighted Participation in School Courses Relevant to the Stated Vocational Objective) are needed to achieve an *r* of .50.

Five vocational maturity measures are needed to achieve an r of this size. Added variables (two in the case of the conventional measures and three in the case of the vocational maturity measures) achieve a modest increase to .53 and .55 respectively. Better results are obtained when both types of measures are used. Grades correlate .44 with the criterion, and the addition of Information about Hours of Work and Participation in Avocational Activities boosts this figure to .50. It can be raised to .60 by adding four more variables and to .66 by adding yet another four.

	Standard Measures	Vocational Maturity Measures	Combined Measures
Multiple r	.53	.55	.66
Number of measures	5	8	11
Number of measures needed to achieve multiple r			
$r = .40$	1	2	1
$r = .50$	3	5	3
$r = .60$			7

The Combined Measures. All of the criteria are better predicted by a combination of the two types of measures than by either type alone. This is most evident in the case of the least well predicted Job Getting and Holding and Economic Self-Sufficiency criteria. By using both types of measures the highest obtained r with either type of measure is raised from .41 to .58 in the case of Times Unemployed, from .39 to .51 in the case of Months Unemployed, and from .37 to .49 in the case of Months of Self-Support.

The r's for the combined measures and the sixteen criteria range from .49 (Months of Self-Support) to .80 (Educational Level at Age 25) with a median of .63. The number of measures needed to achieve these r's ranges from 6 to 17 with a median of 11. Also, r's of .60 and above were obtained for nine, or slightly more than half of the sixteen criteria; the number of vocational maturity and conventional measures needed to achieve these r's ranged from 1 (in the case of Educational Level at Age 25) to 14 (in the case of Career Satisfaction) with a median of 6, suggesting that important career behaviors and outcomes can be predicted quite well with a relatively small number of measures even when seven years separate the predictors and the criteria.

If the two types of measures were equally reliable and easy to derive, the question of which to use would pose no problem, since, as the data show, better results are obtained when both are used. Unfortunately, however, the novel vocational maturity measures which have been shown to contribute to improved predictions are based on interview data which are time-consuming to collect and difficult to quantify. Recently, more economical and objective methods of assessing vocational maturity have become available: Super and associates' multifactor Career Development Inventory (Super, 1974; Super & Forrest, 1972); Crites's Career Maturity Inventory (Crites, 1973, 1974) and Competency Tests, and Westbrook's Cognitive Vocational Maturity Test (Westbrook & Parry-Hill, 1974). Until scores on these instruments have been related to appropriate occupational and career criteria, those who are interested in predicting adult vocational behavior will have to weigh the additional increments of validity yielded by interview-derived vocational maturity measures against the results which can be at least temporarily achieved more economically and reliably by conventional measures. But those who wish to understand adult and especially vocational behavior will, clearly, need to take vocational maturity into account.

The Best Predictors. The measures which were found to be most consistently related to early adult vocational behavior — that is, contributed significantly to the prediction of more than half of the criteria in a given cluster (2 out of 2, 2 out of 3, and 3 out of 5) — are also of interest.

Among the conventional measures, high school grades, after school work experience, and the pursuit of avocational activities appear to be the best predictors. All are related to at least three of the five criterion clusters.

Intelligence, parental occupational level, school curriculum, summer employment, and stability of occupational preference during the high school years, are also useful predictors: each contributes significantly to the prediction of most of the variables in two of the five criterion clusters.

The most useful vocational maturity measures are those which assess the wisdom of the subject's occupational goal (Agreement between Ability and Preference) and his knowledge about the occupation (how to prepare for it, what the hours of work are, and what the important employment prospects are). These are positively associated with favorable outcomes. Attempts to implement or give substance to a preference by engaging in occupationally relevant extracurricular activities are associated with *unfavorable* outcomes, perhaps because most adolescents are not ready to commit themselves to a specific occupational goal. Premature attempts at implementation may inhibit the kind of wide-ranging exploration which many adolescents appear to need.

Crystallization of Interests, shown by having a primary interest pattern on Strong's Vocational Interest Blank and by possessing interests like those of persons in the preferred occupation, also has utility. So does Independence of Work Experience, evidenced by obtaining part-time and summer jobs on one's own or by being self-employed.

Best Measures Regardless of Type. Up to this point we have been looking at the two types of predictors separately. A stepwise regression analysis involving all 34 predictors provides a basis for selecting the most promising predictors from both lists.

It shows that the most promising predictors are:

Conventional
    Parental Occupational Level
    Participation in School Activities
Vocational Maturity
    Agreement between Ability and Preference (sometimes negative)
    Occupational Information: Supply and Demand
    Occupational Information: Material Conditions of Work (sometimes negative)
    Implementation of Preference through Extracurricular Activities (consistently negative)

They are related to most of the criteria in three or more of the five clusters. Except for Implementation of Preference, Agreement between Ability and Preference, and Information about the Material Conditions of Work, they are all associated with positive outcomes.

Only slightly less promising than the aforementioned and consistently positive in their relationships are:

Conventional
    Grades
    After School Employment
    Participation in Out-of-School Avocational Activities
Vocational Maturity
    Occupational Information: Preparation Required
    Occupational Information: Hours of Work

To summarize these data for the light they throw on the relative utility of our conventional and novel measures of adolescent status and behavior, three of the best and two other good predictors are among the novel vocational maturity measures, and two of the best and three other good predictors are conventional measures such as parental status and grades. Two other vocational maturity measures make unique contributions to predicting young adult career behavior, sometimes through positive, sometimes through negative, relationships.

THE ADOLESCENT WHO BECOMES A SUCCESSFUL ADULT

On the basis of the foregoing it is possible to construct a tentative picture of the kind of high school student who is most likely to have achieved success, satisfaction, and a place for himself in the world of work by age 25, as judged both by what he says about himself and by how judges evaluate his work history. He is more likely to come from a middle- than from a lower-class home, gets good grades, is active in school activities, has hobbies and pastimes which he pursues out of school, has goals which are in keeping with his intellectual level, and knows something about the occupation which he thinks he might follow. In short, he uses resources to good effect, both his own and those provided by the school and community. He is active and involved: he not only engages his environment but actively explores it.

Some of these characteristics are interrelated: for example, grades, parental occupational level, and participation in school and out-of-school activities. But the correlations are generally modest, the highest being .40 between Participation in School Activities and Participation in Out-of-School Avocational Activities. High School Grade Point Average (highly correlated with mental ability) and Parental Occupational Level (an equally valid measure of socioeconomic status) correlate only .38 with each other, and in the low .20's and .30's with some of the other characteristics. Correlations of this size obviously leave a good deal of the variance unaccounted for; they certainly cannot be taken as evidence that "good things go together" and that one of these measures is sufficient for the understanding of behavior and development. Furthermore, the fact that a stepwise multiple regression analysis uses only those variables which contribute significantly to the prediction, after their relationships to other predictors have been taken into account, ensures that the variables which emerge furnish not only useful but unique information. Although certain of the variables which we have identified as promising predictors are, as one would expect, related to one another, they do furnish important additional information.

Since multiple correlations typically shrink upon replication and variables which at first look promising may subsequently prove to be less promising and even invalid, these findings need to be replicated with a second group of subjects. Previous analyses of the Career Pattern Study data (Super et al., 1967), using element scores and standard correlation procedures instead of the present factor scores and multiple regression techniques, have yielded important consistencies as well as some inconsistencies between the present group of subjects and a second but comparable group of subjects reserved for replication purposes. The results of the present analysis are generally in accord with those of the less refined but replicated earlier analysis, suggesting that a replication study involving stepwise multiple regression techniques is likely to confirm the major findings of the present analysis.

Conclusions

The results of the longitudinal study discussed in this paper have brought out the manifold nature of vocational maturity in adolescence, the manifold nature of young adult vocational behavior and success, and the complexity of the relationships between these constellations of antecedent and consequent characteristics and behaviors. They have thrown light on the frequency of floundering after leaving high school, whether for the labor market or first for college and then for the labor market. They have illuminated the characteristics of the adolescent who, in early adulthood, copes well with the developmental tasks of that life stage.

Vocational maturity in twelfth-grade boys was found to consist of having crystallized vocational interests, being informed of those aspects of the preferred occupation which bear on the decisions which will soon need to be made (training, entry, supply and demand, duties), having work experiences which demonstrate and develop independence, aspiring to an occupation for which one has the necessary abilities and capital or contacts, weighing alternatives, and accepting responsibility for choice making and planning. Underlying these characteristics, not brought out by the type of factor analysis used in this study but identified by an earlier factor analysis of the same boys in the ninth grade (Super & Overstreet, 1960), and by a subsequent study of tenth-grade boys and girls (Super & Forrest, 1973), appears to be a planning approach to life, a future time perspective, knowledge and use of resources that may be useful, and knowledge of decision-making principles and practices.

Adult success, as seen in the mid-twenties, was shown by the Career Pattern Study to be reflected in six clusters of vocational behaviors which range from occupational status criteria, such as economic self-sufficiency and job getting and holding, to career criteria such as satisfaction with progress made toward an occupational goal and with establishment in an appropriate occupation. Of special interest are career criteria, such as floundering or stabilizing as one copes with the role demands of society, and realism in moving from one position to another. That one third of the subjects, a typical group of American youth, floundered between school leaving and the age of 25 provides useful normative data in judging the vocational coping behaviors of late adolescence and early adulthood.

The prediction of early adult by adolescent behavior is the principal focus of the paper. Vocational behavior being the topic of the Career Pattern Study narrows the focus still more, but the central importance of occupational expectations in industrial societies, the critical importance of occupational roles in the lives of adults, and the scope given for both the development of personality and for the impact of personality on behavior in the selection and playing of occupational roles make this focus anything but narrow.

The best adolescent predictors of vocational behavior in early adulthood were shown to be the measures of vocational maturity, those which reveal in the adolescent a future orientation, planfulness, and responsibility in the acquisition of information relevant to choosing, training for, and entering an occupation. Most of the measures used for this purpose were novel measures useful in pioneering research but awkward and expensive. It was seen that later work, building on this, has developed more practical instruments for larger-scale research and practice.

Conventional measures, those generally used in public schools, also have good predictive value. Unlike most surveys, which combine the advantage of larger numbers with the defects of more superficial methods, the Career Pattern Study found significant relationships between school grades, extracurricular activities, and leisure activities, on the one hand, and young adult vocational success on the other. It makes theoretical sense that the adolescent's coping with the developmental tasks of school and community predicts his success and satisfaction in coping with the developmental tasks of early adulthood.

Finally, the adolescent who copes successfully with his later developmental tasks was shown to be one who has access to the resources of society through his middle-class home, who uses his personal and social resources well, who sets realistic goals, and who in a planful and responsible approach to life acquires information relevant to his career.

COMMENTARY

SCHOOLER. I'm struck by the fact that Jordaan and I are looking at the same phenomena from somewhat different angles. I'm involved in a fairly large-scale study of sociopsychological consequences of occupations. In order to understand these consequences we have had to deal with the question of causal relationships. We have had to examine the characteristics of who goes into what occupation, in order to see the degree to which the job affects the individual or the individual affects the job. To do this we have had to use path analysis and two-stage least-squares analysis. Looking at your data, I was struck by the applicability of such techniques to the particular questions you are asking. You seem to be comparing a theoretically derived set of predictors with a vaguely empirical, generally accepted set of predictors. It seems possible to me, instead, to take those things which you know to be temporally prior — for instance, social class of origin, race, original test scores — and to look at their effects. I'm struck by the fact that you have data for Ss from the eighth grade until they are 36 years of age. Start with their original test scores. Breaking your data down into temporal stages, you can use the data from each stage to predict the next point in time, and so on. You can then have not merely a correlational study, but that rare thing, a causal study. You have all the data.

JORDAAN. This is certainly worth bearing in mind in future analyses. The final Career Pattern Study follow-up is scheduled for 1973 when our original ninth-graders will be about 36 years old, making the kind of analysis which you suggest very feasible. The only researchers who have done something along the lines you suggest are Gribbons and Lohnes, who have applied Markov chain analysis to longitudinal data gathered at six different points between the eighth grade and age 25. At times their focus has been on the subjects' occupational choices in successive time periods, at other times on whether the subjects were floundering or getting established. The usefulness of Markov chain analysis derives from the fact that since this type of analysis is performed without the aid of any external predictors, it can indicate whether or not there is a need for such predictors and also what they might be expected to contribute. Gribbons and Lohnes feel they have demonstrated the usefulness of Markov chain theory for studying changes over time, but correctly point out that in most instances, and especially with respect to choices in successive time periods, there is enough unexplained variance to demonstrate the need for external variables.

SCHOOLER. Markov chains are a much more elaborate procedure than I have in mind. In the standard path analysis you predict time B from time A, time C from time A and time B, time D from time A, B, and C. It is done with basically the same multiple correlation techniques you have used. It would not merely be a matter of predicting which of two occupational positions or attitudes you have but would make it possible to look back to see which things initially predicted the final outcome.

ZUBIN. If you are willing to accept outcome as your final criterion, perhaps a Bayesian approach working backward might be a way of doing it. And perhaps a canonical correlation could give you the universes in which you could make your predictions most powerful. Another point:

I wonder in connection with some of your findings whether it isn't possible that what we are seeing is a generational effect. Maybe this generation doesn't know what it wants, and if so could it be because their adolescence has been so protracted? Are there any data on previous generations?

JORDAAN. Our subjects don't seem to be very different from those studied by other investigators in the past. The evidence is fairly clear that the post–high school years are for many subjects years in which movement from one job to another is horizontal rather than vertical and random rather than purposeful. This has been a fairly consistent finding over the years. All of the studies, even those which go back many years, show that most young people do not move directly into the line of work they will pursue for the rest of their lives. This is, of course, much less true of individuals who enter the labor market with fully qualifying work experience or training. Such individuals move more expeditiously into or toward their regular adult occupation. To comment on another point which you raised: We found that the typical twelfth-grader about to leave school was still actively considering several occupations. His list of occupational possibilities was shorter than it was in the ninth grade, but only slightly shorter. The occupations under consideration were frequently very different from one another with respect to field and level. Thus, a subject might say in the twelfth grade that he was considering becoming a doctor, a mechanic, a forest ranger, or an accountant. Not surprisingly, there was usually not much commitment to, or investment in, any of these "choices." The typical twelfth-grader knew more about these preferred occupations than he did when he was in the ninth grade, but the amount of information possessed, even about the occupation he was considering most seriously, was nevertheless quite limited. The typical 18-year-old is not so ready to specify and implement a vocational preference as is commonly supposed.

VAILLANT. I would like to add some confirmation, from our study of 18-year-olds followed to age 50, of some of the predictors at age 19 of occupational success at 50. First, career success and psychological success are highly correlated. Secondly, at age 19, lack of being rated as having definite purpose or values or very clear ideas of what you are going to do in life did not correlate very well with career success, but being rated as practical, or organized, or pragmatic at age 19 did correlate well with later success. In other words, knowing what you want to do at 19 isn't good, but knowing how you are going to do it is good. Finally, all of our subjects had the advantage of being chosen because they were sophomores in a competitive liberal arts college, and socioeconomic status was factored out altogether in terms of predicting occupational success. In terms of their success, their politics in terms of Democrat versus Republican from 1960 to 1970 didn't differ. But the occupationally unsuccessful men tended, if they were Democrats, to be for Stevenson, and Republicans for Goldwater, whereas the more occupationally successful men, if they were Democrats, were for Kennedy, if Republicans, for Rockefeller. These observations underscore the method of action versus contemplation.

128

RICKS. Any generalization about human beings based on a Harvard sample has to be questioned. That is a very special group.

ROLF. What you seem to be saying here may in fact be partly a function of social background. Parental occupation is one of your better predictors. The middle-class kid can afford to engage in extracurricular activities, to have free time after school for hobbies, and so on. They don't necessarily need to know what their final job outcome may be. They say I want to be a professional, but if I can't, I can be a mechanic, because I am clever with my hands. People of lower social class may not have the opportunity to go out for band or clubs. They may work, and they may find out a lot about some vocational activity. They may find out they don't like it, or the pay isn't too good, so they may get satiated or extinguished on that job. Or they may want to become an accountant, but not have the money for the training, so they take a temporary job. If they switch jobs, this may look like lack of job success.

JORDAAN. An important feature of stepwise multiple regression analysis is that variables which are so highly correlated with other variables that they do not add any fresh information are washed out. Thus, for example, participation in school activities, work experience, and GPA emerge as useful predictors of later success and satisfaction *even* when their relationship to socioeconomic status has been partialled out. Socioeconomic status is an important part of the story but it is not the whole story.

ROLF. I think that you have touched on an important point, but before I can agree with you, I must know the following things: (a) Could it make a difference whether or not it was a forward or backward stepwise multiple regression solution? (b) Were all the correlations generated from the same matrix or were new matrices derived each time a variable was dropped? (c) Is it not also possible that a suppressor variable may have hidden the correlation between social class and occupational outcome? If I am to understand your data fully, I must know your answers to these questions.

REFERENCES

Berlyne, D. E. *Conflict, arousal, and curiosity.* New York: McGraw-Hill, 1960.

Crites, J. E. *The Career Maturity Inventory.* Monterey: California Test Bureau, 1973.

————. The Career Maturity Inventory. In D. E. Super (Ed.), *Measuring vocational maturity for counseling and evaluation.* Washington, D.C.: National Vocational Guidance Association, in preparation.

Elder, G. H., Jr. Adolescent socialization and development. In E. F. Borgatta & W. W. Lambert (Eds.), *Handbook of personality theory and research.* Chicago: Rand McNally, 1968. Ch. 5.

Flavell, J. H. *The developmental psychology of Jean Piaget.* New York: Van Nostrand, 1963.

Ginzberg, E., Ginsburg, S. W., Axelrad, S., & Herma, J. L. *Occupational choice.* New York: Columbia University Press, 1951.

Gribbons, W. D., & Lohnes, P. R. *Emerging careers.* New York: Teachers College Press, Columbia University, 1968.

————. *Career development from age 13 to age 25.* Washington, D.C.: U.S. Department of Health, Education, and Welfare, Office of Education Bureau of Research, 1969.

Havighurst, R. J. *Human development and education.* New York: Longman, 1953.

Jordaan, J. P. Exploratory behavior: The formation of self and occupational concepts. In D. E. Super, R. Starishevsky, & N. Matlin (Eds.), *Career development: Self-concept theory.* New York: College Entrance Examination Board, 1963.

————. Life stages as organizing modes of career development. In E. L. Herr (Ed.), *Vocational guidance and human development.* Boston: Houghton Mifflin, in press.

———— & Heyde, M. B. *The high school years.* Career Pattern Study Monograph N. 3. New York: Teachers College Press, Columbia University, in preparation.

Osipow, S. H. *Theories of career development.* New York: Appleton, 1973.

Roe, A. *Psychology of occupations.* New York: Wiley, 1956.

Smith, M. B. Explorations in competence. *American Psychologist,* 1966, 21, 555–566.

Super, D. E. *The dynamics of vocational adjustment.* New York: Harper, 1942.

————. Vocational adjustment: implementing a self concept. *Occupations,* 1951, 30, 5–9.

————. A theory of vocational development. *American Psychologist,* 1953, 8, 185–190.

————. *The psychology of careers.* New York: Harper, 1957.

————. Vocational development theory: Persons, positions, and process. Paper presented at the Symposium on Vocational Development Theory, Washington University, St. Louis, July 30, 1968.

————. Career development. In J. R. Davitz & S. Ball (Eds.), *Psychology of the educational process.* New York: McGraw-Hill, 1970.

————. (Ed.) *Measuring vocational maturity for counseling and evaluation.* Washington, D.C.: National Vocational Guidance Association, in preparation.

————, Crites, J., Hummel, R., Overstreet, P., & Warnath, C. *Vocational development: A framework for research.* New York: Teachers College Press, Columbia University, 1957.

Super, D. E., & Jordaan, J. P. Career development theory. *British Journal of Guidance and Counseling,* 1973, 1, no. 1.

Super, D. E., Kowalski, R. S., & Gotkin, E. H. *Floundering and trial after high school.* New York: Teachers College Press, Columbia University, 1967.

Super, D. E., & Overstreet, P. L. *The vocational maturity of ninth-grade boys.* New York: Teachers College Press, Columbia University, 1960.

Super, D. E., Starishevsky, R., Matlin, N., & Jordaan, J. P. *Career development: Self-concept theory.* New York: College Entrance Examination Board, 1963.

Tiedeman, D. V., & O'Hara, R. P. *Career development: Choice and adjustment.* New York: College Entrance Examination Board, 1963.

Vroom, V. A. *Work and motivation.* New York: Wiley, 1964.

Westbrook, B. W., & Parry-Hill, J. W., Jr. The measurement of cognitive vocational maturity. *Journal of Vocational Behavior,* 1973, 3.

White, R. W. *Lives in progress.* New York: Dryden, 1952.

————. (Ed.) *The study of lives.* New York: Prentice-Hall, 1963.

MERRILL ROFF *Childhood Antecedents of
Adult Neurosis, Severe Bad Conduct,
and Psychological Health*

THE PURPOSE of this project, which is a part of a larger life history
research program, was to validate child guidance clinic data as a source
of predictive information for adult neurosis, severe bad conduct, and
relatively good adjustment. The use of childhood case histories in comparison with adult outcome information eliminates some of the faults
inherent in retrospective studies of persons who exhibit adult maladjust-
ments. This case history information is subject to various biases, but the
multiple sources of information commonly used tend to balance each
other and to give, as a whole, a more accurate picture than is obtained
from any single source.

This specific project is concerned with the analysis of 150 male child
guidance clinic cases drawn from a much larger data pool who had three
different kinds of adult outcome: neurotic, severe bad conduct, and control. Since earlier work of this same kind had indicated that there was a
greater structuring of behavior in the direction of adult outcome during
the teen-age period than was true earlier, only those cases were employed in our samples whose first contact with the child guidance clinic
occurred at the age of twelve or younger. Earlier work with schizophrenic
cases (Roff, 1963) and with adults diagnosed as schizoid personalities
(Roff, 1965; Roff, Mink, & Hinrichs, 1966) had indicated clearly that
retrospective studies could fail to penetrate beyond teen-age status to

NOTE: The research reported here has been supported in major part by USPHS
Contract No. HSM-42-69-50 with the National Institute of Mental Health. This
paper is a condensation of the Final Contract Report. A few copies of this report
are available to persons planning to do work of this kind. Specific parts of this
report, such as scales and their instructions or the eleven-page bibliography, can
be duplicated and sent to those interested.

behavior occurring during childhood. One result of this was that boys who were acting out fairly vigorously at the age of seven or eight could have become much more quiet and withdrawn during their teens, so that the erroneous impression developed that adults in these two categories had been quiet and withdrawn all through their childhoods, which was not the case. This error is a common one.

A further aim of the project was to review the literature on parent and parent-child behavior and family functioning as it might contribute to an understanding of the development of psychopathology, and to develop a set of codes and rating scales based partly on this literature review, appropriate for use with child guidance clinic records. Studies of normal children in this area, including the few available longitudinal studies, tend to focus more on the behavior of average parents than on potentially maladjustment-producing parental behavior. An illustration of this is given in the Kagan and Moss (1963) follow-up of the Fels Study. In discussing maternal hostility as a variable, they observed that "Major sources of data included (a) criticism of the child's behavior and derogation of his skills and personality, (b) statements of preference for another sib, and (c) active rejection or neglect. *The latter behavior was infrequent*, and this variable was measuring primarily an openly critical attitude toward the child" (pp. 205–206; emphasis added). In contrast with this, for one of our three groups maternal neglect, even to the point of abandonment, was almost usual. That set of mothers was more or less off the end of the scale developed for a normal sample of mothers.

The many kinds of information contained in child guidance case histories provide a highly multivariate situation, both when considered from a purely predictive point of view and when an attempt is made to assess their importance as potential influences. In the present project we were primarily concerned with analyzing the cases into their component parts. An adequate reassembling of these parts was not yet a target. Although some elementary multivariate manipulations of the data have been made to clarify specific points, a thorough-going multivariate treatment of these data awaits replication on additional samples with the resulting increased sample size. Additional child guidance cases with accompanying adult outcome information are available for this purpose.

The Earlier Literature

An intensive search of the relevant literature on the antecedents of adult neurosis and adult severe bad conduct was made; this included variables relating both to the family and general setting and to the child. This had two main purposes: (a) the obvious one of getting everything that could be obtained from the existing literature, and (b) the collection of information for developing our instruments and scales and for constructing a priori keys for these. If we have sixty or seventy items which could be keyed empirically to make scales for the prediction of our three adult outcome groups (50 *S*s per sample — neurosis, bad conduct, and control), it would be possible to overkey by capitalizing on all the chance differences which occurred in the course of analysis. In order to avoid this, where possible we used the literature as a guide to a priori keying of scales.

Since too rigid an adherence to this procedure would have required the throwing away of potentially new information which was generated in the course of this study, we have also used information newly obtained here to make keys or guides which contained information we had not found in the literature. With awareness of the possibility of our overkeying while doing this, these are presented partly as hypotheses which can be tested on other samples, by ourselves or other investigators. For new samples, these would become a priori keys. We have attempted to make full use of the existing literature, without being artificially restricted to information which had already been mentioned there.

Use has been made of a list of 175 references (some 13 pages) which were selected from a larger pool as being more nearly factual than a few more speculative articles or some of those which were devoted primarily to the presentation of one or two case histories (Roff, 1971). There were wide differences in the amount of information which could be found on different topics in relation to different outcomes. Almost the earliest study we found on family factors in relation to juvenile delinquency (Rhoades, 1907) noted that when the family situations of a sample of delinquent youths were examined, they seemed to present an unusual number of broken homes. This finding has been replicated again and again. However, it is also true that most youngsters from broken homes do not become delinquent, so that further information about these parents is needed.

On the other hand, there is hardly a single competent article which relates factors operative during childhood, *which were recorded at the time*, to later adult neurosis. Retrospective case histories, with a psychoanalytic or other orientation, are common. It is a poor clinician indeed who cannot take a retrospective case history and explain how the patient developed the difficulty he now shows. If we take information recorded during childhood and predict forward from that, the apparent complete determinacy of the retrospective study vanishes, and we are left only with a probabilistic prediction, often not too impressive in its accuracy. It is extremely difficult to find good information of a prospective kind about factors leading to adult psychoneurosis.

As a way of getting an independent reading on this apparent fact, we examined the MMPI, the most comprehensive of all the personality inventories, to see what the keying of that had turned up in the way of parental and intra-family items in relation to the diagnosed outcomes of the patients on which the keys were constructed. When all the items which seemed clearly related to the patient's family and his attitudes toward it were isolated and counted, there were eight items each in the Psychopathic Deviate (4) and Schizophrenia (8) scales, and four items in the Hypomania (9) scale. On the other hand, the Hysteria scale (3) contained one item which referred to family, while the Hypochondriasis (1), Depression (2), Psychasthenia (7), and Social Introversion (0) scales contained no family items at all. This agrees with the relatively negative result of our search for firm information on the family background and attitudes toward other family members of adult neurotics.

Although the study of background factors in schizophrenia was not a part of this project, there is substantial literature on parent behavior in relation to schizophrenia. This was also analyzed as part of our parent behavior survey in order to determine whether parental characteristics reported as related to delinquency and to neurosis were specific to those outcomes, or were related to other major behavior disturbances as well. This procedure also suggested additional items which could be included in the child and parent rating scale we were constructing.

The delinquency literature deals mainly with relatively objective data about the parents (e.g., economic status, broken home and absence of a parent, court history of either parent). Much of this information applied to the family rather than to either parent specifically.

On the other hand, studies of parental characteristics of children diagnosed as neurotic (to be distinguished from childhood information for adult neurotics) tend to deal more with abstract personality characteristics of the parents than do the delinquency studies. They also tend to focus on one parent or to consider each parent separately.

A detailed tabulation was made of the literature on the family characteristics of these three types of maladjustment (Roff, 1971). A search was made for family information in 46 bad conduct sources, 19 neurotic sources, and 21 schizophrenic sources. Like the case histories themselves, the different articles tended to contain information on some topics and not on others. A count was made of the number of these sources which reported a positive relationship, no relationship, or a negative relationship for these maladjusted groups. The families of delinquents, as contrasted with the other two groups, tended to be characterized as having a broken home or absent parent, financial inadequacy, a parental history of trouble with the law, and parental harshness, cruelty, and punitiveness. As mentioned above, the literature on the families of neurotics contained much less information. In about a fourth of the articles the families were characterized as warm, affectionate, and loving, whereas this was hardly mentioned for the bad conduct or schizophrenic groups. Both dominant-aggressive-demanding behavior and passivity were mentioned as positive factors among the schizophrenic families with significantly greater frequency than in the other two groups. Parental rejection, conflict, friction and fighting, and parental neglect and lack of supervision were mentioned as characteristics of both schizophrenic and delinquent families but not of neurotics.

Method

Terminology and Checklists. One problem to which we gave a good deal of attention was the possibility of using one or two word checklists. This was of interest in its own right; it is also a problem in the coding of cases, to determine the extent to which coding can be done in terms of one or two words without loss of the information which would accurately reflect the meanings of these terms.

It was found that some terms commonly used in referring to parental behavior or parent-child interactions were unsatisfactory because they could actually refer with equal accuracy to two different kinds of situation. Reflection indicated that this duality was inherent in the terms themselves. One clear-cut case of this is *autonomy* of the child. This applies with equal accuracy to a child who is totally neglected and does whatever he wants to, and to a child who has been reared so that he acts within socially accepted limits without much in the way of external controls.

A second kind of term which caused some difficulty is one whose significance in relation to the parent is dependent on what the child's behavior is like. Two terms which were found to be of limited usefulness when used with reference to a parent alone were *anxiety induction* and *guilt induction.* If a mother exhibited what seemed to be anxiety-inducing or guilt-inducing kinds of behavior, and if the child's behavior appeared unaffected by this, as sometimes happens (since he did not seem to have had either guilt or anxiety induced in him), the outcome expected would be markedly different than if he became anxious or guilt-ridden. Such terms were not too helpful in prediction without also having information about the child. Again, the statement that a mother *worries* is of uncertain significance unless a judgment can be made as to what she is worrying about, how realistic the worry is, and whether or not the worry can lead to any constructive action.

This is an important point, since it is related not only to the kind of case analyses that we were doing, but also to attempts at computerized treatments of case history materials. This problem arises with a number of terms which imply a negative affective tone in the mother. *Resentful, disturbed,* and *afraid* acquire different meanings when followed by phrases such as "about his truanting and running away," "about his asocial tendencies," "that he does not prefer herself to father," or "about his femininity."

Unless the source of concern is indicated, it is difficult to evaluate the appropriateness of the mother's reaction. If the source of concern is indicated, information about the boy as well as the mother is included.

An analysis of the research literature corresponding to that discussed above for parents was made for childhood symptoms relating to childhood neuroses, severe bad conduct, and "problem" behavior independent of these other two. The resulting symptom list — including disobedience, defiance of authority, theft, and running away from home for bad conduct cases; chronic anxiety and depression for those with a neurotic trend; and speech disturbance and enuresis for other problems — in general parallels the symptoms listed under appropriate headings in the *Diagnostic and Statistical Manual of Mental Disorders* (1968). Childhood symptoms are more definitely describable than parental behavior which may be associated with them.

Sampling and Procedure. The sample consisted of 150 males who had dealt with child guidance clinics during childhood (first contact at age 12 or younger) and for whom adult adjustment information was available from records of the military services and related organizations. As adults, 50 of these were diagnosed neurotic, 50 were severe bad conduct cases as indicated either by their disciplinary record and disposition in service or by their confinement in a civilian penitentiary or by both of these, and 50 had made adequate social adjustments in one of the military services. Adequate adjustment was defined as reaching and keeping non-commissioned or commissioned status without significant disciplinary or psychiatric records.

This made three definite adult outcome groups. Any cases diagnosed as neurotic who also showed severe bad conduct at the adult level were excluded. Consideration was given to matching of these cases on other variables. For example, juvenile delinquents and adult felons both occurred with somewhat greater relative frequency in lower socioeconomic groups. Matching the bad conduct cases and the neurotics on, for example, SES would have made either the neurotics or the bad conduct cases atypical. If a compromise had been made, both samples would have been somewhat different from unmatched samples taken as they occurred. It was thus decided to avoid any attempt to match the cases on such variables, with the realization that factors such as SES might need to be taken into account in the interpretation of results. One variable on which the neurotic and bad conduct cases varied somewhat was in age at first clinic contact, the bad conduct cases being slightly older. Again, if we had matched the two groups on this variable, we would have obtained groups which were not wholly representative of the original samples from which they had been selected.

Both those who had entered one of the military services and those who had been rejected because of neurosis or severe bad conduct were included in these groups, to include the broadest possible samples of both neurotics and bad conduct cases. Many of those with very unfavorable disciplinary records in service also had trouble in civilian life; the severe bad conduct group was not a group that merely found military service not to their liking, while getting along perfectly well in civilian life. The control group included only those who had been in military service, because there was positive indication of good adjustment for these which was not available for those who were not in service. The ages of first clinic contact ranged from three to twelve years. There were only five cases younger than five years of age.

Childhood IQ's were available for all but ten of the cases. The mean IQ's of the control, neurotic, and bad conduct groups are 104, 100, and 98, respectively. These differences are not large enough to affect the interpretation much. One point of interest is that four of the five with childhood IQ's below 80 were in the adult neurotic group. A high IQ is not, as is sometimes believed, a prerequisite to the development of neurosis.

Other Descriptive Statistics. How the three groups compare on various other objective and readily available dimensions is also of interest. In one of these, age at first clinic contact, there was enough difference among groups to influence the interpretation of some data, but not enough to be very predictive of adult outcome. The mean ages at first clinic contact of the control, neurotic, and bad conduct groups were 8.0, 8.2, and 9.4 respectively. The higher average age at first clinic contact of the adult bad conduct cases was associated with a tendency for these cases to be grouped more at the ages of 11 and 12 than the other two groups.

From a purely predictive point of view, two face sheet items differentiated the bad conduct cases from the neurotics and controls. (a) The bad conduct cases were referred either by or at the suggestion of a court or probation office much more frequently than the others. (b) Almost three times as many of the bad conduct cases as of the other two groups were referred by welfare or social service agencies. These boys were rarely brought to the clinic by the mother without prodding or a strong suggestion from the agencies mentioned or by the school. Neurotics exceeded controls in the number of medically initiated referrals, either directly by the doctor or through the mother, eleven to three.

A second set of differentiating values from the face sheets concerns the number of Central Registration Bureau items for the families. This included all contacts known to the Central Registration Bureau from social and welfare agencies, corrective agencies, and so on for any family member. More than half of the controls and neurotics had either no referral or not more than two referrals; only six of the bad conduct families had such a low frequency. On the other hand, more than half (27) of the bad conduct families had ten or more referrals as contrasted with eight neurotic and five control families. Again, the bad conduct cases are differentiable from the other two groups on face sheet information alone, but the neurotics and controls are not appreciably different.

Other objective items do not discriminate nearly so sharply. One of these is family size — the number of only children is essentially the same in the three groups, but the bad conduct group includes somewhat more families with five or more children than the other two. It also exceeds the other two groups slightly in the number of half-siblings and step-siblings — a function of the greater frequency of instability in the bad conduct families.

Socioeconomic status was obtained from place of residence and school attended, as determined by the income and education of adults in the census tracts served by the schools. The SES of the schools was divided into quartiles (1 high, 4 low); the results for the three outcome groups in quartiles 1–4 are contained in the accompanying tabulation. The controls (C) were high in the first quartile and relatively low in the fourth, whereas the bad conduct (BC) cases were relatively low in the first quartile and high in the fourth.

	C	*N*	*BC*
1	16	13	7
2	10	9	10
3	12	12	9
4	5	8	18

The SES of the neurotics (N) is particularly interesting. Studies of neurotics who are treated by private psychiatrists show that they tend to be among the more prosperous members of the community, because only the more prosperous can afford such treatment. In the present situation, persons at all income levels could be diagnosed as neurotic, and there was no great difference among the numbers falling in the four SES quartiles. Similarly, they were not as a group higher in SES than the controls. It is believed that this is a function of the fact that their diagnosis as neurotic was not in any way dependent on their financial status.

A final set of values for information of this kind are the parents' ages at the time of the patient's birth. For mothers, there is little difference; the means for the three groups fall at either 25 or 26 years. For fathers, the situation is different, as is shown in the accompanying tabulation. Just

	C	*N*	*BC*
Range of ages	18–44	21–57	21–52
Mean age	29.5	34.2	30.6
No information	7	6	15

what significance the higher age of the fathers of neurotics has is not clear, but this is presented as an interesting bit of information which can be checked by other investigators.

Categories of Case Abstracts (COCA). One main purpose of this project was to study the effectiveness of childhood case history information in predicting adult outcomes of various kinds and to find out by analysis what parts of the childhood information were contributing most to the prediction. A second purpose was to focus sharply on parental behavior and interactions with the patient, on the assumption that there was a possibility of more than a merely predictive relationship for these. To accomplish both these purposes, it was necessary to take the cases apart, as it were, by abstracting information under different categories so that it became possible to evaluate a single category, such as the characteristics of the father or of sibling interactions, without being influenced by all the other information contained in the case histories. The categories used in this abstracting are listed in Table 1.

Table 1. Categories of Case Abstracts (COCA)

1. Patient's symptoms
    A.   Age and reason for referral
    B.   Source of referral
    C.   Symptom information from remainder of case
    D.   Duration of clinic contact
2. Various objective items relating to family
    A.   Number of Central Bureau Registration items
    B.   Adults in home
    C.   Education of mother and father
    D.   Father's occupation and family's SES
    E.   Sibling structure
    F.   Number of schools attended
3. Characteristics of mother
4. Characteristics of father
5. Parental interaction
6. Patient
    A.   Characteristics of patient and interactions with parents
    B.   Interaction of patient with school
        1.   Scholastic (including IQ)
        2.   Interpersonal
            a.   Teacher
            b.   Peers
7. Sibling characteristics and interactions
8. Health and growth
    A.   Health of parents and children
    B.   Retrospective developmental information
9. Contacts with the law
10. Psychiatric prediction

For all case materials being used, all identifying information had been blacked out and photocopies were made, so that the cases being analyzed were completely anonymous and unidentifiable. Cases were labeled by long, nonsense numbers, which eliminated the identification of an abstract with one clinic or another and also eliminated the cues given by the original case numbers that some cases had preceded others in time.

A detailed discussion of this case history outline and the specific instructions which were used in processing the cases has been presented elsewhere (Roff, 1971). In abstracting information from cases, earlier experience had indicated the desirability of retaining both the chronological sequence of events in the history and the category of the informant quoted. Thus, every entry was supposed to indicate the person from whom the information had been obtained and its date. This practice was also found desirable by Eiduson et al. (1967) as their PsyCHES system was developed. More emphasis was placed on making the abstracted information for each category self-contained than on eliminating all overlap with other categories. For example, in the information abstracted about the mother, too rigorous an elimination of all information about the child resulted in too great a loss of meaning of the description of the mother's attitudes and actions.

The "Mother" abstracts were commonly among the longest, for she was the parent seen most by the clinic. The abstracts offer a wealth of information on the problems of mothers of children of grade school age. The clinics ordinarily made successful efforts to interview the father at least once (if he was available).

The "Patient" abstract included both specific symptomatic behavior and information on the context in which the behavior occurred, with particular emphasis on two important settings, family and school.

Referral Study. While we were still working on our review of the literature and on the abstracting of the cases by different categories, a preliminary study was made of the predictability of the cases based solely on referral information at the beginning of each case. This was used because it was quickly available and because it was brief enough that workers, using the predictive guide which was furnished them, could make predictions for a set of cases in a relatively short period of time. A consideration of the *Diagnostic and Statistical Manual of Mental Disorders* (1968) indicated that the implicit consensus underlying that presentation was better for our purposes than an attempt to summarize a somewhat fragmentary literature. A predictive guide, adapted from the *Manual* with slight modifications, would represent an a priori rather than an empirical key, as far as our particular cases were concerned. Such an a priori guide would probably also reflect a consensus of current psychiatric thought more closely than any other single source.

Items to be weighted positively for severe bad conduct outcomes were taken from the sections "Unsocialized aggressive reaction of childhood (or adolescence)" and "Group delinquent reaction of childhood (or adolescence)." The section "Runaway reaction of childhood (or adolescence)" contributed its main characteristic, "running away from home for a day or more without permission."

For the neurotic guide, "Overanxious reaction of childhood (or adolescence)" contributed most, and all its characteristics were taken. The section "Withdrawing reaction of childhood" was omitted, since it was cross-referenced to schizophrenia and schizoid personality.

Two categories taken from the *Manual* were to be regarded as both non-neurotic and non-delinquent as reasons for referral. These were "Special symptoms not elsewhere classified" and "Transient situational disturbances," including "Adjustment reaction of childhood" and "Adjustment reaction of adolescence." The resulting list was an a priori guide for evaluating reasons for referral; it has been given elsewhere (Roff, 1971). As a predictor, it gave obviously non-chance results utilizing only a fragment of the total information available. It could be used by intelligent clerical workers not trained in psychology. As first used, the control cases were omitted, to see to what extent the two adult problem groups could be discriminated on the basis of this easily obtainable childhood information alone. When this was found to work, the control group was included along with the other two.

Another point which was raised and settled in connection with this particular administration concerned the age at first clinic contact in relation to predictability. This procedure was administered using two groups of cases, those whose initial clinic contact occurred before the age of 9, and those whose first contact occurred between 9 and 12. It was found that those in the later initial referral group could be predicted somewhat more accurately than those in the earlier. Age seemed to be something that might have to be taken into account in subsequent work. However, when a breakdown was made between the earlier and later referrals among either the bad conduct cases or the neurotics, there was not much difference in predictability between the earlier and later neurotics, or between the earlier and later bad conduct cases. The bad conduct cases both were more predictable than the neurotic cases and tended to be older at the time of first referral. The apparent difference between early and later referrals was attributable largely to the difference in the predictability of these two groups rather than to age of referral as such.

Predictions were made in the two-outcome situation by twelve raters. The predicted outcome is the pooled choice of the majority of the twelve. The relation between the predicted adult outcomes and the actual outcomes is shown in the accompanying tabulation. Inspection indicates that relatively few adult bad conduct cases had not been predicted bad con-

	Actual *N*	*Actual* *BC*	*Total*
Predicted N	31	6	37
Predicted BC	19	44	63

142

duct outcomes. The total by rows indicates an overprediction of bad conduct outcomes.

When the control group was added and a new set of predictions made by five other raters, the results (again by a majority of the raters) were as in the accompanying tabulation. In this situation, the neurotics

	Actual *C*	*Actual* *N*	*Actual* *BC*	*Total*
Predicted C	28	18	2	48
Predicted N	14	15	1	30
Predicted BC	8	17	47	72

were again underpredicted, and the bad conduct cases were overpredicted. The bad conduct outcomes were identified, but those with neurotic outcomes were scatterd almost evenly over the three predictive possibilities. Control outcomes were between the other two in accuracy of prediction. When the control cases were added, the predictability of the bad conduct cases was not affected much, but the neurotic cases tended to be confused with the control cases, so that their predictability got substantially worse. This agrees with other parts of this study in indicating that the bad conduct cases differ much more sharply from the other two groups than the controls and neurotics do from each other. Analysis of the predictions for each case indicates that inter-rater agreement (reliability) was higher than inter-rater validity. That is, in some cases, the information pointed the wrong direction, and there was inter-rater agreement which was predictively erroneous.

An interesting incidental finding of the inter-rater comparisons just described was that with a highly structured guide of this kind, intelligent clerical workers could predict as well as persons with substantial amounts of training in clinical psychology. In this particular situation, the amount of interpretation required was narrowed down to a point where a psychologically untrained person, who followed the procedure intelligently and conscientiously, could do as well as persons with much more psychological training. This annoyed some clinicians, but it was so. This might not hold under many other circumstances.

The Child and Parent (CAP) Scale

One of the main aims of this project was to construct and validate a comprehensive rating scale which could be used for the comparison of adult "normal," neurotic, and severe bad conduct cases. The result was a two-part rating scale. Part 1 was based almost exclusively on the literature, with some trial testing for appropriateness on cases not included in this study to see how applicable it was to case history materials. It was used primarily to evaluate abstracts for the mother, the father, and their interactions. Part 2 was developed later, following use of Part 1 with the case abstracts, to include material present in the abstracts which seemed inadequately covered by Part 1. In Part 2, evaluations were sometimes required of the family as a whole. Otherwise, either *mother* or *father* was included in the item, so that a rating of both parents was not required.

PART ONE

Instructions for use of the CAP Scale recommended reading the complete Mother and Father abstracts for each case before checking the different kinds of behavior judged characteristic of the mother or father. The scale items were checked for all 150 cases by four raters, all blind as to adult outcome. Although there was some uncontrolled variation in the readiness with which a specific rater would check items, there was relatively little difference in the validity of their ratings. Different ways of combining these ratings were tried out, without much significant difference among different procedures. It was decided that, in view of their approximately equal validities, a meaningful (and adequate?) score could be obtained by counting each case for which an item was rated present by one or more workers. Results obtained with the most differentiating items of Part 1 of the CAP Scale are presented in Table 2. Instead of making a precise comparison of every possible pair of proportions, a general set of significance values are provided as a rough guide which the reader can use to decide which differences seem to be both non-chance and large enough to be worth attention.

The numbers in the columns in Table 2 are the numbers of cases checked out of a total of fifty possible. Doubled, each of these becomes the number out of one hundred possible, or a percentage. By using the procedure for estimating the standard error of a percentage, and transforming these back so that they will fit the numbers in the table, rough approximations to the difference between the numbers of cases, which would be at about the .05 level of significance, are shown in the accompanying tabulation. Since our sample of cases is not really a random sam-

Frequencies		*Differences Significant*
25 and 15	. . . .	10 cases
15 and 5	. . . .	8 cases
10 and 2	. . . .	6 cases

Table 2. Selected Item Frequencies on Child and Parent (CAP) Scale for Mothers and Fathers in the Three Groups[a]

Comparison and Item	C	N	BC
Mothers			
Bad conduct compared with control and neurotic			
Neglect in Important Areas	11	18	*32*
Inadequate Parental Control	9	12	*23*
Wish to Be Rid of Child	3	12	*27*
Abandonment and Repudiation of Child	4	3	*24*
Physical Cruelty	3	3	*11*
Negative Evaluation of Child	9	12	*19*
Babying/Overhelping	17	21	*10*
Annoyance/Impatience, etc.	16	17	*8*
Pressing for Achievement	14	12	*5*
Neurotic compared with control and bad conduct:			
Anxiety or Guilt Induction	9	*19*	13
Control compared with neurotic and bad conduct			
Approval	*16*	7	7
Helping	*11*	6	0
Attention	*15*	6	2
Defensive Behavior	*13*	21	22
No discrimination (approximately equal frequencies)			
Submission to child	12	17	13
Martyrdom	13	13	10
Affection	12	12	13
Fathers			
Bad conduct compared with control and neurotic			
Wish to Be Rid of Child	2	0	*13*
Abandonment and Repudiation of Child	6	8	*21*
Passivity	15	15	*5*
Attention	20	14	*6*
Neurotic compared with control and bad conduct			
Negative Evaluation of Child	3	*10*	5
Sees Child as Inferior	—	7	—
Control compared with neurotic and bad conduct			
Helping	*8*	2	1
Neglect	*13*	21	26
Physical Cruelty	*8*	14	20
No discrimination (approximately equal frequencies)			
Defensive Behavior	6	9	8
Annoyance/Impatience, etc.	10	9	6
Detachment/Coldness	3	4	4
Pressing for Achievement	3	3	5

[a]Italics indicate significant values.

ple drawn from any total universe of cases (any other clinic will inevitably use a somewhat different method of case selection), there is no use pretending that these are precise values. They may, however, be of some help in interpreting Table 2. The values which appear significant by this approximate test are italicized.

Inspection of the item validities for the mothers and fathers on the CAP Scale, Part 1, indicates that the bad conduct cases were more clearly discriminated from the other two groups than were the neurotics and controls from each other. A coherent cluster of items clearly separates the bad conduct mothers and similarly (although not in the same order) the bad conduct fathers. These are Neglect, Inadequate Parental Control, Wish to Be Rid of Child, Abandonment and Repudiation of Child, and Physical Cruelty.

One of the items which had been expected to be more discriminating was Defensive Behavior. One common instance of this consisted of the mother's taking the child's part and denying to someone outside the family either that he had done anything wrong, or that his wrongdoing was of any importance. This differentiated the bad conduct mothers from the controls, but there were almost as many neurotic as bad conduct mothers checked on this item. There were few items which clearly characterized the neurotic mothers or fathers. This was not too surprising in the light of the literature survey. The control parents were most clearly differentiated from one or both the problem groups by positive items such as Approval, Helping, and Attention.

There were some items in which the lack of difference among mothers or among fathers is interesting. Annoyance/Impatience did not discriminate among the fathers at all — annoyance with children apparently occurs as often among the parents of the later normal subjects as among parents of the other two groups. Passivity was noted as characteristic of control and neurotic fathers, though it was hardly noted at all as a characteristic of any set of mothers. Since we had a large number of variables in relation to our sample size, including both the CAP Scale and other variables, it was considered undesirable to attempt to produce empirical keys which would give scores for each of the three groups. An empirical key involves the use of all items meeting some test of significance, whether there is any rational reason for their inclusion or not. With our sample size of fifty cases in each of the three groups, the inclusion in a key of all items of any kind showing a presumed non-chance difference between any two groups could have resulted in an overkeying so substantial as to make almost certain a marked shrinkage when applied to other samples.

PART TWO

The second part of the CAP Scale consists of items derived from work with the cases, which had not emerged from our search of the parent-child literature. They do cover material, such as Markedly Unhappy Marriage which has appeared in earlier psychiatric discussions, but had not been adequately treated in Part 1. This second part contained more items which referred directly to characteristics of the parents by themselves and their interactions, which might, as with Drunkenness, affect their parenting behavior. They required some judgment by the person marking them. The full scale, with instructions, has been presented elsewhere (Roff, 1971).

An attempt was made to base these items on actual behavior descriptions or comments by those involved, from the abstracts of mother, father, and family. The first item was Markedly Unhappy Marriage. This was to be checked if either the mother or father talked about divorce or separation, or if they were constantly quarreling. It was also checked for any really unhappy continuing emotional atmosphere in the home; one indication of this might be the statement of either parent of a wish that he or she had never been married at all. The term Running Around was adopted as being more nearly based on direct observation than the term promiscuity. Drunkenness was to be checked only when alcohol was used to an extent that it interfered with the family's functioning in some way. Other similar rules are presented in the instructions.

The item frequencies for Part 2 are given in Table 3 for the three groups. The two items showing the greatest difference between the bad conduct cases and the other two groups are Drunkenness, which is a factor in almost half the cases, and Running Around. An item which is high for both the bad conduct and neurotic cases is Mother Says She Has No Control. This was included on the hypothesis that there would be some mothers who said they had no control as contrasted with an item in Part 1, Inadequate Parental Control. Mothers of bad conduct cases who said they had no control generally did have a real control problem. Mothers of neurotic cases sometimes had reasonable control but unreasonable expectations (see p. 152).

Differences among the boys as control problems *outside* the home is shown vividly by the number of contacts with the law which were reported in the case histories for the three groups: 43 of the 50 neurotics and 44 of the controls had no record of contact with the law, but only

Table 3. Selected Item Frequencies on Child and Parent (CAP) Scale, Part 2, for the Families of the Three Groups[a]

Comparison and Item	C	N	BC
Bad conduct compared with control and neurotic			
Running Around	8	4	*16*
Drunkenness	6	9	*22*
Mother Sickly	15	15	*4*
Neurotic compared with control and bad conduct			
Mother Seems Overburdened, Ineffective	4	*12*	4
Mother Nervous	17	*27*	3
Father Nervous	3	*19*	2
Neurotic compared with bad conduct			
Parents Disagree about discipline	12	*19*	9
Parents Disappointed in Patient	4	*8*	0
Control compared with neurotic and bad conduct			
Competent Mother	*11*	5	0
Parents Try to Control Their Anxiety/Worry about Patient	*8*	1	0
Mother Says She Has No Control	9	18	22
Control compared with bad conduct: Parents Consider Themselves Happy	*9*	5	3
No discrimination (approximately equal frequencies)			
Markedly Unhappy Marriage	7	13	10
Conflict Caused by Other Person in the Home	7	6	8
Religious Conflict or Marked Overemphasis	2	3	5
Father in the Home But Not Involved in Family Life	4	6	3
Parents Prefer Siblings to Patient	9	7	5

[a]Italics indicate significant values.

6 of the 50 bad conduct cases were clear; only 1 each of the neurotics and control groups had more than three contacts with the law, though this was true of 27 or more than half of the bad conduct group.

Some items in Part 2 were successful in discriminating the neurotic from both the other groups or from the controls alone. The items Mother Nervous and Father Nervous were particularly effective in this. Father Nervous was checked much less frequently for the controls. Another item which differentiated the parents of neurotics significantly was Parents Disagree about Discipline.

Items which were checked more frequently for controls than for the other two groups included Competent Mother, Parents Try to Control Their Anxiety, and Parents Consider Themselves Happy. These are all in the expected direction, but they were not checked so frequently as the main items for the neurotic or bad conduct groups.

To summarize, the parents of the bad conduct cases themselves exhibited more delinquent behavior than either the control or neurotic families and said that they had problems controlling the subject significantly more than did the control parents. The presence of more problems of control *outside* the home is indicated by the greater frequency of contacts with the law for the bad conduct boys as compared with the other groups.

For the neurotics, the most effective items are Father Nervous and Mother Nervous. This is a matter of limited family resemblance (Roff, 1950). Other items are disagreement about discipline and about other things, in unhappy marriages where the parents remain together.

The controls show more competence, contentment, and maturity in dealing with a child about whom they are concerned.

GROSS FAMILY HISTORY

A third family scale was constructed for use with the parent abstracts. This contained objective items which required a minimum of judgment, relating to the marital history of the mother and father; illegitimacy of subject or a sibling, and marriages forced by pregnancy; broken home, abandonment by mother, history of foster homes or adoption; father's absence from home owing to his civilian work or military service; mother's employment; and court history of father and mother as shown in the case.

Results for the three groups are shown in Table 4. In general, these items do not differentiate the controls from the neurotics. Several items differentiate the bad conduct sample quite sharply from the other two groups. Among these are divorce, desertion by either parent, illegitimacy, broken home, separation of mother from child, and residence in more than one foster home. The most sharply discriminating item is Mother Abandons. This included both abandoning the subject (and the rest of the family) and removing him from the home, often by arranging for placement. There were 21 such mothers of the bad conduct cases, with only 1 in the other two categories combined.

Items from All Sources in Relation to Bad Conduct for Non-Abandoning. Attention was directed to the items most predictive of bad conduct from CAP, parts 1 and 2 from the Gross Family History, and a count was made of the item frequencies for the 29 non-abandoning mothers of bad conduct cases. The frequencies are shown in the accompanying tabulations. A count was made of families or mothers who had checks on any of the five most frequent items in this list (drunkenness, neglect,

Table 4. Frequency Counts for Items of Gross Family History

Item	C	N	BC
1. Marital history			
a. One marriage and still married			
Mother	37	35	17
Father	33	23	15
b. Deserted or divorced and not remarried			
Mother	4	2	8
Father	3	2	10
c. Divorced and remarried			
Mother	1	2	11
Father			6
2. Patient illegitimate	5	3	8
3. Mother has had an illegitimate child other than patient	4	3	13
4. "Forced" marriage (record whether child had arrived or not at time of marriage)	2	3	13
5. Broken home	11	11	27
6. Mother abandons (record when mother leaves family or when she is instrumental in forcing the child out of the home into a training school or other institution)	1		21
7. History of foster homes			
a. One	4	6	10
b. Two	2	1	7
c. Three			2
d. Four			2
e. Patient shifted among relatives several times, then put into a foster home or County Home School	1		5
8. Mother's employment			
a. Full time	4	2	8
b. Part time	6	6	6
c. Apparently none	41	42	36
9. Court history of father			
a. Juvenile	1		2
b. Minor		3	6
c. Major/not imprisoned			3
d. Major/imprisoned	2	2	6
e. Apparently none	47	45	33
10. Court history of mother			
a. Juvenile			1
b. Minor	1		3
c. Major/not imprisoned			2
d. Major/imprisoned			
e. Apparently none	49	50	44

broken home, wished to be rid of, and running around). There were none of these 29 without at least one of these checked. When "broken home," which differs somewhat from the other four, was counted by itself, it was found that 3 of the 29 cases had "broken home" only. Of these, 1 was a case with precociously early development, where this fac-

	Frequency
Drunkenness	16
Neglect (mother only)	15
Broken home	13
Wished to be rid of (mother only)	12
Running around	11
No control (mother only)	10
Unhappy marriage	9
"Forced" marriage	6
Mother has had illegitimate children other than patient	6
Patient illegitimate	5

tor came to be central in his life, the second had a brutal stepfather who beat him, and the third was an early adoption case who was a serious behavior problem throughout childhood, although the behavior of his adoptive parents did not seem at all clearly responsible for this. Of the 29 mothers, 5 were checked for Babying/Overhelping; none of these wished to be rid of the boy. In 4 out of 5 of these cases, there was severe physical cruelty by a father or stepfather. The fifth was the physically precocious boy.

Characteristics of Patient and Interaction with Parents. With the CAP Scale the workers frequently felt frustrated by descriptions of parent behavior which did not tell how the child was reacting. Although we did not attempt to reach absolute purity by deleting every reference to the child's behavior in an analysis of the parent behavior, only a fragment of the available descriptions of the child and of the total interaction were covered by the parent abstracts with which the CAP Scale was used. The analysis of the abstracts covering the characteristics of the subject and his interactions with parents came as time was running out on this project, and received only a fraction of the time spent on the analyses of parent behavior. The most interesting result was the prediction of outcome based on these abstracts by a senior research assistant who was blind with respect to adult outcome. This treatment consisted of subjective predictions of adult outcome based on the patient abstracts alone. The results of these predictions, for the three outcome groups, are given in the accompanying tabulation. Here, as elsewhere, the adult bad conduct cases were easier to separate from the neurotic and control cases than the neurotic and

	Actual C	*Actual* N	*Actual* BC	*Total*
Predicted C	41	16	6	63
Predicted N	6	30	1	37
Predicted BC	3	4	43	50

control cases were from each other. The frequencies with which different outcomes were predicted varied somewhat so that there was an overprediction of controls (63 cases) and an underprediction of neurotics (37 cases). Most of the unsuccessfully predicted neurotics were predicted control, not bad conduct. For those who were predicted neurotic, there were more with control outcomes than with bad conduct outcomes.

Along with these global predictions from the patient abstracts, notes were taken of factors operative in the prediction of different outcome groups. The kind of statement which most differentiated the controls from the other two groups was, "He is described as a good boy by mother or father." This was characteristic of almost one third of the control cases and of only one of the bad conduct group.

A type of statement which differentiated the neurotics from the other two groups was "the mother seems 'neurotogenic,' and the patient seems to be giving in" (if the patient seemed to resist successfully, the result was frequently a problem of control, with a different outcome). The term *neurotogenic* was used for such behavior as the mother still dressing or bathing or feeding the boy when he was 10 or 12 years old, unrealistic threats of jail by the mother, or marked overcontrol of the boy's behavior *which he accepted.* Statements of this kind occur much more frequently about the parents of neurotics than in the other two groups. As one worker noted, "it is impossible to tell in most cases how the 'neurotic' interaction got started, but in these cases both mother and patient seemed to be feeding into it." Earlier work on the outcomes of the siblings of child guidance cases (Roff, 1956, 1970) had indicated that although it was possible (though unusual) for a family to turn out a whole set of bad conduct cases, it did not seem possible for a family to produce an entire set of neurotic children. The most discriminating kind of statement for the bad conduct boys was that "his behavior seems to be out of control of parents (or foster parents)." An item in the CAP Scale, Part 2, Mother Says She Has No Control, had frequencies of 18 and 22 for the neurotic and bad conduct groups. In the present context the judgment was made, based on the child's behavior, whether the parents did or did not have control, and the frequencies of the neurotic and bad conduct cases are 5 and 24, respectively. This separates sharply the cases where there was a serious control problem from those where the mother simply complained that the child did not do what she wanted. Another type of statement which separated the bad conduct group sharply from the other two was that the boy was "tough," "proud of misdeeds," and so forth.

Additional intensive work could lead to a more structured scale for dealing with the patient's behavior and interaction with his parents. These interactions would include both generations more comprehensively than was done in the CAP Scale, which was focused primarily on the behavior of parents.

Sibling Interactions and Characteristics. An analysis was made of sibling interactions (Category 7, COCA) to see what predictive significance these might have. The abstracts relating to siblings included not only the interactions but also the characteristics of the siblings. Occasionally, a sibling characteristic might have some predictive value by itself. If a brother, several years older, was in the penitentiary, this might have some predictive value on a probabilistic basis for the patient. This could happen even if the age difference between the two was large enough so that there was little interaction.

The relatively small number of successful blind predictions were largely based on indicative information other than the sibling interaction itself — "patient and his brother stole together," "patient and sibling ran away from their boarding home," and "patient said he wouldn't let his brother in on the stealing because 'he would tell.' " In one case, conflict with the siblings was so great that it suggested serious disturbance in the patient: "Patient, age 10, beats his twin brothers, two years younger, so that the neighbors call the mother because they are afraid he will kill them." Instances of sibling conflict within a "normal" range did not differentiate the three groups well enough to lead to an intensive analysis of this information.

Interaction with the Schools. The number of schools attended, an index of the movement of the boy from place to place, showed that the controls on the average attended a smaller number of schools and the bad conduct cases a larger number of schools with the neurotics in between. There was little difference in the number of grades repeated. The controls were a little higher than the other two groups in the number tutored. This is a consequence of the fact that more of the controls than of the other two groups were referred for learning problems only. In line with the intelligence results presented above, there were slightly more neurotics than others who had been in special classes than the other two groups.

Five school-related items differentiated the bad conduct cases sharply from the other two groups. These have been tabulated here according to the number of times each of them was mentioned at least once

	C	*N*	*BC*
Behavior problem (so described by school)	12	14	30
Dishonesty (stealing, lying)	4	7	23
Truancy	11	15	36
Expelled	1	0	13
Training schools	2	2	19

for each case. The number of times that any of these five was mentioned for a boy was also tabulated. There were 34 controls but only 4 bad conduct cases with none of these in their histories. There were 5 controls as compared with 32 bad conduct cases with two or more of these in their histories.

Discussion

With three groups, two "maladjusted" and one "normal," we may have items which differentiate the normals from the two maladjusted groups or we may have variables on which the normals and one of the maladjusted groups differ from the other maladjusted group. All of these possibilities are of interest.

It has been known since the early days of this program that global predictions by trained clinical psychologists, based on the entire case, could differentiate adequately between groups with good and poor adult outcomes (Roff, 1956). This knowledge was one of the factors which led to continuing work along this line, and to a constantly increasing appreciation of the worth of qualitative descriptions of human behavior made by persons, such as teachers, who were well acquainted with the child being described. On the other hand, global predictions based on the entire case did not tell what specific factors were operating in the predictions and, potentially, were contributing to the development of different kinds of maladjusted behavior. The plan of the present project involved an intensive review of the literature on parent and child behavior and family functioning, and the development of a set of ratings and codes for use in analyzing the case materials so that the specific factors involved could be pinpointed more accurately.

The controls consisted of boys and their families who had been dealt with by a child guidance clinic, so that they were not a random sample of the total population. Random samples of the total population are not studied in clinics and do not have case histories like these. We do have, in connection with a different project, some condensed quasi–case histories of a large sample of normal families of children from grade school populations (Roff, Sells, & Golden, 1972). The better-adjusted children there tend to come from relatively problem-free families with many more assets than liabilities. There were a few families in the control groups of the present study which approximated the "good" families obtained through the general school population, but this was not, of course, true of all the control families.

Our neurotic group consisted of fifty boys who received adult psychiatric diagnoses as neurotic, in general when they were in their early twenties. The families of these boys were similar to the control families in many objective characteristics, such as socioeconomic status, family size and intactness, and history of contact with social welfare agencies; they were also similar on many of the items on the CAP Scale.

The bad conduct cases were, as a group, much more serious and long-lasting offenders than the individuals included in ordinary delinquency studies, many of whom turn out all right as adults. They were differentiable from the other two groups on a wide variety of characteristics, many of which have been reported in the earlier literature. It has frequently been reported that the incidence of broken homes is greater among delinquents than among control groups. However, it is also true that large numbers of boys from broken homes do not become seriously delinquent, so that it is necessary to focus more sharply on the parental characteristics of this group. Parental neglect has been reported frequently in earlier studies. What we have found in many cases is neglect intensified to the "repudiation" found by Robins (1966) in some of her cases, and intensified even beyond that to abandonment of the patient and his siblings by the mother. In most homes broken through separation or divorce, the children ordinarily remain with the mother. In a family situation in which the mother cares so little about the children that she walks off and leaves them, and when the fathers, as commonly happens in such cases, are similarly unconcerned about the welfare of the children, a child or set of children are not only thrown on the support of local welfare agencies, but they have also for years had a mother of the kind who is willing to walk off and leave them, with whatever that implies in the way of earlier maternal care.

The main trends for the different groups, with particular emphasis on the parent-child situation, can be summarized as follows.

Controls. Controls have not been widely studied under this name; they are an approximation to people in general. Studies of parent behavior of normal samples result in scales which do not give sufficient weight to the extreme types of parental behavior of the present cases; some of the parents fall off the end of scales made for normal parental behavior. Our control group families were in some cases characterized by the absence of negative qualities. They tended to remain intact as families, thus differing from the bad conduct, but not from the neurotic, families. They did not show the incidence of nervous fathers which occurred in the families of neurotic cases, but they had a good many nervous mothers. In IQ, the boys were only slightly higher than the neurotic and bad conduct cases. The SES of the families was similar to that of the neurotics, but higher than that of the bad conduct cases. Almost all the control families had two or fewer recorded contacts with social welfare agencies; this was also true of the neurotics. Family size was similar to that of the neurotic cases. The controls, together with the neurotics, differed from the bad conduct group in having had very little contact with law enforcement agencies. Also along with the neurotics, there was a relatively low incidence of serious problems due to the use of alcohol.

As was pointed out, the boys and their families of the control group were not a random sample of the general population, and this study was not so well situated for the intense exploration of the characteristics of normal families as are studies which are set up for that purpose. Control families differed noticeably from the neurotics in the presence of a "competent" mother and on an item described as "parents try to control their anxiety/worry about a patient." This referred to the action of some parents when confronted with anxiety-producing behavior on the part of the patient. Instead of neglecting or avoiding it, or engaging in an unproductive nagging of the boy, they tended to try to present a calm face to the patient and to try to find some way of helping or correcting the behavior involved.

One of the sharpest differences between the control and neurotic parents was on the item "father nervous" (3 to 19). The comparable figures for "mother nervous" were 17 and 27. Apparently, the family situation with a nervous mother but a non-nervous father had a much better prognosis than that where both the father and mother were nervous. Information on parent-child relations from the abstract about the patient tends to supplement this. This is a good illustration of the limited family resemblance concept which holds for many personality characteristics (Roff, 1950).

In all our work with the parents and their characteristics, it was recognized that there was a certain artificiality in looking at the behavior of the parents without at the same time getting as full a view as possible of the boy and his behavior. This artificiality also characterizes the use of parent behavior scales with parents alone. This may be one reason why such scales have not had so much validity as those constructing them had hoped. Owing to the type of analysis made of these cases, where we attempted to abstract the information into different categories, we did not ever get the parental and child behavior fully reintegrated. Work with the abstract about the behavior of the boy himself gave a somewhat different picture of the parent-child interaction. Some parts of this picture are highly consistent with the discussion above. The "good" family occurred more frequently among the controls than among the neurotics. Here the parents seem to approve of the boy in general, no serious discipline problems are present, and the impression is given of relative smoothness in the parent-child relation (15 controls, 5 neurotics). On the other hand, anxiety-inducing behavior on the part of the mother contributes more to discrimination when information about whether or not the patient is anxious is included. Thus, a pattern which is more frequently characteristic of the neurotic mother-child relationship than of the controls was described by a research worker as follows: "patient seems to be giving in (or patient seems to be forcing mother to give in) to his neurotic demands or mother is anxiety-inducing and patient is correspondingly anxious (or mother doesn't discourage patient's anxiety). It is impossible to tell in most cases how the neurotic interaction got started, but in these cases both mother and patient seemed to be feeding into it" (3 control, 15 neurotic).

Much the most effective discrimination between the control and neurotic parent-boy combinations was achieved by global predictions from the abstracts of the patient's characteristics and behavior. These gave an indication both of what the patient was like and of the parent-child relations as seen from the child's point of view. It was the strong impression of the person doing this work that the parent-child relations as seen by the boy were more accurately predictive than the relations reported by the mother. This line of work was initiated relatively late in the project, and it was not exploited so intensively as the CAP Scale, which was used with the parent abstracts. It seems a promising area for further work.

Neurotics. The neurotics and their families have received substantial attention in the discussion of the controls, since they were similar in many characteristics. They were essentially the same in SES and in freedom from social agency contacts. They were somewhat higher than the controls on medically initiated referrals (by family doctor and pediatrician). They had some cases with both low IQ and low SES. When, as here, there is opportunity for diagnosis unrelated to the cost of treatment, the neurotic groups do not appear high in income or SES. There were slightly more individuals with low IQ than there were in the control or bad conduct group. A possible explanation of this is that persons with low IQ were at a disadvantage competitively and thus under more stress in noncombat military life. Among the items of the CAP Scale which characterized the neurotic families were unhappy marriages, but there was little difference from the controls in separation and divorce. The parents might have disagreed more than the control parents about various things, including the discipline of their children, but they stayed together. The boys who were later neurotic had no more contacts with the law than did the control boys. Neither did they exceed the controls on the cluster of school-related items which differentiated the bad conduct cases from the other two groups. In general, the separation of the neurotics from the controls through either objective information or the rating scale items was less adequate than a more subjective and less structured approach which could pick up subtleties in parent-child interactions missed by both objective information and a rating scale approach. It was found that the neurotics could be differentiated adequately from both the other groups by a global prediction based on the abstracted information about the patient and his statements about the parents. This indicated quite clearly that differentiation was possible, and that it is possible to improve substantially on a rating scale approach in separating the childhood characteristics and parent-child interactions of the later neurotics from the later controls.

Bad Conduct Cases. In a preliminary predictive study based on reason for referral to the clinic, it was found possible to identify the bad conduct cases quite accurately in relation to adult outcome in terms of their presenting symptoms and the delinquencies included among these. Further work indicated that many variables, both those relating to the family and those concerning the patient himself, would also distinguish the bad conduct cases from the other two groups. Since there were many of these, they will simply be listed here.

Family and parental variables
    Broken homes
    Mother has had other illegitimate children
    Forced marriage to avoid illegitimacy
    Mother abandons
    History of more than one foster home
    Parental trouble with the law

Low SES
Ten or more Central Registration Bureau entries
Slightly larger families
Parental neglect, repudiation, and abandonment
Parent wishes to be rid of the child
Physical cruelty to child
Inadequate control of boy
Drunkenness
Parental promiscuity
Characteristics of patient
    Frequency of contacts with the law
    Control problems in the school situation (as indicated by expulsion,
       behavior problems, theft, truancy, training school)
    Original referral by court and welfare agencies

To summarize concerning the bad conduct parents and cases in rather broad terms, a frequent family situation was one in which there was a serious lack of normal parental affection and care. This was coupled with the use of overvigorous physical violence in an attempt to assert a control over a misbehaving boy which the parent had not acquired by working at being a parent. The statements made in the public press or in letters to the editor that the problem of delinquency could be brought under control if the parents would simply exercise some discipline miss the fact that by this time the parents have lost control through negligence, abandonment, and other forms of parental delinquency. In this situation, the application of physical force tends to produce resentment and hostility rather than the compliance which is the purported goal of the use of physical force. In many of these cases, by the time the boy had become an early delinquent, the mother realized that she had lost control of him. The loss of control ordinarily came after years of negligence on the part of the parents. It would seem that repressive measures applied late will not substitute for earlier affection and adequate care.

Parent Practices, Intra-family Relations, and Behavior Genetics. Case histories of the kind with which we are working offer a rich source of information about family life and the relation of some family variables to adjustment level at a much later time. These materials are not well adapted to the almost impossibly difficult task of unraveling the relative contributions of genetics and of life experiences to behavioral outcome. I thus retain the agnostic position on this problem which was expressed earlier (Roff, 1950). The parent practices literature has tended to assume implicitly an "environmental" position that the behavior of the child is a direct result of the way he has been treated. On the other hand, the behavior genetics literature is much more explicit about its claims, and sometimes goes beyond its data in the conclusions reached. Family resemblance is not synonymous with heritability. When we consider the interaction of a mother with a child who is later diagnosed as neurotic, it is not possible from this information alone to say either that her treatment of the child was solely responsible or to say that his condition was genetically determined and that he would have turned out much the same no matter how he had been treated. In this situation it is impossible to tell to what extent the parent's behavior is primarily a cause or primarily a reflection of the characteristics of the child. Any genetic contributions will undoubtedly be found eventually to vary markedly from one type of maladjustment to another.

An observation from Mosher and Feinsilver's (1971) review of work on schizophrenia, about the genetics of schizophrenia, gives a picture of the current status of information and theory concerning a type of maladjustment other than those with which we have been concerned. They point out that recent twin studies have found a much lower degree of concordance between identical twins than had been found earlier, and observe, "Thus, the genetic contribution to schizophrenia, which based on the early twin studies was felt to be of over-riding importance, has gradually been whittled down in size. It is ironic that, as concordance rates have fallen, confidence in the existence of a predisposing genetic factor in schizophrenia has paradoxically increased."

Life history work does not depend for its importance on a final solution to the problem of genetic influences. It is possible that we are too impatient in looking for clear and clean-cut solutions to problems such as this. In other parts of science, there are some problems where there is an open conflict between two mutually exclusive theories, each of which is supported by some generally accepted facts. Light is an example of this. In some situations light behaves as if it were a wave (or in accordance with a wave model), in others as if it consisted of particles (or in accordance with a particle model). This open conflict between the two theories of light has been unresolved for a long time. We have more comprehensive studies of genetic influences in relation to measured IQ than it has been possible to get in the area of psychopathology, partly because everyone has an IQ whereas the frequency of, for example, schizophrenia in a population is very small. In adoption studies of intelligence, there are some indications which suggest a strong genetic influence, but there is other information which suggests that over a normal range, heredity is relatively unimportant. This is, I believe, no more contradictory than wave and particle interpretations of light.

Whatever the relative genetic contribution, there is need for careful life history studies. The present project has attempted to contribute information about the life histories of three groups of individuals, adult neurotics, bad conduct cases, and controls, in the belief that information yielded by work of this kind is an indispensable part of the total developmental picture. It is encouraging to realize that the number of persons who share this belief is growing.

COMMENTARY

ZUBIN. What are the conclusions from the table showing the predictions of adult outcome based on the boy's characteristics?

ROFF. Those indicate the number of correct blind predictions made by one trained psychologist in sorting the controls, the neurotics, and the bad conducts. They are based on the material abstracted from the case history about the person himself, with incidental information about the parents and his interaction with them.

BIRCH. Was this done before your analysis? In other words, did this psychologist have the advantage of knowing the nature of the information that you had obtained?

ROFF. Yes, the psychologist knew about the project. In fact, she had been working with me for several years, but was blind as to the specific outcomes of the cases.

BIRCH. I don't mean about the specific cases. Did the one who predicted it know the nature of the relations and factors that you have obtained from the project as a whole?

ROFF. Yes, in general, and, as mentioned, she had several years' experience.

BIRCH. OK. This then is the utilization of your clusterings that you had obtained through the case records.

ROFF. This person had also been in charge of our literature review, but had never seen these specific cases or their outcomes.

QUESTION. That's more the prediction made by the clinic, isn't it, including psychiatric diagnosis?

ROFF. It includes that. However, the clinic made different predictions at different times, and you had to weight those and balance them. In other words, the same child did not always get the same diagnosis in successive years, and he might be seen for a number of years. The predictive significance of psychiatric diagnoses during childhood in relation to adult adjustment has been discussed in an earlier paper (Roff, 1970a). This table is simply a predictive thing. I don't want to make too much out of it. We were interested primarily in the family, the whole family picture.

REFERENCES

Diagnostic and statistical manual of mental disorders. (2nd ed.) Washington, D.C.: American Psychiatric Association, 1968.

Eiduson, B., Brooks, S., Motto, R., Platz, A., & Carmichael, R. Recent developments in the psychiatric case history event system. *Behavior Science*, 1967, 12, 254–267.

Kagan, J., & Moss, H. A. *Birth to maturity.* New York: Wiley, 1963.

Mosher, L. R., & Feinsilver, D. *Special report: Schizophrenia.* NIMH, Center for Studies of Schizophrenia, Publication No. HSM-72-9042. 1971.

Rhoades, M. C. Case study of delinquent boys in the juvenile court of Chicago. *American Journal of Sociology*, 1907–1908, 13, 56–78.

Robins, L. N. *Deviant children grown up.* Baltimore: Williams & Wilkins, 1966.

Roff, M. Intra-family resemblances in personality characteristics. *Journal of Psychology*, 1950, 30, 199–227.

————. Preservice personality problems and subsequent adjustment to military service: Gross outcome in relation in military service. Rep. No. 55–138. Randolph AFB, Texas: School of Aviation Medicine, USAF, 1956.

————. Childhood social interactions and young adult psychosis. *Journal of Clinical Psychology*, 1963, 19, 152–157.

————. Some developmental aspects of schizoid personality. Rep. No. 65–4. U.S. Army Medical Research and Development Command, Contract No. DA-49-007-MD-2015. March 1965.

————. Childhood antecedents in the mental health development of three groups of adult males: Neurotics, severe bad conduct cases and controls. Final Project Rep. NIMH, Center for Epidemiologic Studies, Contract No. HSM-42-69-50. September 1971.

————. Some life history factors in relation to various types of adult maladjustment. In M. Roff & D. F. Ricks (Eds.), *Life history research in psychopathology.* Vol. 1. Minneapolis: University of Minnesota Press, 1970. Pp. 265–287. (a)

————. Some problems in life history research. In M. Roff & D. F. Ricks (Eds.), *Life history research in psychopathology.* Vol. 1. Minneapolis: University of Minnesota Press, 1970. Pp. 10–30. (b)

————. A two-factor approach to juvenile delinquency and the later histories of juvenile delinquents. In M. Roff, L. N. Robins, & M. Pollack (Eds.), *Life history research in psychopathology.* Vol. 2. Minneapolis: University of Minnesota Press, 1972. Pp. 77–101.

————, Mink, W. D., & Hinrichs, G. B. *Developmental abnormal psychology.* New York: Holt, 1966.

Roff, M., Sells, S. B., & Golden, M. M. *Social adjustment and personality development in children.* Minneapolis: University of Minnesota Press, 1972.

MARC A. SCHUCKIT
JAMES A. HALIKAS
JUDITH J. SCHUCKIT
JAMES MC CLURE
JOHN RIMMER *Drug Use and Psychiatric Problems on the Campus: I. Methods and Drug Use at Outset*

THE RATE OF nonmedical drug use among students at American universities may exceed 50 per cent (Berg, 1970). Mailed or classroom-administered questionnaires have shown the average student drug user to be from a large Eastern city, to be Jewish or agnostic in religion, and to have well-educated parents of high socioeconomic status (Eelis, 1968; Hinckley, 1968; Imperi, Kleber, & Davie, 1968; King, 1969; Mizner, Bater, & Werme, 1970; Pearlman, 1967; Rand, Hammond, & Moscau, 1968; Robbins et al., 1970; Subcommittee on Alcoholism and Narcotics, 1971).

Most investigations of psychiatric and emotional problems in college students have drawn subjects from those reporting to the campus health service; few have surveyed emotional problems of the general campus population (Blum et al., 1969; Boyce & Thurlow, 1969; Davie, 1958; Kidd, 1965; Scheff, 1966). Students who seek psychiatric advice demographically resemble those using drugs — they too tend to be agnostic or Jewish, to come from large Eastern cities, and to have well-educated parents of high socioeconomic status (Scheff, 1966).

Few studies have dealt with the interactions between drug use and psychiatric problems among students (Berg, 1970; Blum et al., 1969; Goldstein, 1966; Kidd, 1965; Kleckner, 1968; McGlothlin & Cohen,

NOTE: This study was supported in part by U.S. PHS-NIMH grants nos. MH-09247, MH-7081, MH-5804, MH-K$_3$-18292, and MH-12504-01.

1965; Murphy, Leventhal, & Balter, 1969; Simmons & Winograd, 1966). Our four-year study, employing a prospective model in a college population, is designed to outline factors associated with the development of psychiatric illness and drug use, to evaluate the interaction of the two problems, and to ascertain their possible impact on college experience.

Method

Two campuses in the United States were chosen as study sites: a medium-sized private university in suburban St. Louis, Washington University, and the campus of the University of California in San Diego. Within each university, 100 men and 100 women incoming freshmen, all United States citizens, were randomly chosen and interviewed. The same basic procedure was followed at both campuses.

The initial freshman interview was divided into seven parts, each systematically covering the area in question:

a. *Identifying data.*

b. *School history*, including schools attended, history of failures or truancy, study skills, social adjustment, and relationships with parent-figures.

c. *Family history*, detailing physical and psychiatric illness in each first-degree relative and those second-degree relatives known to the student.

d. *Personal experiences and attitudes*, including job experiences, religious, social and political opinions and activities.

e. *Psychiatric symptom review.*

f. *Drug use history*, outlining for *each drug* the frequency of use, methods of administration, mode of acquisition, physical and psychological reactions, and factors affecting use of and reaction to the drug. For those drugs no longer or never used, reasons for abstinence were obtained.

g. *Alcohol and tobacco use history.*

The follow-up interview will be given to all students still at their original college in each of the three subsequent undergraduate years and to dropouts or transfer students residing within a fifty-mile radius of the original university. To gather follow-up data on the dropout and transfer groups (Harrison, 1958), while staying within the fiscal limitations of the study, a shortened self-administered questionnaire will be mailed to subjects who have moved beyond the fifty-mile radius. Similar in scope and wording to the initial interview, the follow-up will elicit an interval history in each of the outlined areas. The initial interview took one to two hours; the follow-up interview will take one-half to one hour.

An interview promotes the development of rapport between student and investigator, and may increase students' veracity as well as facilitate clarification of ancillary information and assure students' understanding of the questions. In addition, the subject's general appearance, affect, and patterns of interaction can be observed.

Yearly re-evaluation of the students will allow determination of incidence and prevalence rates of drug use and psychiatric illness (Reifler & Liptzin, 1969), facilitate accurate observation of the onset and development of psychiatric symptoms, and set the stage for the measurement of the interactions of mental illness, drug use, and academic performance — relationships not yet clearly established (Lucas & Stringer, 1972; Reinhart et al., 1972). Changes in personal mental status and drug use patterns will be noted promptly, and errors of omission regarding important life events will be minimized (Douglas & Blomfield, 1956).

The initial interview was based upon the Washington University questionnaire, which used symptoms, not intrapsychic events, to outline the lifetime prevalence of specific psychiatric illness (Feighner et al., 1971; Guze et al., 1963; Robins & Braroe, 1964; Robins et al., 1971; Rimmer & Chambers, 1969). The assignment of a diagnosis required fulfillment of pre-established criteria as outlined by Feighner et al. (1971), thus minimizing the need for clinical judgment as a final arbiter (Dohrenwend, Ergi, & Mendelsohn, 1971; Feinstein, 1968). The pre-set definition of each psychiatric diagnosis will enable each reader, regardless of theoretic orientation, to understand what is meant by a specific nosologic entity (Babigian et al., 1965; Zubin, 1969).

The advantages of the structured interview have been discussed by Saghir (1971) and Robins (1966). This format fosters consistency of administration, thereby minimizing variability in the interviewer's emphasis on different questions. Within this framework, interviewers were trained to extract and record all relevant contributory data.

Since information regarding relatives depends solely upon student knowledge and report and a diagnosis is made only when strict symptom criteria are met, the reported figures probably underestimate illness rates (Feinstein, 1968), but should be a fair indication of the *range* of morbidity (Douglas & Blomfield, 1956). The most accuracy probably will be for presence versus absence of illness (Guze et al., 1963), with the general category of illness more accurately determined than the specific diagnosis (Enterline, 1959; Whitney, Cadoret, & McClure, 1971).

Robins (1966), comparing diagnoses made from structured interview material with final categorizations made from a collation of all recorded data, found that 85 per cent of the diagnoses could have been made by interviews alone. She also found that the more distant in time and kinship, the less valid the information on a given relative. The accuracy of data correlated directly with the degree of privacy at interview. Similar results were obtained by Guze et al. (1963), in their work with an alcoholic population.

Underreporting of personal psychiatric illness can also be expected, but owing to the interview format (Robins & Braroe, 1964) the bias is anticipated to be no greater than that for any psychiatric interview. The population self-report of symptoms will be checked against student health service files for recorded illness.

The 400 students in the two-campus sample can be expected to show significant amounts of drug use and emotional illness. Although a larger sample would have been preferable, drug use may be seen in at least 200 students (Berg, 1970) and psychiatric problems in about 75 (Reifler & Liptzin, 1969).

The present interview was administered in St. Louis by two of the authors (M. A. S. and J. J. S.) and by five specially trained lay interviewers. Robins and Braroe (1964) compared the information gained through structured interview by trained lay interviewers and by psychiatrists, and found no differences in duration of interview or in the ability of a psychiatrist to make a final diagnosis from the recorded information.

This paper deals primarily with the demography of the St. Louis sample and drug history at the outset of the study.

First Year of the St. Louis Study

The St. Louis sample consisted of 161 students; the result of a random selection of 200 from whom transfer students were then excluded. Of the 161, 158 completed interviews. Initially, 13 students refused to participate in the study; however, when recontacted by one of the investigators, 12 acquiesced. Comparison of these 12 with the other cooperating students revealed no significant differences in interview content. Two additional students had moved out of the city and could not be located.

The sample of 158 consisted of 84 men and 74 women, almost all of whom were Caucasian (152) and liberal arts majors (117). The most frequently reported religious preferences were Jewish (58), "No Religion" (43), Protestant (28), and Catholic (24). The number reporting religion of upbringing was found to be slightly higher for each religion and 20 per cent lower for the category "No Religion." Students' parents were highly educated: 123 fathers and 104 mothers had at least some college experience.

The sample was weighted for scholastic achievers: more than 90 per cent had a high school average of B or better, 88 per cent won academic or athletic honors in high school, and less than 3 per cent had ever dropped out of school. Some 65 per cent had attended only public schools, and 11 per cent had attended only private or parochial schools.

Truancy in grade school was reported by 2 per cent and in high school by 16 per cent; 6 students (4 per cent) reported receiving school suspensions. Ten subjects (6 per cent) experienced major problems in learning to read or had a history of persistent mirror writing. Almost 20 per cent (29) had been more active, restless, and difficult to control in grade school than their classmates. One person repeated a lower grade, and five reported failing a high school course.

Social adjustment was also estimated: 90 per cent of the people felt that, in general, they were quite happy as children; but in adolescence, 35 per cent reported themselves to have been loners, 8 per cent usually angry, 37 per cent anxious, and 13 per cent rebellious; 80 per cent reported having had many friends in grade and high school.

Upon entering college, most students felt that their study skills would carry them in good stead during their college career. Good or superior skills were indicated by almost three quarters of the group.

GENERAL DRUG INFORMATION

Alcohol and Tobacco. Regular tobacco smoking at any time was reported by 35 per cent of the students; of these almost one quarter were no longer current users and another quarter smoked fewer than 10 cigarettes a day. Virtually no alcohol use was reported by 27 per cent of the total population, whereas 20 per cent listed three or more beers or highballs as the amount imbibed on the average occasion. Five students did report having had problems from drinking — either with family, police, or school.

Illicit Drug Use. Drug use was reported by 53 per cent (84) of the

	No. Using	%		No. Using	%
Marijuana	84	53	Psilocybin	4	3
Mescaline	21	14	Amphetamines	4	3
Hashish	18	12	Opiates	3	2
LSD	14	9	Speed	2	1.5
Medicinal drugs	6	4	STP	2	1.5
MDA	4	3			

students. Most of these had used only marijuana or hashish and, as shown in the accompanying tabulation, employment of other drugs was relatively infrequent and did not occur in the absence of experience with marijuana. Of the 84 users, 61 per cent reported that their mood state influenced drug intake, either in the selection of a specific drug for use (14 per cent) or in the perception of the drug's effects (47 per cent). Both alcohol and drugs had been used by 81 students: 36 indicated that they preferred drugs to alcohol, and 7 preferred alcohol. The remainder were equally divided between those reporting no preference and those who felt their preference changed with the circumstances.

Marijuana. As outlined in Table 1, 38 per cent of the marijuana users reported having used the drug 40 times or more. Most began smoking it after age 17, and 71 per cent used it in the month before interview. Of these, 83 per cent first tried marijuana out of curiosity, and most were introduced to it by a peer (80 per cent) or sibling (7 per cent). All but 17 per cent planned continued use, most often for the pleasant feelings associated with the drug (55 per cent). Marijuana was almost always obtained from friends — usually without charge (60 per cent) — but occasionally through purchase (17 per cent).

All 84 users reported that the usual marijuana effects were pleasant; 75 per cent experienced feelings of euphoria, relaxation, silly behavior, increased empathy, or enhanced mental power. Unpleasant reactions, including nausea, depression, "paranoia," and visual "hallucinations," were reported as occasional occurrences by 22 per cent of the users. Less than 6 per cent noted occasional feelings of dependence, craving, or "Withdrawal symptoms," and 3 per cent reported experiencing flashbacks. Only one third of the 37 per cent of the users who attributed medical or psychological hazards to marijuana had modified their use for these reasons.

Few differences were revealed in a comparison of students using marijuana on fewer than 40 occasions during the previous year (light users) with those who used it 40 or more times (heavy users). More of the heavy users had introduced marijuana to friends (53 versus 6 per cent) and more of this group projected continued use themselves (85 versus 60 per cent). The drug effects were felt within 15 minutes by more heavy users (73 versus 44 per cent), and they were more aware of ever having had an outstandingly pleasant experience (74 versus 40 per cent). More heavy users felt marijuana had been helpful in relieving physical or mental distress (47 versus 20 per cent). Reports of unpleasant episodes associated with drug use, awareness of medical or psychological hazards, mode of introduction to the drug, presence or absence of friends while taking the drug, length of drug action, and reasons for drug taking were similar for the two groups.

Mescaline and LSD. Of the sample, 21 students reported taking mescaline and 14 LSD, with all but 3 of the LSD users having also taken mescaline. Current involvement was reported by 6 of the mescaline and

Table 1. Patterns of Use of Marijuana ($N = 84$)

Patterns of Use	Percentage
Number of times used	
1–3	18
4–10	16
11–20	12
21–40	15
41–70	5
70	22
Too numerous to count	12
Age first used	
16–17	42
18–19	58
Usual time until effects felt	
Never felt effects	12
15 min or less	55
15–30 min	19
30 min or more	9
Unable to estimate	5
Usual length of high	
Never felt effects	11
Less than 1 hour	8
1–3 hr	51
4–6 hr	18
Unable to estimate	12
Drug usually taken with	
Alone	0
1 or 2 friends	43
3–5 friends	46
More than 5 friends	4
Unable to say	7

Table 2. Patterns of Use of Mescaline and LSD

Patterns of Use	No. Using Mescaline[a]	No. Using LSD[b]
Number of times used		
1–3	12	5
4–10	6	5
11 or more	3	4
Age first used		
15 or under	1	0
16–17	8	10
18 or more	12	4
Times most used per month		
Less than 1	1	1
1–4	20	12
5 or more	0	1
Major drug effect[c]		
Euphoria	8	2
Enhanced mental powers	6	7
Visual hallucinations	10	9

[a]$N = 21$.   [b]$N = 14$.
[c]More than one drug effect was reported by some.

5 of the LSD users. Self-reports of ingestions per month and lifetime rates (Table 2) indicated no regular mescaline or LSD users.

As with most of the drugs, the manner of procurement was most often from friends without cost. The drugs were taken in the presence of one or more friends by 86 per cent of the mescaline and LSD users. First ingestion was motivated by curiosity for 14 mescaline and 9 LSD users; the remainder began to "go along with friends," to "enhance the mind," or just "as a lark."

Half of the hallucinogen users had no plans for continued use of mescaline or LSD. Although no strong pattern emerged, the largest group stopped because they didn't enjoy the effects. Those who planned future use did so because they either liked the effects or felt the drug enhanced their mental powers. Each of these students anticipated fewer than five future ingestions per month.

The overall mescaline and LSD experience was rated as "pleasant" by 86 per cent, and 93 per cent, respectively. Not all the mescaline effects were pleasant, however; negative experiences included depression, nausea or dizziness, silliness, and a feeling of decreased empathy. Loss of self-control from mescaline, where regretted acts were carried out while high, were reported by 3 students. For LSD, unpleasant effects were also noted: anxiety or depression was experienced by 9, decreased empathy by 1, and flashbacks by 5; 4 reported carrying out either physically or verbally aggressive acts.

No user reported having felt physically or psychologically dependent on the drugs. Drug dangers were recognized by 38 per cent of the mescaline and 86 per cent of the LSD users, of whom 50 per cent and 75 per cent, respectively, modified their use of these drugs as a result of the recognition of dangers. Most frequently mentioned were fears of gene damage, future habituation, and precipitation of psychosis.

Other Drugs. Frequency of consumption of other drugs is listed on page 168. The number of students in each category is too small for detailed analysis, but some general comments can be made. All drug use began at age 16 or older, most often after the age of 17. No student had taken any of these drugs in excess of 4 times per month or any more than 10 times in their lives. Most first took the drugs out of curiosity, and continued because they enjoyed the effects. Users of peyote, speed (intravenous amphetamine), STP, and other amphetamines all felt they would not take these drugs again; about half the users of hashish, MDA, and psilocybin planned future use. Feelings of physical or psychological dependence were denied by all except one amphetamine user.

Discussion

The data presented here must be viewed with some reservations. Analysis of illicit drug samples has shown that users often do not receive the drug they believe they have purchased (Marshman & Gibbins, 1970; Srole, 1962). Also, except for marijuana and hashish, the number of drug users in each group was small and of limited value in a statistical analysis. The most useful information dealt with general attitudes and drug experiences.

Slightly more than half the population had some experience with illicit drugs; a rate exceeding that for regular use of tobacco. The drug taken most often was marijuana, rarely on a daily basis. The first drug experience was often the result of curiosity, continued use arose from enjoyment of drug effects. Most students avoided certain drugs because of their perceived medical or psychological consequences. Only a minority gave legal dangers as a reason for abstention, an indication that programs designed to decrease student drug use should concentrate on real medical dangers and avoid legalistic or moral arguments.

Unpleasant drug effects were not uncommon. Flashbacks were reported by one third of the LSD users, but were rarely mentioned in connection with any other hallucinogen. The most common unpleasant reactions were feelings of depression or anxiety. Few students, including five marijuana users and one amphetamine user, reported experiencing physical withdrawal symptoms — occurrences that may be in doubt (Goodman & Gilman, 1966).

Although the percentage of students engaged in illicit drug use is large, the depth of individual involvement appears to be minimal. This indicates, perhaps, that most students are able to show moderation after satiation of their curiosity. It may well be that the greatest peril of drug use is for a subpopulation of students with emotional problems. The case reports of "drug-related" suicide, psychosis, anxiety-laden panic reactions, and severe paranoia, although possible for all users, may be especially dangerous for those who are psychologically ill (Blacker et al., 1968; Keeler, 1967; Pillard, 1970; Smart & Batemon, 1967; Weil, 1970).

This important relationship should be documented. The resulting data could then be used by administrators and mental health workers to caution high-risk students to avoid drug contact. It is hoped that the present investigation, through its phenomenologic definition of illness similar to that used in a psychiatric interview, its emphasis on objective data, and its yearly re-evaluation of the population, will be able to demonstrate the presence or absence of a clear relationship between drug use, psychiatric illness, and academic performance.

COMMENTARY

ROLF. I assume you were at Washington University because the questions you're asking indicate that this particular sample of students is unique— hard driving, fairly straight. In fact, it's a loaded population.

SCHUCKIT. Not really. Most studies of either high users of psychiatric health services (which doesn't necessarily mean they are the most ill) or high users of drugs show them to be exactly *my* population. They were Jewish or agnostic, they were from urban areas, they were liberal arts majors, they had highly educated high socioeconomic parents — so they should have been high risk, and they were, for my use.

MACK. How would they compare with the population at a state school? Are they Harvard or Kent State?

SCHUCKIT. I don't know how to answer that. Probably more like Harvard. But the point is that it's a special population. That is one of the reasons we wanted a state school for comparison.

RICKS. David, how would you compare it with Columbia freshmen? I have a special advantage here in having a son who is a dormitory counselor, a senior with Columbia freshmen to look after.

D. J. RICKS. Before Christmas vacation the Columbia freshmen are like Schuckit's Ss. They mostly talk about drug experiences they had in high school, and they haven't had time yet in college to learn where to pick up drugs. A lot of guys are away from home for the first time. I think if the interviews were done three months later, the results would be quite different.

SCHUCKIT. You might be interested in what our first-year follow-up showed. Out of 157 that we initially interviewed last year, 153 were just reinterviewed. I got the data last night from St. Louis. The population showed an increase in drug use, but interestingly enough showed a decrease in the heavy users, although the average number of people who had tried marijuana was higher.

D. J. RICKS. A lot of guys think they are getting mescaline when they are getting other things. I would put all the mescaline users in with the LSD users.

SCHUCKIT. We are basing this study on self-reports. Street analyses show that marijuana is usually marijuana, LSD is often LSD, and mescaline is usually LSD.

D. KLEIN. Here is a suggestion. We were doing a study on psychiatric patients in relationship to drug abuse (Cohen & Klein, 1973). In analyzing the data, when we contrasted all patients who were drug users with the patients who weren't drug users, we didn't get too much. When we stratified the drug users into three levels — occasional users, fairly heavy users, and heads — and split the patients between heads and everybody else, we got substantial differences. Apparently, all of the relationships with drug abuse that we got both cross-sectionally and prognostically relate to extremely heavy users.

For instance, we did a six-month follow-up on these patients after they were out of the hospital. In the first two groups, using drugs seemed not to matter. But the severe drug users had dismal prognoses.

Also, I wonder whether you are using any measure of deviant associations. Apparently that was the question that got you interested — whether deviant associations were predictive of drug abuse and later psychiatric illness, or whether psychiatric illness and drug abuse led to deviant associations. We have a small bit of data there. Allan Willner, who works at Hillside Hospital, developed a test for rare deviant associations and gave it across the board to patients at Hillside. When the patients were divided into three groups, there were very significant differentiations (Willner, 1972a & b). The non-schizophrenic sample had little in the way of rare deviant associations, but patients with toxic psychosis that we attributed to LSD or dextro-amphetamine had the most, by far the greatest. It might be interesting to use some such measure.

SCHUCKIT. On our drug analyses, we did compare those who never used any drugs with those who had used any in various quantities; for example, of the marijuana users, those who used it fewer than 10 times, 11 to 40, more than 40; and then we made a tripartite comparison of none to marijuana or hashish only to others. Basically, when we used the less heavy marijuana users (there was a strong correlation between degree of marijuana use and use of other drugs), we got the same type of correlations for no use to any use, but the correlations were stronger.

ZUBIN. Clearly, the number of psychopathological people is nowhere near the number of drug users.

SCHUCKIT. Definitely.

ZUBIN. So the question arises, If psychopathology doesn't explain it, what does? I suppose you have some ideas about that. Is it like the case of heroin, with a kind of epidemic spreading, as happened in England? There, one person fed the heroin to two or three others, and the epidemic spread through actual contacts. Or is this something else?

SCHUCKIT. I think it's more like bathtub gin, a social phenomenon. The subjects indicated as much by saying they never smoke alone. Of course, that is my guess.

ZUBIN. I have suspected that for a long time. Most of us have, and the head of our Family Research Section in the Biometrics Research Unit, Denise Kandel, is finding that peers are more important than parents in drug abuse. I have wondered why the entire pressure of the government is to study the biochemistry rather than the sociology and the epidemiology of drug use.

ROLF. Wouldn't one useful method be a test of personality? Why not the MMPI? It is virtually free. *S*s can complete it on their own. Or, also in terms of reliability statements, why not use a nonpersonal interview? You may get more accurate information on drug use in a completely anonymous situation where *S*s are filling out a questionnaire, just as you may get more reliable information from female *S*s if you don't ask them face to face if they had had sexual intercourse.

SCHUCKIT. We feel that the structured interview gives accurate diagnosis and that the time necessary to administer the MMPI is prohibitive. I don't think there's any solid evidence that you get more valid information from an anonymous questionnaire and such an instrument would destroy follow-up.

ROLF. Do you use male and female interviewers for the appropriate sex?

SCHUCKIT. Yes and no. We used both for both and compared to see if there were any differences on any of the major incidence indices, and there weren't. So we used both male and female interviewers for both males and females.

ROLF. On certain items, a match in sex may be helpful. And if a personal interview is too expensive in time, why not give the same structured interview in questionnaire form to the same sample, for replication?

SCHUCKIT. We're trying to devise a form which would do that. I have feelings that we're getting more valid data with the personally administered interview, but I would like to check that. The hardest part of devising a form that we can hand out to people is the family history.

REFERENCES

Babigian, H. M., Gardner, E. A., Miles, H. C., & Romano, J. Diagnostic consistency and change in a follow-up study of 215 patients. *American Journal of Psychiatry*, 1965, 121, 895–901.

Berg, D. F. The non-medical use of dangerous drugs in the United States: A comprehensive view. *International Journal of Addition*, December 1970, 5.

Blacker, K. H., Jones, R. T., Stone, G. C., & Pfefferbaum, D. Chronic users of LSD: The acidheads. *American Journal of Psychiatry*, 1968, 125, 341–351.

Blum, R. H., et al. *Drugs II: Students and drugs.* San Francisco: Jossey-Bass, 1969.

Boyce, R. M., & Thurlow, H. J. Characteristics of university students with emotional problems. *Canadian Psychiatric Association Journal*, 1969, 14, 481–491.

Cohen, M., & Klein, D. F. Post-hospital adjustment of psychiatrically hospitalized drug users. Paper presented at the meeting of the American Psychiatric Association, Honolulu, 1973.

Davie, J. S. Who uses a college mental hygiene clinic? In B. M. Wedge (Ed.), *Psychosocial problems of college men.* New Haven: Yale University Press, 1958. Pp. 15–140.

Dohrenwend, B. P., Ergi, G., & Mendelsohn, F. S. Psychiatric disorder in general populations: A study of the problem of clinical judgment. *American Journal of Psychiatry*, 1971, 127, 1304–1312.

Douglas, J. W. B., & Blomfield, J. M. The reliability of longitudinal surveys. *Milbank Memorial Fund Quarterly*, 1956, 34, 227–252.

Eelis, J. Marijuana and LSD: A survey of one college campus. *Journal of Counseling Psychology*, 1968, 15, 459–467.

Enterline, P. E. A validation of information provided by household respondents in health surveys. *American Journal of Public Health*, 1959, 49, 205–212.

Feighner, J. P., Guze, S. B., Woodruff, R. A., Winokur, G., & Munoz, R. Diagnostic criteria for use in psychiatric research. *Archives of General Psychiatry*, 1971, 26, 57–63.

Feinstein, A. R. Clinical epidemiology: II. The identification rates of disease. *Annals of Internal Medicine*, 1968, 69, 1037–1061.

Goldstein, R. *1 in 7: Drugs on campus.* New York: Walker, 1966.

Goodman, L. S., & Gilman, A. *The pharmacological basis of therapeutics.* New York: Macmillan, 1966. P. 298.

Guze, S. B., Tuason, V. B., Stewart, M. A., & Picken, B. The drinking history: A comparison of reports by subjects and their relatives. *Quarterly Journal of Studies on Alcohol*, 1963, 24, 249–260.

Harrison, R. W. Leaving college because of emotional problems. In B. M. Wedge (Ed.), *Psychosocial problems of college men.* New Haven: Yale University Press, 1958, Pp. 95–112.

Hinckley, R. G. Non-medical drug use and the college student. *Journal of the American College Health Association*, 1968, 17, 35–42.

Imperi, L. L., Kleber, M. D., & Davie, J. S. Use of hallucinogenic drugs on campus. *Journal of the American Medical Association*, 1968, 204, 1021–1024.

Keeler, M. H. Adverse reactions to marijuana. *American Journal of Psychiatry*, 1967, 124, 674–677.

Kidd, C. B. Psychiatric morbidity among students. *British Journal of Preventive and Social Medicine*, 1965, 19, 143–150.

King, F. W. Marijuana and LSD usage among male college students. *Psychiatry*, 1969, 32, 265–276.

Kleckner, J. H. Personality differences between psychedelic drug users and non-users. *Psychology*, 1968, 5, 66–71.

Lucas, C. J., & Stringer, P. Interaction in university selection, mental health, and academic performance. *British Journal of Psychiatry*, 1972, 120, 189–195.

McGlothlin, W. H., & Cohen, S. The use of hallucinogenic drugs among college students. *American Journal of Psychiatry*, 1965, 122, 572–574.

Marshman, J. A., & Gibbins, R. J. A note on the composition of illicit drugs. *Ontario Medical Review*, 1970, 37, 1–3.

Mizner, G. L., Bater, J. T., & Werme, P. H. Patterns of drug use among college students: A preliminary report. *American Journal of Psychiatry*, 1970, 127, 55–64.

Murphy, B. W., Leventhal, A. M., & Balter, M. B. Drug use on the campus: A survey of university health services and counseling centers. *Journal of the American College Health Association*, 1969, 17, 389–402.

Pearlman, S. Drug use and experience in an urban college population. *American Journal of Orthopsychiatry*, 1967, 38, 503–514.

Pillard, R. C. Marijuana. *New England Journal of Medicine*, 1970, 283, 294–303.

Rand, M. E., Hammond, J. D., & Moscau, P. A survey of drug use at Ithaca College. *Journal of the American College Health Association*, 1968, 17, 43–51.

Reifler, C. B., & Liptzin, M. B. Epidemiological studies of college mental health. *Archives of General Psychiatry*, 1969, 20, 528–540.

Reinhart, M. J., Lohr, N. E., Schaefer, D. L., Berlinger, N. T., & Huddlestone, J. R. Evaluation of academic performance in a neuropsychiatric hospitalized population. *Archives of General Psychiatry*, 1972, 26, 68–70.

Rimmer, J., & Chambers, D. S. Alcoholism: Methodological considerations in the study of family illness. *American Journal of Orthopsychiatry*, 1969, 39, 760–768.

Robbins, E. S., Robbins, L., Frosch, W. A., Stern, M. College student drug use. *American Journal of Psychiatry*, 1970, 126, 1743–1751.

Robins, L. N. *Deviant children grown up*. Baltimore: Williams & Wilkins, 1966.

———— & Braroe, N. W. The lay interviewer in psychiatric research. *Journal of Nervous and Mental Disease*, 1964, 138, 70–78.

Robins, L. N., Murphy, G. E., Woodruff, R. A., & King, L. J. Adult psychiatric status of black schoolboys. *Archives of General Psychiatry*, 1971, 24, 338–345.

Saghir, M. T. A comparison of some aspects of structured and unstructured psychiatric interviews. *American Journal of Psychiatry*, 1971, 128, 180–184.

Scheff, T. J. Users and non-users of a student psychiatric clinic. *Journal of Health and Human Behavior*, 1966, 7, 114–121.

Simmons, J. L., & Winograd, B. *It's happening*. Santa Barbara, Calif: Marc-Laird, 1966.

Smart, R. G., & Batemon, K. Unfavorable reactions to LSD. *Canadian Medical Association Journal*, 1967, 97, 1214–1221.

Srole, L. *Mental health in the metropolis*. New York: McGraw-Hill, 1962.

Subcommittee on Alcoholism and Narcotics of the Committee on Labor and Public Welfare, U.S. Senate. *Marijuana and health*. Washington, D.C.: GPO, 1971.

Weil, A. T. Adverse reactions to marijuana. *New England Journal of Medicine*, 1970, 282, 998–1000.

Whitney, W. W., Cadoret, R. J., & McClure, J. N. Depressive symptoms and academic performance in college students. *American Journal of Psychiatry*, 1971, 128, 766–770.

Willner, A. E. Associative disturbance and toxic psychosis. *Proceedings of the 80th annual convention*. Washington, D.C.: American Psychiatric Association, 1972.

————. Different types of impaired abstraction among schizophrenic and non-schizophrenic hospitalized patients. *Proceedings of the 80th annual convention*. Washington, D.C.: American Psychiatric Association, 1972.

Zubin, J. Cross national study of diagnosis of the mental disorders: Methodology and planning. *American Journal of Psychiatry*, 1969, 125, 12–20, Supp. 1.

MAURICE LORR
RICHARD P. YOUNISS

The Interpersonal Styles of Outpatient Neurotics and Prison Inmates

THIS PAPER represents an effort to establish a system for classifying neurotics and personality disorders into mutually exclusive classes or types on the basis of their interpersonal behaviors. The term *type* is used to refer to a subgroup of individuals all members of which share a common pattern of characteristics. Since the characteristics to be studied are ways of relating interpersonally, the pattern that distinguishes members of a type is called an *interpersonal style*. Thus, the goal is to identify and to compare on the basis of self-report data, any interpersonal types to be found among samples of normals, neurotics, and personality disorders.

Typing and taxonomic grouping have long been of interest to scientists in many fields. The use of statistical approaches and the computer for type-searching has been fairly recent, however. Zubin (1938) applied agreement analyses to differentiate psychiatric patients from normals. Thorndike (1953) proposed a procedure for grouping jobs into families. McQuitty (1961) has developed numerous techniques. Sokal and Sneath (1963) offer a wide review of procedures applied by biologists in numerical taxonomy. Broadly speaking, typological analysis techniques have been developed and applied by biologists. statisticians, archaeologists, anthropologists, psychologists, and many other researchers.

A common aim of typological analysis is to identify any natural groupings of objects under study with respect to the similarities among them. Another aim, conceptual in nature, is to establish a taxonomy for grouping large numbers of objects into a smaller number of mutually exclusive classes. From the latter viewpoint, a type is a scientific construct useful for comprehending data. Types facilitate communication by making it easier to recognize, remember, and differentiate members from non-members. For example, to label a person a psychopath immediately suggests a broad set of characteristics and expected behaviors. Obviously, a typology reflects an increased understanding of a field. Knowledge of morphological structure is increased when people can be classified as mesomorphs, endomorphs, and ectomorphs. The use of homogeneous subgroups may lead to the discovery of laws and relationships obscured or unobservable within a mixed sample. Members of a type are more homogeneous than people in general. It follows that type members should be more similar relative to behaviors outside the basis of classification. In this way accuracy of prediction can be improved.

Our assumption is that a limited number of types can account for similarities among individuals in the domain of interpersonal behavior. The problem is whether normals, neurotics, and personality disorders may be allocated to the same subgroups. Neurotics manifest symptom syndromes, and persons labeled behavior disorders are more antisocial than normal individuals. One hypothesis of this study is that the same types will be found among these three groups. These groups will differ mainly in the relative incidence by which they are represented in the various interpersonal types found. They will also differ with respect to *level* of scores that defines the type profile. In other words, although (say) neurotics can be categorized as similar to normals in interpersonal style, they are more extreme in these patterns.

Leary's interpersonal scheme (1957) resembles the viewpoint sketched here. He describes eight modes of interpersonal adjustment and eight modes of maladjustment on the same variables. He regards the Kraepelinian type categories as synonyms for his maladjustive types. A hysteric, for instance, corresponds to his overconventional personality, and a psychopath resembles the sadistic personality. The major basis for a diagnosis is the individual's interpersonal interaction pattern and not his symptoms. Foulds and Caine (1965) propose comparable conceptions for relating personality and "personal illness." Their investigations indicate that hysteroids and obsessoids do not necessarily manifest hysteric or obsessive-compulsive syndromes. Their findings suggest that a double classification system is needed for neurotics — one system covering interpersonal style, and the other the symptom syndromes. The conceptual approach in this study is thus by no means new. It is novel in that a multivariate technique, typological analysis, is applied to search and to identify interpersonal types.

178

The aims of the study were (a) to identify any types to be found among samples of male and female outpatient neurotics and correctional institutional inmates, and (b) to compare the types found among neurotics and correctional cases with those found among normals of the same sex.

METHOD OF PROCEDURE

The Measures. The principal measuring device was the Interpersonal Style Inventory (ISI; Lorr & Youniss, 1969). The ISI (Form B) measures 14 bipolar factors. The first-order dimensions are Directive versus Nondirective, Attention Seeking versus Attention Avoiding, Sociable versus Detached, Succorant versus Help Rejecting, Nurturant versus Help Withholding, Conscientious versus Expedient, Trusting versus Suspicious, Tolerant versus Hostile, Independent versus Yielding, Rule Free versus Rule Bound, Orderly versus Disorderly, Deliberate versus Impulsive, Admitting Frailties versus Defensive, and Stable versus Neurotic. Norms for the ISI-B are based on 370 men and 471 women drawn from university and working adult samples. The five more inclusive or second-order factors, also established for men and women, are Extroversion-Introversion, Socialized-Unsocialized, Independent-Dependent, Structure Seeking–Avoiding, Stable-Neurotic (see Table A*). The median value of the first-order scale reliabilities is .82. Correlations indicate reasonably adequate concurrent validity for many of the scales (Lorr & Youniss, 1973).

The ISI-B is used to differentiate normal individuals from outpatient neurotics and prison inmates. Thus, some evidence is needed to indicate that the ISI scales are indeed sensitive to anticipated differences among these three groups. For this reason four groups of men and four groups of women were compared with one another by means of discriminant function analyses. The women compared consisted of 120 working adults, 150 college students, 114 neurotics, and 141 prisoners. The men compared included 86 working adults, 150 college students, 135 prisoners, and 102 psychiatric outpatients. Each analysis yielded three highly significant dimensions of group difference. The percentage of variance accounted for by the first two artificial variates was 86 for the men and 88 for the women. The working adults, the neurotics, and the prisoners were significantly separated by the ISI scores in both the male and female samples. Neurotics were characterized by low emotional stability, help-seeking, and rule-free

*For Tables A–F, order NAPS Document 02197 from ASIS/NAPS, c/o Microfiche Publications, 305 East 46th Street, New York, New York 10017, remitting $1.50 for microfiche or $5.00 for photocopies. Make checks payable to Microfiche Publications.

tendencies. The prisoners were characterized by mistrust and lack of moral scruples (low conscientiousness). The working adults were significantly more trusting, conscientious, emotionally stable, and rule-bound. The college students were located between the neurotics and working adults. The findings thus provide support for the construct validity of the ISI.

The Sample. The cases selected for study ranged in age between 18 and 55. All had completed at least two years of high school or its equivalent. Psychotics and brain-injured and drug-addicted persons were excluded from the study. The outpatient cases were all diagnosed neurotic but some also were given secondary diagnoses of personality disorder. The correctional institution cases consisted of 135 men from three state prisons, and 141 women from one federal and two state institutions. The neurotics included 102 men and 114 women. The normal subjects were drawn from the universities and from working adults who belonged to parent-teacher associations.

Typological Analysis. In typological analysis one is given a collection of N objects each measured with respect to K attributes or variables. The ordered set of measures representing the object is called a profile. The objects may be conceptualized as points (or vectors) imbedded in K-dimensional attribute space. The first problem is to assess the degree of closeness, nearness, or similarity between objects. The relationship may be quantified in terms of some index. If the attributes have been metricized, two classes of similarity indices may be used. The first is the familiar Euclidian distance measure D between the two objects. D^2 is simply the sum of squared differences between the scores of the two objects. The second is a measure of the angular separation between the vectors representing the two objects. A vector, of course, has direction and magnitude. The cosine of the angular separation is the function most commonly used. The congruency coefficient (Cohen, 1969) and the ordinary product-moment correlation coefficient are such measures. Both measures equalize the dispersion of scores represented by the vector lengths. However, the congruency coefficient includes information about the means of the object scores which is removed from the scores in the correlation coefficient. The measures used in our analyses were the congruency coefficient and the distance measure.

To search for types it is necessary to establish an inclusion criterion L_i for type membership — that is, to shift from a quantitative index of similarity to a categorical criterion of belonging. A link between two objects is defined either as (a) a correlation coefficient above an arbitrary or natural minimum, or (b) a distance less than some arbitrary maximum. If the relations (links) among objects are symmetric but not necessarily transitive, then the subsets or types to be found are called compact (Rice & Lorr, 1969). If the object relations are transitive (e.g., greater than, preferred to, dominated by), then the subsets are called ordinal or extended. Only compact types are of concern here.

Two methods of typological analysis were applied in the study, the Buildup and the Ward Hierarchical procedure. In the Buildup algorithm (Lorr & Radhakrishnan, 1967), the procedure begins with a nucleus consisting of the three most highly correlated objects in the aggregate. A fourth object is added to the nucleus if it is on the average within the limit L_i of all objects in the subset. The process continues until no other object can be found which correlates on the average L_i or more with other members of the subset. The limit L_i is usually set at the value at which a correlation based on K independent measures is significant at the 2 per cent level.

Next an upper limit of exclusion L_e is set to remove objects that lie between two or more types and thus prevent overlap. Any profiles in the residual matrix that correlate on the average L_e or more with the first subset are deleted and not considered for inclusion in subsequent types. The second subset is generated from the reduced matrix in the same manner as the first. The process is continued until no type with at least four members can be formed. The types that are formed are mutually exclusive. The final step is to compute the mean correlation of each profile with each type and the mean correlation among members of each type.

The hierarchical procedure applied differs from the Buildup in several ways. First, in the hierarchical procedure, objects are sorted on the basis of distance rather than angular separation. Second, the Ward procedure does not require nuclei for potential groups. Third, the partitioning into mutually exclusive groups at any level of the hierarchy is exhaustive, since every object is allocated somewhere. In the Buildup procedure a fair proportion of the objects analyzed are excluded as mixed types.

Hierarchical analysis is a method for generating an ordered arrangement of mutually exclusive subsets into more inclusive subsets at successive levels. The Ward (1963) grouping procedure is based on an objective error function. The goal at each stage is to form a subset that minimizes the sum of squared within-group deviations about the group mean of each test variable for all variables, for all groups at the same time. The procedure begins with each object constituting a subset and combines the two that are closest. At each succeeding step two groups are combined so that a minimum increase in the objective function occurs. The function is the sum, taken over all subsets, of the distances of all objects from their subset means (centroids). The process continues until all groups are combined and yields a binary tree hierarchical structure. However, it is possible to identify a level of the hierarchy which yields an optimal number of groups. Values of the error function are plotted against the number of groups. An abrupt change in the slope of the error curve indicates a sharp increase in error when two subsets were combined. The subsets found at the level just preceding a sharp rise in error are those retained.

Each individual in the study was represented by twelve standard scores. The raw scores were transformed into standard scores derived from the means and dispersion of normative samples of men and women. The male sample scores were standardized on the male norms, and all the female sample scores on the female norms. Two of the scale measures, Stability and Defensiveness, were suppressed in computing distances or correlations among profiles on theoretical grounds. The Stable versus Neurotic scale was excluded because it is the major variable that differentiates normal persons from neurotics. The study itself is focused on differences in interpersonal style rather than on dystonic reactions. Thus, it appeared best to identify subgroups on the basis of normal traits only. Since the Defensive (Lie) scale represents a measure of response distortion, it also was excluded.

Because of computer limitations the samples analyzed consisted of not more than 120 cases. The equivalence of types identified in several samples was evaluated in two ways. One method consisted of combining all members included in each of the types identified in several analyses into a single stratified sample. Members of the pooled sample were then searched for subgroups by the Buildup procedure. Types that were allocated to the same subgroup were judged typologically equivalent. On the other hand, subgroups that failed to emerge were regarded as mixtures. The logic of this process is that the subgroups should be invariant under changes in the sample of persons analyzed. The second procedure for appraising the equivalence of the sample subgroups was to apply the hierarchical grouping procedures to their mean standard score profiles. Subgroups from two or more samples that were grouped together were judged to be similar. The number of groups selected was determined by inspecting the error function previously described.

THE FINDINGS

The Typological Results. Members of a type may be described in terms of their mean standard score profile. However, the differentiating scales are those on which all members agree fairly closely and on which members lie significantly above or below the norm sample mean. Scales on which members differ widely may be ignored as undifferentiating. Since all members must satisfy the same conditions to belong, type membership implies the joint presence of all defining characteristics. It should be remembered that measures of Stability and Defensiveness were excluded in the process of identifying types. However, the mean standard scores of all type members on these two scales (computed after the analysis) are recorded along with all other profile measures.

The normal sample consisted of 360 men and 360 women drawn from the normative sample used in standardizing ISI-B. Each block of 360 cases was randomly divided into three subsamples of 120 cases. Analyses of these subsamples yielded seven male and nine female types. To what extent are types found among men the same as those found among women? To answer this question, the hierarchical grouping procedure was applied to the mean score profiles of these men and women. The analysis indicated that six subgroups were equivalent. The equivalent sets are presented in parallel columns in Table 1. The letters *M* and *F* hereafter refer to the male and female types.

Typological analysis of the 120 male prisoners disclosed six male prisoner subgroups. All of the twelve variables differentiated among the types at highly significant levels ($p<.001$). Analysis of the female prisoner sample profiles disclosed only four types. Again, *F* ratios for each of the twelve scale variables indicated significant differentiation among the four types at $p<.001$. The mean profiles are presented in Tables C and D.

The same process of typological analysis, applied to a sample of 102 male outpatients, disclosed six subgroups. Each of the twelve scales, except Deliberate-Impulsive, discriminated among the types at significant levels. Analysis of the female sample of outpatients disclosed six types. Each of the measures discriminated among the subgroups at highly significant levels. The mean profiles appear in Tables E and F.

Comparison with Normals. As stated earlier, a hypothesis of the investigation is that neurotics and the personality disorders are similar to normals in the kinds of interpersonal styles they manifest, but are different in profile level and in percentage distribution within the various types. Now that we have identified a variety of subgroups within each of the three

Table 1. Mean Standard Scores of Normal Male (M) and Female (F) Types

Scale[a]	M1	F1	M3	F9	M5	F4	M6	F5	M2	F6	M4	F2
Dir	.38	−.12	.13	1.02	.59	.97	.07	−.66	−.71	−.10	−.35	−.95
Att	1.58	.69	−.41	1.27	1.12	−.14	−.39	−.92	−.98	−.90	.56	−.70
Soc	.68	.21	.55	1.00	1.17	.97	−.10	−1.69	−.71	−.65	−.57	−.98
Suc	.87	.08	.55	.70	.66	.95	−1.34	−1.36	.00	−.77	−.10	.03
Nur	.07	−.45	.97	.93	.53	.58	−.02	−.42	−.02	.35	−2.14	−1.22
Con	−1.17	−1.94	.58	.55	.46	.73	−.26	−.02	.49	.60	−1.58	−.07
Trs	−.52	−1.75	1.09	.39	.04	.91	−1.22	−.50	1.09	.91	−.94	−.78
Tol	−1.12	−1.58	.84	.66	−.09	.91	−1.14	−.46	1.08	1.36	−.56	−.21
Ind	.57	.89	.84	1.07	.20	.80	.90	.36	−1.30	−.68	−1.30	−1.74
Rlf	.87	1.51	1.51	.53	−.88	.16	.83	.36	−1.60	−.31	.12	−.91
Ord	−1.49	−1.05	−.90	−1.45	1.22	1.23	.16	.85	1.14	.16	−.16	.64
Del	−.94	−.99	−.15	−.84	.16	−.03	−.05	.52	1.11	.76	−.18	.35
Sta	−.31	−.44	.69	.08	.11	.70	−.82	−.85	.06	.29	−1.21	−.77
Def	−.87	−.90	.71	.43	.68	1.09	−.64	−.15	.09	.37	−.06	−1.03

[a] Dir = Directive vs. Nondirective; Att = Attention Seeking vs. Attention Avoiding; Soc = Sociable vs. Detached; Suc = Succorant vs. Help Rejecting; Nur = Nurturant vs. Help Withholding; Con = Conscientious vs. Expedient; Trs = Trusting vs. Suspicious; Tol = Tolerant vs. Hostile; Ind = Independent vs. Yielding; Rlf = Rule Free vs. Rule Bound; Ord = Orderly vs. Disorderly; Del = Deliberate vs. Impulsive; Sta = Stable vs. Neurotic; Def = Admitting Frailties vs. Defensive.

184

populations, some evaluation of the assumption can be made. The hierarchical (H-group) method was used to compare outpatients with normals and prisoners with normals, after separation by sex. In each analysis the grouping procedure was applied to the mean score profiles of all the types involved. For example, the seven male normal types were analyzed with the six male prisoner types.

The results for men and women are presented separately in Table 2. Each row of the table indicates the type code numbers of roughly equivalent subgroups. (For example, normal male no. 1 is similar to outpatient male no. 3; normal female no. 1 to female prisoner no. 3 and female outpatient no. 2.) Nine H-groups accounted for the male prisoner and normal types. Four of the prisoner types could be grouped with normals, but types no. 1 and no. 6 were unequal. However normal types nos. 1, 3, 6 and 7 had no equivalent within the prisoner sample. Seven H-groups accounted for the male outpatient and male normal profiles. In this respect male outpatient neurotics are more like normals than are prison inmates.

Nine H-groups were sufficient to account for the female normal and female prisoner subgroups. Five of the six female outpatient subgroups were classed as equivalent to five of the normal female types. Thus it is possible to conclude that except for two male prisoner subgroups and one neurotic female subgroup, the same interpersonal types appear among normals, prisoners, and neurotics. On the other hand, there are fewer types to be found among prisoners than among normals.

Differentiation and Overlap. The subgroups isolated by the Buildup procedure are discrete and non-overlapping by virtue of the inclusion-exclusion limits. The Ward H-group method also generates mutually exclusive subgroups since every profile is assigned to one group. Yet there

Table 2. Equivalent Groups for Normals, Prisoners, and Outpatients

Group	Type Code Numbers								
Men									
Normals	1	2	3	4[a]	5	6[a]	7		
Prisoners		3,5[a]		4	2[a]			1[a]	6[a]
Outpatients	3	2[a]	5[a]	1[a]	6[a]	4[a]			
Women									
Normals	1	6	9	2[a]	4	5[a]	7	8	3
Prisoners	3	2[a]		4[a]		1			
Outpatients	2	3[a]		1[a]		6		5	4[a]

[a]Subgroups with high scores on neuroticism.

still is the question, How differentiated are the type profiles? In the case of the Buildup types, one basis for judging the extent of differentiation is to determine the average correlation within and between types. Each analysis yields a table of mean correlations (a) among members of each type and (b) between members of a type and members of every other type.

Table F presents these means for the pooled normal samples. The average between-type coefficients ranged from .28 to —.62. The within-type coefficients ranged from .64 to .78. Unrelated profiles tend to have negligible correlations. Similar profiles tend to be positively correlated, whereas dissimilar profiles tend to be negatively correlated. The coefficients in Table F indicate high consistency among score profiles within subgroups and low consistency between subgroups. The correlations within and between the prisoner subgroups and within and between the outpatient subgroups were at comparable levels. For this reason no data need be presented.

Type Sizes. Typological analysis is concerned with the number and nature of subgroups present within a nonhomogeneous sample. The problem of resolving mixtures when subgroups are unknown a priori should not be confused with classification. Classification is concerned with the assignment of new cases to already established subgroups in accordance with certain rules of decision-making. Once subgroups have been established, appropriate rules can be formulated by means of multiple cutting score techniques, discriminant function analysis, and other procedures.

The relative size of the subgroups or types is thus a problem not to be confused with the percentage of cases classifiable. There were 120 cases in each of the normal samples analyzed. Among men, 43 per cent were allocated to one of the subgroups in the analyses. Within the subsample of women, 37 per cent of all cases were found in the types isolated. However, 53 per cent of the pooled sample of 112 men and 69 per cent of the pooled sample of 118 women were allocated to one of the types. Less than half of the cases analyzed provided the definition of the types found among normals.

The Normal Types. To simplify the interpretations, the six types common to normal men and women will be described in terms of the higher-level factors. The first four scales listed in Table 1 represent extroversion-introversion, the next four socialization, the next two independence-dependence, followed by two scales descriptive of impulse control. The last two scales represent the stability versus neuroticism factor.

The first six columns present the mean profiles of the extroverts, and the last six columns the profiles of the introverts. M1 and F1 are extroverted, unsocialized, and independent but relatively disorderly and impulsive. M3 and F9 are extroverted, socialized, and independent but relatively disorderly and impulsive. The third extroverted set (M5 and F4) are moderately socialized but orderly and systematic in living habits. Stability fails to differentiate the three subgroups, although the first is most neurotic and willing to admit frailties.

The first introverted type (M6 and F5) is mistrustful and hostile, somewhat independent, and moderately neurotic. The second set (M2, F6) are definitely socialized (but average in nurturance), yielding-conventional, as well as orderly-deliberate. The third subgroup (M4, F2) is unsocialized, strongly yielding, and neurotic. It should be noted that the unsocialized subgroups, whether extroverted or introverted, tend to have low stability scores.

Neuroticism and Interpersonal Style. An important issue is whether certain interpersonal styles are more strongly associated with neurotic reactions than others. The ISI Stability scale correlates —.78 with the 16 Personality Factor Questionnaire (Cattell & Stice) second-order measure and —.71 with Eysenck's measure of neuroticism. In addition, the Stability scale differentiates neurotic outpatients from normal samples. Thus, the measure's construct validity is fairly strong. A standard score of —.50 will be used as a rough index to the presence of neurotic behavior. By this criterion normal types M6-F5 and M4-F2 evidence neurotic behavior. Also, four of the male neurotic types (1, 2, 3, 4) and three of the female neurotic types (1, 2, 4) evidence neurotic behavior. Among the prisoners, three of the male subgroups (1, 2, 6) and one of the female subgroups (4) score at or above the criterion.

The question still remains whether any particular subgroups are consistently neurotic by our criterion. Each row in Table 2 lists the subgroups judged equivalent by the H-group procedure. Only M6-F5 and M4-F2 and equivalents among outpatients and prisoners of either sex manifest significant neurotic scores. Both of these interpersonal styles involve introverted and unsocialized personality patterns. By contrast, M3-F9, who are extroverted, socialized, and independent, have only one doubtful equivalent in male outpatient no. 5.

The Prisoner Inmate Types. As was stated earlier, the prisoner subgroups, unlike the outpatient types, are more often unique and more limited in range. Only four types were isolated in the women's sample and of the six identified among the men, two (1 and 6) are not found among normals and outpatients. In both male and female samples, the first and largest type identified can be characterized as extremely introverted and unsocialized. In addition, the men report themselves as extremely impulsive (deliberate versus impulsive: —1.05). The social history data indicate that the men tend to be unmarried, had few close friends in school, are estranged from their families, and had trouble in school. The women report that they belonged to few groups or clubs and that they were often in trouble in school.

CONCLUSIONS

Our aim was to determine, in an exploratory fashion, the number and nature of personality types into which normals, outpatient neurotics, and prison inmates could be classified using the Interpersonal Style Inventory.

This paper thus offers a tentative conceptual scheme for classifying outpatient neurotics and prison inmates. Since the findings are tentative and must be duplicated on new samples, no effort has been made to develop decision rules for classifying new cases.

COMMENTARY

ZUBIN. The problem of diagnosis is not an easy one, especially in the behavior disorders. Why it is so much more difficult to diagnose mental disorders is an interesting question. Lorr has spent a good deal of his professional life on this problem, and his attempt at introducing typological approaches into diagnosis is indeed stimulating even though success thus far has not been extensive.

There are at least three aspects to the behavior of the mentally disordered person which need to be kept in mind in making diagnoses, even though we do not yet know how to separate them pragmatically: (a) the premorbid personality; (b) the disorder; and (c) the illness.

a. It is obvious that the behavioral repertoire of the patient antedates his psychopathology — that is, that a premorbid personality exists and varies from patient to patient even in groups of patients suffering from the same disorder.

b. The disorder from which the patient suffers can sometimes be objectively specified clearly as to etiology and process, as is the case for example with general paresis, PKU, and other conditions of known etiology. But even in disorders of unknown etiology, there is provided at least a description of the underlying characteristics which are fundamental to the disorder.

c. To distinguish the illness from the disorder with which it is associated, we must remember that the illness from which the patient suffers consists of the focal disorder plus the penumbra of specific situations surrounding the disorder, as well as the patient's idiosyncratic responses to the disorder and to treatment. That is why two patients suffering with the same focal disorder often behave differently.

This illness will vary considerably from patient to patient, even when the etiology and process of the disorder is known. It will be most variable, however, in disorders of unknown origin, because we still do not know how to separate the components of the disorder from the peripheral components of the illness. It is the illness rather than the disorder which provides the "bewildering complexity of the psychiatric patients." Perhaps one of the most important components of the illness is the interaction between the premorbid personality and the disorder. The specific situation surrounding the disorder has recently been scbjected to a definitive examination by Holmes in his study of the relation of changes in life events.

In considering the effect of therapeutic intervention on the patient, we may have to consider not only the disorder but also the illness, since it is still debatable whether the observed changes in behavior reflect changes in the focal disorder or changes in the peripheral aspects of the illness. Thus, drug effects may cut across the various disorders, if they bring relief from symptoms which, though not germane to the focal disorder, nevertheless frequently accompany it.

In view of these difficulties in arriving at a diagnosis, it becomes necessary to specify operationally the specific signs and symptoms which have to be exhibited by the patient before he is placed in a given category. Thus, a certain amount of arbitrariness must enter in order to render diagnoses comparable from one diagnostician to another. For this purpose certain glossaries have been developed which spell out what kinds of behaviors entitle a person to a given diagnosis. Even with a specification of these requirements, diagnosis often still depends on some still undefinable subjective quality, even as is the case with the definition of species in biology. Only in mathematics do we have ironclad definitions. In biology we must depend upon certain specified indicators plus a little *flair*, as Julian Huxley tells us, in order to define a species. Similarly, in schizophrenia we can not do without a similar *flair*.

However, with the availability of systematic structured interviews, which give rise to specific dimensional profiles, we can leave temporarily the standard diagnostic approach in which we try to classify symptoms and signs into syndromes and enter the typological area in which we classify individuals in accordance with the similarity in their profiles. This typological approach has prospered in recent times. We can still deal with the standard diagnosis but try to cluster the like-structured individuals within each diagnostic category into subgroups. Should we find a group with the same profile which cuts across diagnostic categories, we can separate out this group and exclude it from the standard diagnosis by giving it a new designation. This typological approach has to be validated by finding certain underlying characteristics which separate the subgroups — such as different common fates with regard to outcome, duration of illness, and response to different therapies. Lorr has been one of the chief contributors to the typological approach, and he is to be admired for the tenacious way in which he pursues this approach.

Returning to the application of the typological approach to schizophrenia, it is well to remember that while searching for the subgroups, we can still hold on to our overall diagnostic category — our core disorder — until we can determine what it consists of, or give it up, if we find no common link between our subgroups.

The typological approach also has implications for outcome of treatment. One of the most baffling problems in treatment of schizophrenia is prognosis. The only factor which seems to be prognostic in schizophrenia, and has been so from the very beginning, is that of premorbid personality. Good premorbids tend to improve, poor premorbids do not. All other findings, such as the relation of marital status and education to outcome, can be subsumed under this general heading. Why should this be so? If we assume that the basic feature of schizophrenia is a relatively high degree of vulnerability to stressors, either endogenous or exogenous, and that when an episode occurs, it has time limits, then we may conclude that when the episode is over, the patient returns to his premorbid personality. If that was good to begin with, he is rated as recovered; if it was poor to begin with, it is difficult to know just when the episode is over, and another episode may soon develop because of his inability to cope.

Thus, types with poor premorbid personalities can become the targets for personality remolding. We can shift our focus from trying to cure the patient to concentrating on his personality, so that when the episode is over, he will be able to cope with life's exigencies.

I have devoted my comments purposely to the psychoses because it is in these disorders that typology has been found of some use. There is no reason to believe that similar approaches separating the premorbid personality from the focal disorder and from the illness should not eventually prove useful in the nonpsychotic aspects of the behavior disorders. To quote an old adage: It is not the disease itself that is the important thing, it is the person who has the disease that makes all the difference.

LORR. You are following an anachronistic mental illness model. These are not disorders like the old psychoses, even if you could assume those models were true. I'm talking about character disorders, and about neurotics, not about schizophrenics. And I think you are going to find very few people working with neurotics or prisoners who think they are prey to some kind of core disorder.

ZUBIN. You are not considering a genetic element in neurosis at all?

LORR. Sure, there is a genetic element in any individual.

ZUBIN. Do you accept the evidence that compulsive neurotics often breed compulsive neurotics in their families?

LORR. No, I don't, if by *breed* is meant genetics.

ZUBIN. You don't.

LORR. I don't accept that.

ZUBIN. There are some convincing data on that.

D. KLEIN. The problem with clustering techniques is that because of the way a type is defined, everybody in a type is more like the others in that type than like anybody outside. This is reasonable, except for the word *like*. How you define *like* results in quite different types. Lorr should be commended for using several different definitions of *like* and cross-checking one against the other. If I understood correctly, he used a correlational definition of *like*, using Cohen's pattern analysis, and he also used a distance measure of *like*. That is a marked methodological advance that actually Lorr could have made more of, because not many people are that stringent in their definition of *like*. But the headache is still with us because any of these measures, whether correlational or distance, must utilize all the dimensions that go into the measure of likeness. If it is conceivable that certain dimensions are noise, irrelevant to basic typologies that are important in the sphere that Lorr is interested in, he has gotten himself into trouble.

I think there is a certain circularity in the problem of cluster analysis. We can best cluster analyze when the dimensions are known to be relevant to the typology. To the degree that you have dimensions irrelevant to the typology that you are concerned about, to that degree it's hard to cluster analyze. But of course to the degree that you know the dimensions in advance, to that degree you don't need to cluster analyze. For these reasons, I prefer multivariate approaches that explicitly relate to a validity criterion such as follow-up, rather than try to develop all-purpose clusters.

VAILLANT. I'm delighted with Klein's first remark, and suggest as an alternative to Lorr's scheme, the approach of Washington University to psychiatric problems. Scales are individual, and you become dependent in data processing on what the person said on the scale. People respond to scales at different times in different ways, and a great deal of ambiguity gets built in, which sophisticated statistical manipulation simply compounds. This perhaps leads to typologies that are perfectly clear and rational to people who understand the statistics but are difficult to carry out effectively in everyday research. The people at Washington University have described typology in terms of overt observable behavior that occurs over time, so that you don't need a scale; what you need is a history and selected items of data which you then put together as a cluster. Whether or not you are dealing with a unitary concept of sociopathy or schizophrenia, you have a descriptive entity that is easily checkable from one center to another. This prevents the babble of nomenclature that we saw earlier when one person was talking about minimal brain dysfunction and somebody else was talking about hyperkinetic children. Are infantile autism in Baltimore and atypical children in Bostom simply the same disorder in different cities? Or are they really very different disorders? The elegance of the Washington University approach is that it avoids such confusion. I would suggest it either as an alternative to Lorr's or as a supplement — Lorr and the Washington University groups might get together and use his analysis on their types of data.

BIRCH. Maybe we can get an argument going. It seems to me that what Lorr has been doing for many years with quite conspicuous success is something extremely interesting. That is, can you indeed, across quite functionally diverse groups of individuals, develop a set of measures with respect to their modes of function in social interactions which in fact are describable and which in fact result in certain types? All that is required to validate that concept is replicability. He has replicated these measures within the United States, outside the United States, and so on. The next question, and one that he has not dealt with, except in the negative, is that he has clearly told us today that this typology is irrelevant to differences between modes of function in clinically or socially defined groups. He says that these typologies are as manifest in prisoners as they are in normals, they are as manifest in neurotics as they are in non-neurotics. This doesn't mean that neurotics, prisoners, and normals are the same. In general, we know from other criteria that they're different. It means that they are the same on his measures. For example, if I were to do blood pressure studies, I could develop typologies of blood pressure across populations which would have no relationship to their clinical status in a psychological sense. Therefore, there is no validity criterion with respect to psychopathology that necessarily stems from Lorr's typology. He is explicitly denying that it has such a criterion value. Therefore, why do we make such a demand of the man? We may think that it is useless to us as a typology because it does not discriminate among the particular entities we are interested in. But that is not his problem, it's ours.

RICKS. I got the impression that there were more ways to be normal than there are to be disturbed. For those of us who have been working on disturbance for years, that means that there is an awful lot that we don't know about normal people.

LORR. That's right. There are more numerous explicit classes among the normal groups. It is as though some types were just wiped out, particularly among the prison groups. They just weren't present.

REFERENCES

Cohen, J. A profile similarity coefficient invariant over variable reflection. *Psychological Bulletin*, 1969, 71, 281–284.

Foulds, G. A., & Caine, T. M. *Personality and personal illness.* London: Tavistock, 1965.

Leary, T. *Interpersonal diagnosis of personality.* New York: Ronald Press, 1957.

Lorr, M., & Radhakrishnan, B. K. A comparison of two methods of cluster analysis. *Educational and Psychological Measurement*, 1967, 27, 47–53.

Lorr, M., & Youniss, R. P. The Interpersonal Style Inventory — Form B. Washington, D.C.: Catholic University of America, 1969.

————. An inventory of interpersonal style. *Journal of Personality Assessment*, 1973, 37, 165–173.

McQuitty, L. L. Typal analysis. *Educational and Psychological Measurement*, 1961, 21, 677–696.

Rice, C. E., & Lorr, M. An empirical comparison of typological analysis methods. Washington, D.C.: Office of Naval Research, 1969. Contract N0014-67-A-0214.

Sokal, R. B., & Sneath, P. H. *Principles of numerical taxonomy*. San Francisco: Freeman, 1963.

Thorndike, R. L. Who belongs in the family? *Psychometrika*, 1953, 18, 267–276.

Ward, J. H., Jr. Hierarchical grouping to optimize an objective function. *Journal of American Statistical Association*, 1963, 58, 236–244.

Zubin, J. Socio-biological types and methods for their isolation. *Psychiatry*, 1938, 1, 237–247.

NORMAN F. WATT

Childhood and Adolescent Routes to Schizophrenia

THERE IS AN interesting schism in the psychological literature on child development that bears upon the childhood roots of schizophrenia. On the one hand is a large and growing body of research on the antecedents of schizophrenic disorder (Erlenmeyer-Kimling, Rainer, & Kallmann, 1966; Heston, 1966; Lane & Albee, 1964; Ricks & Berry, 1970; Robins, 1966; Roff, 1963; Rosenthal et al., 1968; Wittman & Steinberg, 1944; Zigler & Phillips, 1960) conducted by clinical psychologists, psychiatrists, and social workers and usually published in clinical journals.

On the other hand is a sizable number of studies by educators, psychologists, and psychiatrists concerning the early identification of emotionally disturbed children in school (Bower, 1960; Cowen et al., 1966; Kellam & Schiff, 1967; Khleif, 1964; Mensch et al., 1959; Mitchell, 1949; Rubin et al., 1966; Ullmann, 1952).

The two camps have seemed to ignore each other, as if there were no communality in their missions. But they indeed have a great deal in common. In 1970, some 51,600,000 children attended secondary schools in the United States, 89 per cent of them public (Simon & Grant, 1970).

NOTE: The research reported here was supported by the Schizophrenia Research Program of the Supreme Council 33° A. A. Scottish Rite, Northern Masonic Jurisdiction, by Public Health Service Research Grant MH-13280 from NIMH, and by Office of Education Research Grant OEG-1-71-0021 (059).

The author gratefully acknowledges the research assistance of Maxine Frohwein, Nathan Riley, Roberta McGovern, Joy Corsi, Bruce King, Emily Serkin, Mary Goethals, Judy Pekarsky, Sona Stork, Rick de Friesse, Sally Ives, and Barbara Kupferman, and the generous cooperation of Dr. Thomas F. Pugh, Director of Evaluation, Research, and Statistics in the Massachusetts Department of Mental Health, and the public school authorities and filing personnel in the high school in "Maybury." Bob Stolorow, Amy Lubensky, and David McClelland were primarily responsible for developing the coding system for analyzing the content of the school records.

The general consensus in the educational camp is that about 5 million of those children (10 per cent) are emotionally handicapped *right now*, they can be identified readily, and something can and should be done about it. The general consensus in the clinical camp is that about a million (±500,000) of those children (1–3 per cent) will become schizophrenic someday, but it won't happen for twenty years or so and they can't be identified in advance, so there's nothing we can do about it now. I believe that many, if not most, of tomorrow's schizophrenics are emotionally handicapped children today. If we are bold enough to study and follow such vulnerable children, including those with clear genetic vulnerability, it is possible that we might turn up some answers of value to both camps.

METHOD

The clinical studies of the antecedents of schizophrenia are characterized by Garmezy (in press) as follow-up and follow-back studies, relying heavily on case records and especially valuable for generating hypotheses about the historical roots of schizophrenia. The intellectual offspring of this literature is the high-risk or follow-through study (Anthony, 1968; Garmezy, in press; Mednick, 1970). The advantages of the follow-through method with high-risk populations are obvious and large. The measures for assessment may be chosen by the investigator to suit his purposes, thus freeing him from the limitations of institutional records. The children may be observed clinically by the same observers both before and after onset of schizophrenic symptoms. And most important, instead of the 1–3 per cent rate of schizophrenic outcome (Yolles & Kramer, 1969) to be expected in any random sample of children, the rate may go as high as 9 per cent (Kety et al., 1968) or 15 per cent (Mednick, 1970) for children of one schizophrenic parent or even as high as 35–45 per cent for children of two schizophrenic parents (Rosenthal, 1970).

The follow-through method with high-risk populations represents an important breakthrough for research in schizophrenia. However, I should like to point out that the method is not sufficiently exploited if risk is measured solely by a genetic criterion. (*Genetic criterion* is used here descriptively, as Mednick uses it: a child with a schizophrenic parent is empirically more likely than average to become schizophrenic himself. No assumption is made about the mechanism(s) by which the pathology of the parent is causally related to the pathology of the child.) The genetic criterion of risk is too narrow for the purposes of developing a general theory of etiology in schizophrenia. A very small proportion (10–15 per cent) of people who will be schizophrenic in their lifetime can be so identified by the criterion of having a schizophrenic parent. A comparable proportion (85–90 per cent) of children identified as being at risk for schizophrenia by this genetic criterion will not become schizophrenic, although perhaps as many as half of them will become psychiatrically deviant. In short, using the genetic criterion, the number of false positive predictions and false negative predictions will be six to nine times as large as the number of true positives.

Subjects. Preliminary results for about half of the schizophrenics in this project have been published (Watt et al., 1970, 1972) with details of the methodology employed. The present report is based on the entire sample of 54 schizophrenics and 143 matched controls. The patients were schizophrenics 15–34 years old first admitted to mental hospitals anywhere in Massachusetts between 1958 and 1965, who had attended public schools in a large Boston suburb ("Maybury"). Their cumulative school records were located, and three control records for each were drawn from the files. The controls were matched individually for sex, race, age, and parental social class. Eight of the schizophrenics had nonpsychotic diagnoses at first admission, and only one control record was drawn for each of these (we learned subsequently that the 8 were unequivocally schizophrenic at later admissions). Three control records were unusable. Therefore, 43 schizophrenics had three controls, 3 had two controls, and 8 had one control. None of the 143 controls had ever been hospitalized for mental illness in Massachusetts before 1970.

Measures. A cumulative school record usually consisted of three parts, one for the elementary school grades through six, one for the junior high grades seven through nine, and one for the senior high school years. The results of periodic intelligence tests and physical examinations were recorded on separate forms. As the child progressed through the Maybury school system, his cumulative record followed him, and it remained on file at the last Maybury school he attended, typically the high school.

One side of the elementary school card contained primarily demographic information about the pupil, his family, siblings, birth residence, and some crude estimates of his standing and progress to the sixth grade. The rest of the elementary record form consisted mainly of comments written each year by the principal teacher under three broad headings: first, scholastic performance in skill subjects; second, personal characteristics, such as social, emotional, mental, and physical growth, and special abilities, interests, and disabilities; and third, special help and guidance used during the year and recommendations for the next year.

The format of the junior high school record was somewhat more structured. About half of the record contained information primarily of a scholastic nature, such as attendance, curriculum, parents' and pupil's plans for the future, and school marks for the three grades. The other half listed the student's special abilities, intramural activities, clubs, outside activities, vocational experiences, use of money earned or allowed, offices held, and general health, and provided a substantial space for the principal teacher each year to write notes concerning mental health, social adjustment, work habits, subject matter achievement, and the like.

The format of the senior high school record was similar to that for junior high, but contained in addition eight 5-point rating scales of personality traits to be filled in independently by each of the pupil's teachers in the tenth and eleventh grades.

Comparisons in this report are based upon four kinds of measures derived from the total cumulative school records. Listed from simplest to most complex, these were: (a) standardized school marks for English and math in grades 7–12 (they were not available for grades K–6); (b) standardized IQ scores on the Kuhlmann-Anderson Test in grades 3 and 6 and on the Otis Test in grades 8 and 10 or 11; (c) the personality trait ratings from the high school record; and (d) systematic analysis of the ad lib comments written annually by the homeroom teachers.

Primary emphasis here will be given to the teachers' comments. A system for coding the comments was devised comprising 37 bipolar dimensions, each with a positive and negative category. These were further combined into five rational factors based on D'Andrade's (1965) cross-cultural research. About two thirds of the records were coded blindly by a research assistant using this system. The interjudge reliability coefficients (Spearman rank correlations) for the principal coding factors were satisfactory, except Factor 4 Negative, Passivity (.51). The coefficients for the other factors ranged from .68 to .91 with a median of .80. The coding system was revised for the scoring of the last third of the records by a different assistant. Infrequently used coding categories and redundant ones were collapsed to yield a revised system of 23 bipolar dimensions, still combined in the same five factors. The revised system had better reliability than the original one, and when the two coding systems were correlated for 24 random records, the reliability cofficients for the principal factors ranged from .61 to .90 with a median of .81. Therefore, all of the records coded with the original system were converted to the revised system for the final analysis. A summary of the revised coding system is presented in Table A.* A total of 8,396 comments were coded for the 197 subjects, an average of 43 coded comments apiece.

These data were analyzed by adding all the teachers' comments in each category for every child's total cumulative record and dividing that sum by the number of years for which comments were written. This ratio score indicated the average number of comments per year for each category. Also, the category sums within each factor were combined and divided by the number of years of comments to give a positive ratio score and a negative ratio score for each factor. A difference score was then computed by subtracting the negative score from the positive score for each factor.

Treatment of the Data. It was generally presumed that any differences to be found would show greater maladjustment by the pre-schizophrenic children probably in the areas of introversion and passivity. Therefore, all statistical comparisons of the pre-schizophrenic groups and their matched control groups were based upon one-tailed tests of significance if the difference indicated greater maladjustment in the pre-schizophrenics. A secondary objective was to compare the behavior of the pre-schizophrenic boys and girls by means of direct comparisons because the direction of difference could not be specified in advance. With one exception (indicated below) the major findings were corroborated by non-parametric (sign test) analysis of the same scores.

RESULTS

Table 1 presents the means and group comparisons for all the coding factors of the teachers' annual comments. These means were computed by dividing the number of comments for each coding factor in the total cumulative record by the number of years for which comments were written. That ratio was then multiplied by 8, the overall average for years of comments written. Thus, a mean of 6.73 for the pre-schizophrenic boys on Scholastic Motivation indicates that the teachers described them as being motivated scholastically 6.73 times on the average in the entire course of their schooling at Maybury; the male controls were so described 9.71 times. The means of the controls for each subject were combined to

*For Tables A–F and Figures 1 and 2, order NAPS Document 02197 from ASIS/NAPS, c/o Microfiche Publications, 305 East 46th Street, New York, New York 10017; remitting $1.50 for microfiche or $5.00 for photocopies. Make checks payable to Microfiche Publications.

Table 1. Means[a] and Statistical Comparisons of Pre-Schizophrenic Children and Matched Controls for the Coding Factors of Teachers' Annual Comments ($N = 27$)[b]

Coding Factor	M Schizophrenics vs. Controls		F Schizophrenics vs. Controls		M vs. F Schizophrenics (t test)[c]	M vs. F Controls (t test)[c]	Sex x Diagnosis Interaction (F test)[c]
	Mean	Mean by Triads	Mean	Mean by Triads			
1. Conscientiousness	6.73	9.71**	8.54	9.24			
Nonconscientiousness	5.74	7.69	3.85	4.28		<.025	
Difference	0.99	2.02	4.69	4.96			
2. Emotional Stability	1.10	2.01*****	2.49	2.86	<.025	<.10	
Emotional Instability	6.32	3.09****	4.00	2.90*			<.20
Difference	−5.22	−1.08*****	−1.51	−0.04*	<.05		<.20
3. Extroversion	2.73	3.75	3.02	3.99*			
Introversion	3.34	3.44	3.83	2.30***		<.10	<.20
Difference	−0.61	0.31	−0.80	1.69***			
4. Assertiveness	1.26	1.06	1.17	1.29			
Passivity	2.60	2.74	2.62	1.57**		<.05	<.20
Difference	−1.34	−1.68	−1.45	−0.28*		<.05	
5. Agreeableness	2.88	6.15******	5.42	5.79	<.01		<.025
Disagreeableness	3.71	1.52***	2.06	1.34			<.20
Difference	−0.83	4.63******	3.36	4.45	.005		<.01
Composite Positive	14.70	22.68****	20.64	23.17	<.10		
Composite Negative	21.71	18.48	16.35	12.39**		<.025	
Difference	−7.01	4.20***	4.29	10.78**	<.10	<.10	

[a]Based on average number of comments per year in school and prorated for 8 years of usable comments, which was the overall average.

[b]M = male; F = female.

[c]All based on two-tailed tests of significance. All the comparisons of the pre-schizophrenic groups against their respective control groups report one-tailed probability values.

*p<.10. **p<.05. ***p<.025.

****p<.01. *****p<.005.

******p<.001.

199

yield a mean that was treated as a single score. For this reason, although the control sample comprised 72 boys, the size of the control sample for statistical purposes was 27. Similarly, although there were 71 control girls, they were treated statistically as 27.

The boys differed most sharply from their controls on Factor 5, having fewer comments indicating agreeableness ($p<.001$) and more comments indicating disagreeableness ($p<.025$). The teachers described the pre-schizophrenic boys as significantly less stable emotionally than their controls ($p<.005$) and more emotionally unstable ($p<.01$). They were also less motivated scholastically than their controls. There were no differences on the extroversion or assertiveness factors. The composite scores at the bottom of Table 1 show that teachers expressed their criticisms of the pre-schizophrenic boys primarily by withholding positive remarks ($p<.01$), damning them with faint praise.

By contrast, teachers' criticisms of the pre-schizophrenic girls were more direct, as shown by the composite negative score difference ($p<.05$). The pattern of maladjustment in girls was also dramatically different from that in boys. Like the boys, the girls were somewhat more emotionally unstable than their controls ($p<.10$). As a result of this there was a trend ($p<.10$) toward significant difference on the Factor 2 difference score (emotional stability — emotional instability) for the girls. This Factor 2 difference is the *only* factor score (excluding the composite difference score) on which the schizophrenics differed from the controls with the sexes combined ($p = .01$). An analysis of these data that ignored the breakdown by sex would report only that pre-schizophrenic children are more emotionally unstable than normal children. However, even here the pre-schizophrenic boys and girls differed sharply in the quality of their emotional instability. The girls were slightly less extroverted ($p<.10$) and much more introverted ($p<.025$) than their controls. The parametric analysis showed them also to be significantly more passive than the controls ($p<.05$, $p<.10$ on the assertive — passive difference score), but this result must be discounted because neither score approached significance by nonparametric analysis (sign test and Wilcoxon matched-pairs signed-ranks test). What can be said with confidence is that a quarter of the pre-schizophrenic girls were extremely passive. Their high passivity scores inflated the group mean to the point of violating the distributional assumptions for the *t* test.

Sex differences are indicated in the last three columns of Table 1. Two-tailed *t*-test comparisons showed the pre-schizophrenic boys to be significantly less emotionally stable than the girls ($p<.025$), but since this paralleled a similar trend among the controls ($p<.10$), the sex $\times$ diagnosis interaction was not significant. The boys were clearly less agreeable than the girls ($p<.01$), and since the controls did not differ, the sex $\times$ diagnosis interaction was significant $p<.025$). The pattern of scores for disagreeableness was complementary, producing a highly significant sex difference among the schizophrenics on the agreeableness — disagreeableness difference score ($p = .005$) and a reliable sex $\times$ diagnosis interaction ($p<.01$). One further impression of the pervasiveness of the sex differences can be gained from the interaction trends in parentheses in the last column. On four of the five negative factors there were slight sex $\times$ diagnosis interaction trends ($p<.20$). The pre-schizophrenic boys had the higher scores for emotional instability and disagreeableness, but the lower scores for introversion and passivity.

Table A summarizes the analysis of the categories within the factors where significant differences were found. The category data were analyzed in the following way. A subject's ratio score for a negative category (e.g., underachieving) was subtracted from his score for the corresponding positive category (e.g., achieving) to arrive at a difference score. The same was done for his control(s), and the control scores were averaged. A paired t test was computed to measure the difference between the pre-schizophrenics and matched controls on each category. The one-tailed probability values associated with each test of the difference are reported for boys and girls separately. The results are that the boys were slightly lower than their controls on self-control and significantly less achieving, dependable, cheerful, adjusted, pleasant, cooperative, considerate, and well behaved. They would have encountered difficulty in the Boy Scouts. It is equally clear that the majority were not shy and withdrawn — the shut-in personality type was the exception among the boys.

On the other side, the girls were slightly more immature and egocentric than their controls, and significantly more insecure, maladjusted, unsociable, and quiet. They were also *less* nervous than the control girls ($p<.01$, two-tailed test), which produced a significant sex interaction. This apparently complimentary trait, however, seemed to covary with others (quiet, passive) that indicate a generally inactive pattern. Moreover, the difference on this category rested primarily on the teachers' descriptions of nervousness in the controls. Thus, it appears that the norm for girls was to be nervous, restless, and worried, and the pre-schizophrenic girls deviated from that pattern.

201

The principal sex differences appeared under Factor 5. Relative to their normal counterparts, the boys were more unpleasant, negativistic, and antisocial than the girls.

Developmental Trends. The results of an extensive analysis of longitudinal changes in the school behavior of 39 pre-schizophrenic children and their matched controls can be summarized briefly. The factor scores for each subject were broken down and analyzed for two time periods: grades K–6 and grades 7–12. Some evidence of introversion, passivity, and emotional instability in the pre-schizophrenic girls emerged in the early grades, but the boys were indistinguishable from their controls during this period. The clearest signs of introversion in the girls were reported in grades 7–12. The only indication of emotional instability and a dramatic turn toward disagreeableness characterized the pre-schizophrenic boys in the adolescent years. The major developmental trends are shown graphically in Figures 1 and 2 (deposited with NAPS). From this I conclude that incipient behavioral deviations may appear in the primary school years, at least those of the introverted kind shown by the girls. However, from the point of view of *efficient* early identification, the optimum time to begin screening for behavioral signs of risk is in the junior high school years, age 12 to 15.

Personality Trait Ratings in High School. In the grades 10 and 11 and occasionally in grade 12, 4–6 teachers independently rated the children on 8–10 personality rating scales. Two different rating systems were used, the first for 1941–1955 and the second for 1955–1964. Of the schizophrenics, 30 (13 males, 17 females) had data only for the "old" coding system, and 17 (7 males, 10 females) had ratings only in the new system; 4 males had some ratings in both systems. All ratings for each subject were averaged to give a single score for each variable, keeping the systems separate. The same was done for the matched controls. The groups were then compared with the Wilcoxon matched-pairs signed-ranks test. The results are summarized in Tables B and C.

The results for the old system are quite consistent with the previous analyses of the teachers' qualitative descriptions. The pre-schizophrenic boys were rated lower on personality, reliability, and general promise for success. The pre-schizophrenic girls were rated lower for personality, initiative, and leadership. The results for the new system were surprising. Predictably, the pre-schizophrenic boys were lower on emotional stability. However, the girls were higher than their controls in industry and responsibility and slightly higher in motivation. These differences all produced significant sex interactions. Indeed, the 10 "new" schizophrenic females, relative to their respective controls, were significantly ($p<.025$) more industrious than the 17 "old" schizophrenic females. This unexpected result could be considered a sampling anomaly, but I'm inclined to think not. All three of the rating scale differences rested upon the scores of the same 6 (of 10) girls. Of these, 3 girls were otherwise described as extremely (top quartile of teachers' comments) stable emotionally, outgoing, and/or assertive; the other 3 were just as extremely (bottom quartile) unstable, introverted, and/or passive. The first half were obviously exceptional girls who were very bright and pleased the teachers immensely. The second half clearly had more emotional handicaps but were no less conscientious in their schoolwork. I think this pattern of extreme conscientiousness in the girls is worth some attention in prediction studies.

Intellectual Functioning. As a part of this research program, Amy Lubensky (1972) analyzed the childhood intelligence and scholastic performance of the schizophrenics, comparing them with their controls and their own siblings. Combining and standardizing all the test measures of intelligence, she found that the average IQ of the schizophrenics (102.86) was significantly lower ($p<.01$, two-tailed test) than that of their controls (107.66). However, they did not differ significantly from their siblings, a more stringent control group.

School marks were also available for grades 7–12. Lubensky analyzed the marks for English and math. The schizophrenics did not differ from either their controls or their siblings in English, nor from their siblings in math. However, their math grades were significantly lower ($p<.05$, two-tailed test) than their classmate controls'.

From these data, we conclude that, as a group, pre-schizophrenics are somewhat impaired in their intellectual functioning, primarily in the area of quantitative skills. This deficiency seems to be related to low scholastic motivation, but, it seems doubtful that these indices would be powerful predictors of schizophrenic outcome. Such practical considerations should not, on the other hand, detract from their potential significance for theoretical conceptualization of schizophrenic development. Our results are generally consistent with the findings of Lane and Albee (1970).

Other Indications of Risk. From various parts of the school record we were able to glean some evidence about other factors which could logically be expected to contribute to schizophrenic outcome. Since this information was not systematically recorded for all children, these findings must be considered tentative. However, we have no reason to expect systematic bias in the recording for schizophrenics and controls, since our classification was based on subsequent outcome. The findings will be summarized here.

There was a greater frequency of parental death before completion of high school among the schizophrenics (19 per cent) than among their matched controls (8 per cent). That difference was highly significant ($p<.005$, one-tailed binomial test). The difference was also significant ($p<.025$) when the schizophrenics were compared with a random sample of 907 control records for which the parental death rate was 10 per cent. Incidentally, the rate for the 17 manic-depressives (18 per cent) was also larger ($p<.01$) than for their 43 controls (0), but the neurotics (3 per cent) and personality disorders (7 per cent) had rates equal to their controls. These findings are similar to Barry's (1937).

Organic handicaps (sensory impairment, neurological disorders, obesity, heart condition, etc.) were reported more frequently ($p<.005$) for schizophrenics (39 per cent) than their controls' (21 per cent). There was also more evidence of internal family conflict (33 versus 23 per cent, $p<.05$). There were only slight trends toward difference ($p<.20$) for parental separation and long physical illness.

POSTDICTING SCHIZOPHRENIC OUTCOME

Deriving a prediction formula from one relatively small sample of data is at best problematic, and it is especially so in this case, where the vagaries of sampling and the attrition to be expected in cross-validation (Meehl & Rosen, 1955) are compounded by limitations in the quality of the original data. Still, the original data are concrete and relatively unbiased, and tangible, persuasive evidence seems necessary in order to counter the pervasive skepticism about predicting so rare a disorder as schizophrenia. Here, I am less concerned with the specific findings of our study, though these provide the framework for my thinking, than with the larger argument that *schizophrenics are observably maladjusted in childhood.*

Five elements were selected for postdicting schizophrenic outcome: (a) parental death, (b) severe organic handicap, (c) extreme family conflict, (d) extreme emotional instability, and (e) extreme introversion for girls or extreme disagreeableness for boys. The latter two measures were obtained by selecting individuals whose factor difference scores for those variables in the teachers' comments fell in the bottom quartile of the distribution of controls. Conceivably, postdictive efficiency would have been further improved by including the high school ratings, IQ, and math grades, but the results for these measures were less clear and the illustration is emphatic enough without including them.

Each of the indices discriminates substantially between the two groups, and in combination, the discrimination is still more efficient (Table D). Combining the first three indices, 25 schizophrenics (46 per cent) and 25 controls (17 per cent) either had a parent die or had a severe organic handicap or were reared in an extremely conflicted home atmosphere. Combining the other indices, 10 of the schizophrenic males (37 per cent) and 6 of their controls (8 per cent) had scores on the teacher comment codes in the bottom quartile for both emotional stability and agreeableness. Among the females, 9 schizophrenics (33 per cent) and 7 controls (10 per cent) had scores in the bottom quartile for both emotional stability and extroversion. Table E presents the results when all the indices are combined.

The rule for postdicting schizophrenic outcome is as follows: A subject *either* had a parent die *or* had a severe organic handicap *or* suffered extreme family conflict *or* had scores in the bottom quartiles for *both* discriminating factors for his/her sex (i.e., emotional stability and extroversion for girls, but emotional stability and agreeableness for boys). Applying the formula post hoc to this sample of 197 subjects identifies 34 "true" schizophrenics (17 per cent of the total sample) and 105 "true" non-schizophrenics (53 per cent of the total sample). The formula also postdicts 38 "false" schizophrenics (19 per cent of the total sample) and 20 "false" non-schizophrenics (10 per cent of the total sample). Thus, it correctly categorizes seven out of ten subjects. The most important figures in Table E are that 63 per cent of the schizophrenics (correctly) and 27 per cent of the controls (incorrectly) would be designated as at risk for schizophrenia. If the frequencies in the last column are extrapolated to approximate the actual preponderance of non-schizophrenics in an unlimited population (97–99 per cent), a crude estimate of the predictive efficiency of the formula can be computed.

Table F projects the results to be expected from such a predictive study, assuming a prevalence of 2 per cent schizophrenic outcomes in the general population initially sampled. Approximately 5 per cent of the children designated at risk would actually become schizophrenic. If schizophrenic prevalence were only 1 per cent, the proportion of schizophrenic outcomes in the risk sample would be lower (2 per cent), but if the prevalence turned out to be 3 per cent (Yolles & Kramer, 1969), then the "payoff" in schizophrenic outcomes would be higher (7 per cent). An important advantage of such a prospective study is that a substantial portion of the children at risk would become psychologically deviant, though not schizophrenic. Moreover, those children at risk who did *not* become deviant adults would constitute a distinctive control group: emotionally *invulnerable* children (Garmezy, 1970). From the latter we might learn a good deal about the natural forces that work to prevent schizophrenic or other deviant outcomes.

CONCLUSION

As a group children destined to be schizophrenic adults behave differently in school than do other children. A third to a half of them are identifiable in childhood before they show any clear indications of psychotic disorganization. Behavioral deviations are obvious enough that teachers comment on them spontaneously in cumulative school records. The patterns of maladjustment differ for boys and girls. Therefore, any attempts at early identification of emotionally vulnerable children should look for different signs of risk in boys than in girls. Specifically, the boys in this study were negativistic, egocentric, unpleasant, and antisocial, whereas the girls were primarily quiet and introverted though also slightly egocentric. In addition, the boys were scholastic underachievers and were undependable. Both sexes were emotionally unstable, but even here the boys and girls differed qualitatively — the boys were cheerless, emotional, and *actively* maladjusted, whereas the girls were calm, insecure, immature and *quietly* maladjusted.

The introverted tendencies of the girls began to emerge in the primary grades, but the boys were hardly distinguishable from their controls at that time. Sharp differences appeared in both sexes by the early adolescent years. It may be that the longitudinal changes represent only increments in degree of deviation rather than fundamental changes in their modes of adjustment in school. In reading the school records clinically, the continuity of adjustment styles over time was much more impressive than the evidence of dramatic change. For example, the pre-schizophrenic boys were significantly more disagreeable than their controls in the later school years, though they did not differ appreciably in grade school, producing a significant temporal interaction. It is clear from individual inspection that abrasive pre-schizophrenic boys were becoming somewhat more abrasive and well-behaved ones were becoming somewhat less well behaved, but there were no startling transformations with age. The optimum time to identify children with behavioral risk for schizophrenia is in early adolescence.

As a group, the childhood intelligence of schizophrenics is lower than average but not lower than their own siblings'. Impairment of quantitative performance is the greatest, and this may be a subtle prodromal sign of the radical cognitive disruption that occurs in many adult schizophrenics.

Pre-schizophrenic children have an unusually high frequency of parental deaths, organic handicaps, and family conflicts, all of which can be expected logically to affect psychological growth adversely.

Finally, a formula incorporating five of these factors quite efficiently postdicted schizophrenic outcome. I wish to make no extravagant claims about the potential efficiency of such a formula for predicting schizophrenia, but only to emphasize that the majority of schizophrenics are observably, and usually extremely, maladjusted in childhood.

COMMENTARY

MACK. Some of the follow up that Ricks and I and others did at a child guidance clinic ultimately led Ricks to move from following the kids to looking at the therapists. To what degree do the teachers play a role in the phenomena that they are describing? We know the power of expectancy phenomena, and I wonder what kind of role it plays in such things as emotional stability and agreeableness. Did you find any data having to do with teachers' ratings across children and children's ratings across teachers? Are there in fact two kinds of consistency? Teachers have told me, "The child is saucy and what's even worse, he's now becoming nervous." I went to see the child, and yes, he was saucy. The teacher sure was making him nervous. He made me nervous. If I had a chance, I would like to study the teachers.

WATT. I thoroughly agree with you. We are trying now to get a variety of teachers to rate the same children; perhaps in another eight years I can report the results of that study. It is important to take seriously the effect the teacher's behavior has upon the children. That may be of very paramount significance in understanding these elements of alienation, especially in the records of the pre-schizophrenic boys.

ROLF. We found that one thing that differentiated at least the sons of the schizophrenic mothers were peer ratings — their peers really disliked them. The teachers thought they were OK. They rated them a little lower than their matched or random controls in the same classroom, but to teachers these Ss were perhaps the highest, best adjusted, of our four target groups, whereas peers judged the sons of schizophrenic mothers to be almost as bad as the externalizing kids (bullies, etc.) in the classroom. However, teachers were better at discriminating the daughters of schizophrenic mothers at this earlier age in grade school. Even so, both sons and daughters of schizophrenic mothers were rated as being rather aggressive — at least 40 per cent of daughters, and 50 or so per cent of sons being so rated, whereas 3 per cent of the matched control groups were.

WATT. A number of studies (e.g., Roff, 1963; Bower, 1960) have shown the same thing with regard to peer ratings. We found little evidence of aggressiveness in the pre-schizophrenic girls. There were a few aggressive Ss, but I believe that this pattern will show up in any other studies of females.

ZUBIN. I admire Watt's enthusiasm. The last time I saw such enthusiasm displayed was from Franz Kallman on the opposite end of the scale. However, I don't quite understand why you are teetering between genetics and environment. All that you report could be based on the genetic background. It doesn't have to be, but I don't know that any of your data would negate genetic disposition or diathesis.

WATT. I agree with you.

ZUBIN. We used to argue with Franz Kallman about the 15 per cent of the monozygotic twins that are discordant. And he, of course, would say that we shall find a reason for this eventually. What about the 37 per cent that you cannot include in your risk? I think that the literature in this field, and of course the more recent work of Lane and Albee, has put a new view on the matter, but basically your statement that schizophrenics are observably maladjusted in childhood is not borne out by the facts. Not all those who become schizophrenic later can be identified earlier. You yourself point out 37 per cent that you cannot detect. I think we must realize that there are some studies in the field now, dealing not with childhood but later periods, which demonstrate that there is a split or a separation between personality and psychopathology. For example, Essen-Moeller and Ole Hagnelle have demonstrated that you could not have predicted from the personality characteristics of the population in 1947 who was going to develop mental disorder in 1957. So let's not go overboard and say that we can now identify every one of these people ahead of time.

Let me say one more thing about your giving bad marks for schizophrenics. Victor Bergen is just finishing a dissertation in which he demonstrates, using Project Talent tests for verbal behavior, that although in grades nine and ten the subsequent mental casualties are lower than their controls, in grades eleven and twelve they exceed their controls. The data deal with all admissions to mental hospitals and not necessarily with schizophrenics alone. So I think there are some good things about schizophrenics as well as bad things, and we can't always mark them down in this fashion.

Now I didn't mean earlier that there has to be a genetic core to the disorder. In fact, there are now several studies in the field that demonstrate possible nongenetic sources of schizophrenia. For example, H. B. M. Murphy has found in Canada, where they have censuses of ethnic origin, that the Catholics in every ethnic group he has studied have higher rates of schizophrenia than non-Catholics. And although this is only "hospital-ized" data and we don't know the whole story, it looks as if there is at least a potential problem in discovering whether sociocultural forces alone may not be sufficient to elicit a schizophrenic condition.

CHESS. I'd like to raise two questions, one of which was already men-tioned, but I have had some trouble with it. That is the question of using the cumulative records of teachers. About 15 or 20 years ago, a school health survey was done to see whether remedial measures for physical health hazards identified in third grade were taken before the sixth grade follow-up. The question was raised whether there could be any mental health aspect to the follow-up studies. I was elected to find out whether there was indeed a base point in the school records, and I spent days and days and days reading cumulative records to find out whether there were any reliable data that could be used to put markers on the children. What impressed me more than anything else was the degree to which even the very same wording was used by very busy teachers, obviously filling out that time-consuming cumulative record with its lengthy scale of behavioral items. But every once in a while in the middle of this repetition, there would be a teacher's note, "I don't know why these previous teachers put this down, I find this child . . ." — and then would come a string of adjectives contrary to what had been checked off before. I was impressed that the teacher's harassment and lack of time were more important than the question of sitting down and thinking about each individual child. Now, you said that you found a school system with unusually good records and that this method might be applicable only to this system or to this particular school. It would be useful if we could generally, throughout the nation, tag our children. But from my experience in New York City, I wouldn't rely on these records for this purpose, except possibly the very first one, if a child transferred into a school.

Now, for my other question. With regard to scholastic motivation, one question of contamination that we found coming up in our longitudinal study, particularly with the parents of our children but also with the teachers, is that distractability frequently is reported in motivational terms.

WATT. We included it in our factors.

CHESS. Yes, but I'm talking about the teachers' reporting, where the possibility is very great that they would report poor motivation when in fact what they observed was high distractability.

WATT. I'm saying if they said distractable, we coded it as scholas-tically unmotivated.

COMMENT. Then you may have made the mistakes, not the teacher.

REFERENCES

Anthony, E. J. The developmental precursors of schizophrenia. In D. Rosenthal & S. S. Kety (Eds.), *The transmission of schizophrenia.* Oxford: Pergamon Press, 1968.

Barry, H., & Bousfield, W. A. Incidence of orphanhood among fifteen hundred psychotic patients. *Journal of Genetic Psychology*, 1937, 50, 198–201.

Bleuler, E. *Dementia praecox, or the group of schizophrenias*. Leipzig: Deutsche, 1911. English trans.: New York: International Universities Press, 1950.

Bower, E. M. *Early identification of emotionally handicapped children in school*. Springfield, Ill.: Thomas, 1960.

Cowen, E. I., Zax, M., Izzo, L. D., & Trost, M. A. Prevention of emotional disorders in the school setting: A further investigation. *Journal of Consulting Psychology*, 1966, 30, 381–387.

D'Andrade, R. Trait psychology and componential analysis. *American Anthropologist*, 1965, 67, 215–228.

Erlenmeyer-Kimling, L., Rainer, J. D., & Kallmann, F. J. Current reproductive trends in schizophrenia. In P. H. Hoch & J. Zubin (Eds.), *Psychopathology of schizophrenia*. New York: Grune & Stratton, 1966.

Fleming, P. Emotions of children before schizophrenia and before character disorder. In M. Roff & D. F. Ricks (Eds.), *Life history research in psychopathology*. Vol. 1. Minneapolis: University of Minnesota Press, 1970.

Garmezy, N. Vulnerable children: Implications derived from studies of an internalizing-externalizing symptom dimension. In J. Zubin & A. M. Freedman (Eds.), *Psychopathology of adolescence*. New York: Grune & Stratton, 1970.

————. Research strategies for the study of children who are at risk for schizophrenia. In M. M. Katz, R. Littlestone, L. Mosher, M. S. Roath, & A. H. Tuma (Eds.), *Schizophrenia: Implications of research findings for treatment and teaching*. In press.

Heston, L. L. Psychiatric disorders in foster home reared children of schizophrenic mothers. *British Journal of Psychiatry*, 1966, 112, 819–825.

Kellam, S. G., & Schiff, S. K. Adaptation and mental illness in the first-grade classrooms of an urban community. *Psychiatric Research Reports*, 1967, 21, 79–91.

Kety, S. S., Rosenthal, D., Wender, P. H., & Schulsinger, F. The types and prevalence of mental illness in the biological and adoptive families of adopted schizophrenics. In D. Rosenthal & S. S. Kety (Eds.), *The transmission of schizophrenia*. Oxford: Pergamon Press, 1968.

Khleif, B. B. Teachers as predictors of juvenile delinquency and psychiatric disturbance. *Social Problems*, 1964, 11, 270–282.

Lane, E. A., & Albee, G. W. Early childhood intellectual differences between schizophrenic adults and their siblings. *Journal of Abnormal and Social Psychology*, 1964, 68, 193–195.

————. Intellectual antecedents of schizophrenia. In M. Roff & D. F. Ricks (Eds.), *Life history research in psychopathology*. Vol. 1. Minneapolis: University of Minnesota Press, 1970.

Lubensky, A. Intelligence and school performance of children hospitalized for schizophrenia as adults. Ph.D. thesis, Harvard University, 1972.

Mednick, S. A. Breakdown in individuals at high risk for schizophrenia: Possible predispositional perinatal factors. *Mental Hygiene*, 1970, 54, 50–63.

Meehl, P., & Rosen, A. Antecedent probability and the efficiency of psychometric signs, patterns or cutting scores. *Psychological Bulletin*, 1955, 52, 194–216.

Mensch, I. N., Kantor, M. B., Domke, H. R., Gildea, M. C. L., & Glidewell, J. C. Children's behavior symptoms and their relationships to school adjustment, sex, and social class. *Journal of Social Issues*, 1959, 15, 8–15.

Mitchell, J. C. A study of teachers' and mental hygienists' ratings of certain behavior problems of children. *Journal of Educational Research*, 1942, 36, 292–307.

Ricks, D. F., & Berry, J. C. Family and symptom patterns that precede schizophrenia. In M. Roff & D. F. Ricks (Eds.), *Life history research in psychopathology*. Vol. 1. Minneapolis: University of Minnesota Press, 1970.

Robins, L. N. *Deviant children grown up.* Baltimore: Williams & Wilkins, 1966.

Roff, M. Childhood social interactions and young adult psychosis. *Journal of Clinical Psychology,* 1963, 19, 152–157.

Rosenthal, D. *Genetic theory and abnormal behavior.* New York: McGraw-Hill, 1970.

Rubin, E. Z., Simson, C., & Betwee, M. *Emotionally handicapped children and the elementary school.* Detroit: Wayne State University Press, 1966.

Simon, K. A., & Grant, W. V. *1970 digest of educational statistics.* Washington, D.C.: GPO, 1970.

Ullmann, C. A. *Identification of maladjusted school children: A comparison of three methods of screening.* Public Health Monograph No. 7. Washington, D.C.: GPO, 1952.

Watt, N. F. Longitudinal changes in the social behavior of children hospitalized for schizophrenia as adults. *Journal of Nervous and Mental Disease,* 1972, 155, 42–54.

————, Stolorow, R. D., Lubensky, A. W., & McClelland, D. C. School adjustment and behavior of children hospitalized for schizophrenia as adults. *American Journal of Orthopsychiatry,* 1970, 40, 637–657.

Wittman, M., & Steinberg, D. A study of prodromal factors in mental illness with special reference to schizophrenia. *American Journal of Psychiatry,* 1944, 100, 811–816.

Yolles, S. F., & Kramer, M. Vital statistics. In L. Bellak & L. Loeb (Eds.), *The schizophrenic syndrome.* New York: Grune & Stratton, 1969.

Zigler, E., & Phillips, L. Social effectiveness and symptomatic behaviors. *Journal of Abnormal and Social Psychology,* 1960, 61, 231–238.

JEROME K. MYERS
JACOB J. LINDENTHAL
MAX P. PEPPER

Life Events and Psychiatric Symptomatology

THIS IS A report on relationships between changes in life events and changes in psychiatric symptomatology in a community sample of 720 adults in New Haven, Connecticut. It is part of a longitudinal study of the population of a community mental health center catchment area (Lindenthal et al., 1970, 1971; Myers et al., 1971, 1972; Paykel et al., 1969). The major aims of the larger research are (a) to understand relationships between health and social role performance; (b) to determine knowledge and attitudes about psychiatric, health, and social service facilities and the utilization patterns of these facilities for persons within the catchment area; (c) to determine how individuals cope with or handle the crises of family living, including mental health problems, and how these problems develop; and (d) to determine to what extent psychiatric and medical symptoms and social role performance vary over time with situational stress and life crises.

The theoretical framework for this paper finds its roots in two bodies of sociomedical literature, namely, stress research and epidemiological field studies of mental illness. The positive relationship between the occurrence of "stress," "life crises," or "life events" and the onset of physical illness and/or the presence of psychiatric symptomatology has been demonstrated in numerous sociomedical studies during the last two decades

NOTE: The research upon which this paper is based was supported by PHS Contract No. 43-67-743 and Research Grant No. MH-15522 from NIMH, Department of Health, Education, and Welfare. At the time of the research, all of the authors were affiliated with Yale University.

This paper was published, in slightly different form, as J. K. Myers, J. J. Lindenthal, M. P. Pepper, and D. R. Ostrander, "Life Events and Mental Status: A Longitudinal Study," *Journal of Health and Social Behavior*, 1972, 13, 398–406, and appears here by permission of the American Sociological Association.

(Brown & Birley, 1968; Fischer et al., 1962; Graham & Stevenson, 1963; Greene, 1954; Greene et al., 1956; Greene & Miller, 1958; Hawkins et al., 1957; Hinkle & Wolff, 1957; Kissen, 1958; Rahe, 1969; Rahe et al., 1964; Rahe & Holmes, 1965; Weiss et al., 1957). In five recent studies, for example, significant relationships were found between life events and illness in such diverse groups as naval personnel aboard ship, male college students, patients in a university hospital, schizophrenics, and depressed patients under treatment (Brown & Birley, 1968; Paykel et al., 1969; Rahe et al., 1970; Spilken & Jacobs, 1971; Wyler et al., 1971).

The epidemiological literature, in turn, indicates that a significant proportion of the population is psychiatrically impaired (Gurin et al., 1960; Leighton et al., 1963; Myers et al., 1971; Phillips, 1966; Srole et al., 1962). Exact rates vary according to the specific operational definitions of psychological distress, but field studies since 1950 suggest that between 15 and 20 per cent of the population exhibit high symptomatology, with the proportion of mildly disturbed as high as 80 per cent. Some researchers — such as Tyhurst (1957), Dohrenwend and Dohrenwend (1965), and Haberman (1965) — have questioned the meaning of these findings, reasoning that a portion of the symptomatology reported in epidemiological field studies may be induced by stressful events in the contemporary situation and may be temporary rather than a manifestation of basic and persistent psychological disorder.

Most research in stress and mental illness, though provocative theoretically, has been handicapped methodologically in at least four respects: (a) Such investigations have been restricted to very specific populations, such as schizophrenics, college students, and alcoholics. (b) The number of respondents has been relatively small. (c) The range and number of life events examined have been limited. (d) Most studies were made at one point in time, except for the Dohrenwend (1969) and Haberman (1965) panels, which had small numbers. Thus, it has been impossible to determine the stability of the relationships between life events and mental status.

The current study permits for the first time a detailed examination over time of relationships between large numbers of life events and mental status in a large community sample. Myers et al. (1971) reported, on the basis of data in our study, that the greater the number of life events experienced by a respondent in the year before being interviewed, the greater the likelihood of psychological impairment. In this paper we shall determine whether or not changes in the occurrence of life events over time and their patterning are related to changes in the degree of psychological distress.

Methodology

The sample consists of one adult selected at random from each of 720 households in a systematic sample of a mental health catchment area of approximately 72,000 people in metropolitan New Haven. The area includes a changing inner-city section of 22,000 and a more stable industrial town of 50,000. It represents a cross-section of the community's population and includes all ethnic, racial, and socioeconomic groups. Interviews were conducted in person with each respondent between July 1967 and January 1968. A total of 1,095 individuals were contacted. Of these, 12 per cent refused to be interviewed, 2 per cent could not be reached at home, and 86 per cent (938) were interviewed.

Two years later the same population was reinterviewed. Of the original 938, 8 per cent refused to be reinterviewed, 11 per cent had moved out of the area, 4 per cent had died, and 77 per cent (720) were reinterviewed. It is these 720 persons who provided the data on which this paper is based. With one exception, the reinterviewed sample did not differ significantly from the original cohort within any of the major categories of the following variables: social class, race, sex, religion, marital status, mental status, and age. The exception cited above was the *under 30 age group*, which dropped from 25 per cent in 1967 to 19 per cent in 1969.

Information was gathered for each respondent on the following dimensions: (a) basic demographic variables, (b) physical health status, (c) mental health status (as measured by items which have been found to discriminate between psychiatrically sick and healthy populations), (d) social and instrumental role performance, (e) help-seeking behavior and use of community health and social agency facilities, and (f) life crises which occurred during the past year. We defined such crises or events as experiences involving a role transformation, changes in status or environment, or impositions of pain (Antonovsky & Kats, 1967). The respondent was asked whether any of 62 such events had occurred to him in the year preceding our interview. This list of events was based upon selected items developed by Antonovsky and Kats (1967), Holmes and Rahe (Hawkins et al., 1957; Rahe et al., 1964), and an array of other items we developed. These events ranged from a change in residence, a child starting school, marriage, and loss of job *to* divorce, serious illness, and the death of a

214

loved one. In addition, there were open-ended questions to elicit information about events that may not have been covered in the list. If a given event did occur, the respondent was queried systematically about any change in social role performance and physical or mental health status. The events can be analyzed individually or in terms of larger conceptual categories.

Psychopathology is measured by an index of mental status. Although a comprehensive evaluation of mental status requires an extensive clinical examination in which a composite assessment is made of the individual's behavior, thought, and emotional processes, recent studies have employed short screening devices as an alternative to this clinical evaluation (Leighton et al., 1963; Phillips, 1966; Rogler & Hollingshead, 1965; Srole, 1962).

Screening tests are not new (Hunt et al., 1944). They were developed during World War I, and by World War II were widely used in the military services. Among the better known symptom checklists was the Neuropsychiatric Screening Adjunct developed during World War II (Stouffer et al., 1949, 1950). Later, other instruments were developed which could be readily administered in the field by non-psychiatrists to a large number of individuals for epidemiological and community studies of mental illness. In the Nova Scotia studies, MacMillan developed a 16-item scale, the Health Opinion Survey (HOS), which was based in part on the Neuropsychiatric Screening Adjunct (Leighton et al., 1963; MacMillan, 1957). Srole et al. (1962) used a number of the same questions in the Midtown Study, and Gurin et al. (1960) further modified the scale for a nationwide survey of mental health. More recently, Phillips (1966) utilized a similar instrument in a New England study, and Rogler and Hollingshead (1965) used both the HOS scale and a modification of it in their Puerto Rican research.

Although such scales may not be notably successful in identifying a particular individual with a particular set of psychological problems, except perhaps for extremely disturbed or impaired individuals, research indicates that these mental health scales or symptom inventories are reliable and valid in discriminating between groups of psychiatric patients and controls. The scales are suitable for our purpose because we were interested primarily in groups of people, not individuals. In the Stirling County, Nova Scotia, Midtown, and Puerto Rican studies, the scales differentiated between respondents diagnosed by psychiatrists as having psychiatric problems and respondents judged as not having such difficulties. Also, Manis et al. (1964) demonstrated that such a mental health scale distinguished between hospitalized and non-hospitalized groups.

We adopted the instrument developed by MacMillan (1957) and further modified by Gurin et al. (1960). It lists 20 psychiatric symptoms which are scored and developed into an index of mental status. Examples of the questions are: "Do you ever feel that you are bothered by all sorts of pains or ailments in different parts of your body?" "Do you ever have trouble in getting to sleep or staying asleep?" "Are you ever bothered by nervousness (feeling fidgety, irritable, tense)?" A response of often is scored 1; sometimes, 2; hardly ever, 3; never, 4. Scores range from 20 (maximum impairment) to 80 (total absence of symptoms). Previous research indicates that relatively low scores identify individuals with major psychological problems and that the individual scores may be grouped into larger categories (Jackson, 1962; Leighton et al., 1963; Srole et al., 1962). We have examined our data both in terms of individual scores and by categories. When dealing with categories, we have classified those scoring 66 and lower as "very distressed psychologically," those scoring between 67 and 76 as "moderately distressed," and those scoring 77 and above as "relatively symptom free" (Jackson, 1962).

Results

We discovered a significant amount of psychiatric symptomatology in the community, as has been found in other field studies. In 1967, 18 per cent of the adults interviewed were classified as having a high symptom level, 47 per cent as a medium symptom level, and 35 per cent as a low symptom level. In 1969, the corresponding percentage distribution was very similar. During this two-year period, the Gurin scores for 54 per cent of the study population remained at the same symptom level, 21 per cent became worse, and 25 per cent improved by one or two levels. Changes in terms of actual Gurin point scores were similar to those by Gurin category: 58 per cent changed less than 5 points, 18 per cent changed for the worse by 5 or more points, and 24 per cent improved to a similar degree.

In 1967, 20 per cent of the respondents had experienced no events in the year preceding the interview; 28 per cent, one event; 20 per cent, two events; 11 per cent, three events; 6 per cent, four events; and 15 per cent, five or more events. In 1969 the distribution was practically the same. Over the two-year period the changes in the number of events experienced by the study group were as follows: no change, 21 per cent; net increase, 42 per cent; and net decrease, 37 per cent.

Table 1. Change in Number of Events and in Psychiatric Symptomatology,
1967–1969

Net Change in Events	Worse[a]				0[a]	Better[a]			
	15+	6–14	2–5	1		1	2–5	6–14	15+
Increase									
4 or more ...	15	33	62	73	77	84	99	100	100
2 or 3	1	21	52	59	72	76	87	96	100
1	2	18	38	42	50	60	84	99	100
No change	2	11	29	32	45	54	82	96	100
Decrease									
1	0	4	23	26	50	66	86	99	100
2 or 3	0	11	25	33	37	42	66	97	100
4 or more ...	2	9	20	22	27	29	50	85	100

SOURCE: J. K. Myers, J. J. Lindenthal, M. P. Pepper, and D. R. Ostrander, "Life Events and Mental Status: A Longitudinal Study," *Journal of Health and Social Behavior*, 1972, 18, 401, Table 2.
[a]Changes in Gurin scores, in cumulative percentage.

The important question is whether or not there is a relationship between changes in mental status scores and changes in the occurrence of life events. We found that there is indeed such a relationship: the greater the number of changes in life events, the *more likely* are the psychiatric symptoms of the individual to have changed substantially. More specifically, a net increase in life events is associated with a worsening of symptomatology, a decrease with improvement. Of those persons who had a net increase of two or more life events, 21 per cent displayed an improvement in their symptomatology (more than 1-point change in the Gurin scale), whereas, for those who experienced a net decrease of two or more events, 64 per cent improved. In contrast, the corresponding figures for a symptom's worsening were 56 per cent and 23 per cent.

A more detailed picture of this relationship demonstrates that the greater the net change in number of events, the greater the movement on the mental health scale (see Table 1). Thus, 15 per cent of those persons who had a net increase of four or more events changed 15 or more points for the worse on the Gurin scale, whereas only 2 per cent of those who had a net decrease of four or more events did so. The difference between an increase of four or more events and a similar net decrease is seen clearly in the cumulative percentages presented in Table 1: 62 per cent of the former but only 20 per cent of the latter had a 2-point or greater worsening of symptomatology; the cumulative percentages which include no change or a change for the worse in psychological status were 77 and 27, respectively.

We questioned whether this same pattern would hold when the number of events experienced in 1967 and the general symptom level at that time were both controlled. That is, we determined the relationship between changes in events and changes in symptoms for only those persons who had no events in 1967, one event, two events, etc., and for those who had a high, a medium, and a low symptom level. When these controls were introduced, the same pattern held. Likewise, when we examined the data in terms of Gurin category changes (rather than actual point scores as shown in Table 1), we found the same pattern.

INDIVIDUAL EVENTS

We then studied the relationship between change in events and change in symptoms for each event. Three types of statistical testing were employed: tests of significance, correlation, and regression analysis. Of 64 events taken separately, all but 6 were in the predicted direction — that is, a greater proportion of those persons who underwent the event recently (in 1969 but not in 1967) experienced a worsening of symptomatology, whereas those who sustained the event only in 1967 were more likely to improve. The exceptions were pregnancy, birth of child, adopting a child, new person moved into household, out of work over a month, and

Table 2. Changes in Gurin Categories and in Selected Life Events, 1967–1969

Life Event	Improved[a]	No Change[a]	Worse[a]	N[b]
Graduated from school				
Never experienced event ..	24	55	21	605
1967 but not 1969	43	45	12	49
1969 but not 1967	20	51	29	55
Changes in relations with neighbors				
Never experienced event ..	25	55	20	691
1967 but not 1969	36	55	9	22
1969 but not 1967	33	17	50	6
Finances worse				
Never experienced event ..	24	56	20	675
1967 but not 1969	52	36	12	25
1969 but not 1967	13	43	44	16

SOURCE: J. K. Myers, J. J. Lindenthal, M. P. Pepper, and D. R. Ostrander, "Life Events and Mental Status: A Longitudinal Study," *Journal of Health and Social Behavior*, 1972, 18, 403, Table 3.

[a]Changes in Gurin categories in percentages.

[b]Total numbers do not necessarily add to 720 since in a few cases life events were present in both years. Unfortunately, there were not enough cases of this type to include in the analysis.

divorce. Examples of the relationship between change in events and change in symptoms are presented in Table 2.

A major difficulty in research on life crises and mental illness has been that many events treated as independent variables may have been the result of the individual's mental status rather than its precipitant. This can certainly be true for variables such as divorce, job loss, or failure in school. On the other hand, certain kinds of events are relatively independent of the individual's psychological condition, such as a major reorganization at work resulting from the merger of a local company with a national corporation or a child's starting school at the legal age. Of the 64 life events, 13 can be considered independent by this method.* For these events the recency of the occurrence of an event is related to a worsening of symptomatology. Thus, the basic finding of this paper seems to hold for life events independent of one's psychological condition as well as those which may interact with it.

CATEGORIZATION OF EVENTS

The list of events was examined and grouped into categories in three alternative but overlapping ways. The first method employed was to categorize the events in terms of the *area of social activity* which they involved. The following ten categories were developed: education-related events, relocation, marriage, family, interpersonal, health, work, finance, legal, and community crises.† The relationship between changes in number of

---

*Events classified as independent are: family member started to school, serious physical illness, serious injury or accident, death of spouse, death of other loved one, frequent minor illnesses, death of pet, major reorganization at work, retirement at appropriate age, community crisis, family member entered armed forces, family member left home for marriage, school, etc., and started to work for the first time at appropriate age.

†The individual events in each category are as follows: (1) *Education-related event*: started to school, graduated from school, failed school, changed school, problems in school; (2) *Relocation*: moved to same type of neighborhood, moved to better neighborhood, moved to worse neighborhood, built a new house; (3) *Marriage*: engaged, married, divorced, separated, intermarried, major change in relationship with spouse; (4) *Family*: engaged, married, family member entered armed forces, birth of a child, adoption of a child, new person moved into household, member of family left home, change in number of family get-togethers, pregnancy; (5) *Interpersonal*: major changes in relationship with spouse, trouble with in-laws, trouble with boss, change in relationship with friends; (6) *Health*: birth of a child, serious physical illness, serious injury or accident, pregnancy, stillbirth, frequent minor illness, mental illness; (7) *Work*: started to work for the first time, changed to same kind of job, promoted or moved to more responsible job, demoted or changed to less responsible job, laid off (temporarily), expanded business, business failed, trouble with boss, troubles at work, out of work over a month, fired, any big reorganization at work, retirement, success at work; (8) *Finance*: laid off (temporarily), business failed, out

Table 3. Change in Number of Events and Change in
Psychiatric Symptomatology, 1967–1969, for
Event Categories

Type of Event	N	r	F
Area of activity			
Legal	76	.41	16***
Interpersonal	85	.33	11***
Education	280	.32	31***
Finance	236	.29	22***
Marriage	211	.29	20***
Work	338	.27	27***
Community crisis ...	74	.26	6**
Health	424	.19	16***
Family	402	.16	10***
Relocation	177	.12	3 ᵃ
Changes in social field			
Exit	291	.21	13***
Entrance	327	.10	3*
Desirability			
Undesirable	535	.36	80***
Desirable	386	.29	37***

*$p<.10$. **$p<.05$.
***$p<.01$. ᵃNot significant.

events and changes in symptoms within each event category was analyzed
in two ways: (a) actual point-score change, using correlations to determine the direction and strength of the relationship, and (b) Gurin category changes, employing the chi square for testing significance. The results
using correlational measures are shown in Table 3. In all analyses we
found the same pattern that existed for total events, although the level of
significance did not reach .05 for relocation events in either method of
analysis. The strength of the relationship, however, varied greatly: it was
much stronger for legal events, for example, than for family events.

The second categorization of events was *changes in the immediate social field of the respondents*. Two classes of events were so defined:
entrance-related events — entrance of a new person into the social field of
the respondent or someone close to the respondent (engagement, marriage,
birth of child, adoption of child, and a new person moved into the household); *exit-related events* — exit of a person or treasured object from the
social field of the respondent or someone close to him (death of spouse,

of work over a month, improvement in financial status, financial status a lot
worse, foreclosure of mortgage or loan; (9) *Legal*: been in court, detention in
jail, been arrested, lawsuit or legal action, loss of driver's license; (10) *Community crises*: such as fires, burglaries, redevelopment.

death of other loved one, death of pet, divorce, separation, and member of family left home). The same pattern as for total events was found for exit events (see Table 3). In contrast, while there was a trend in the same direction for entrance-related events, it did not reach the .05 level of statistical significance.

A third way of classifying events was by an evaluated dimension corresponding to *social desirability*. In terms of the currently shared values of society, one group of events which was clearly *desirable* includes graduation from school, moved to a better neighborhood, engagement, marriage, promotion in job, success at work, and improvement in financial status. The second and larger group of events was *undesirable* for most persons, such as failure in school, a move to a less desirable neighborhood, divorce, trouble with in-laws, serious injury or accident, death of a loved one, business failure, and detention in jail.* As shown in Table 3, the same relationship previously found held for both these categories, although it was far stronger for undesirable events.

Since factors other than psychological impairment may be related to the appearance of life events, we analyzed our materials further. Specifically, we determined whether seven independent variables, which could conceivably be related to the presence of life events and mental status — race, sex, age, marital status, religion, social class, and number of persons living in the household — were accounting for the relationships we found between changes in life events and changes in symptoms. For both total events and categories of events, we undertook multiple regression analyses, correlation analyses, and contingency controls. The results of all three analyses were similar and in no way negated our basic findings: the greater the change in events, the greater the change in mental status.

Discussion

The findings in this paper demonstrate a clear relationship between changes in the occurrence of selected life events in a two-year period and changes in psychiatric symptomatology: an increase in the number of events is associated with a worsening of symptoms, a decrease with an improvement.

The data shed light on the tenuous balance between the individual's

*Other events in this category include: problems in school, widowhood, separation, departure of family member from home, serious physical illness, stillbirth, mental illness, death of a pet, demotion (job), temporary loss of job, permanent loss of job, worsening of financial status, foreclosure of mortgage, court appearance, arrest, lawsuit, loss of driver's license, crisis in community.

psychic economy and the social milieu within which he is forced to adapt. They demonstrate the importance of social and interpersonal forces frequently external to the individual in influencing psychological status. The sheer quantity of events alone seems to have a striking effect upon one's capacity to maintain a state of mental health. On a more theoretical level, the findings advance our knowledge of the relationship between the challenges of everyday living and an individual's overall well-being. Apparently, not only serious crises, but almost any event requiring attention and/or some form of behavioral adaptation, may be potentially detrimental to one's mental health. Life events thus must be included in considering the coping equipment which the individual can bring to bear in his adaptive processes.

Beyond sheer quantity, the nature of the event seems to have much to do with the degree of subsequent psychopathology (see Table 3). Within the *area of activity* classification, changes in legal, interpersonal, education, finance, marriage, and work events are more strongly related to changes in symptomatology than health, family, or relocation events.

Events which bring the individual into confrontation with the legal system are most closely related to changes in psychological symptoms. Once the judicial process is under way, one has relatively little control over his destiny. Similarly, interpersonal relationships are frequently characterized by uncertainty or fear of uncertainty in terms of reciprocal expectations.* Thus, the degree of control the individual has over his experiences seems to be an important element in the relation to mental status.

Education, finance, marriage, and work all have in common the fact that they represent formal societal institutions which most directly impinge upon the destinies of individuals. Education is potentially the most influential institution in our society, since it is capable of helping the individual maintain and possibly increase his social position and/or that of his offspring (Duncan & Hodge, 1963; Lipset & Bendix, 1957).

Recent studies have demonstrated the relationship between the economy and admission to mental hospitals (Brenner, 1967, 1969). A person's financial status, security, and overall identity are related to his capacity to become integrated into the larger social system. A loss of this capacity is a social embarrassment, and for certain segments of our society it may be perceived as an indication of personal failure (Weber, 1948).

*Sullivan (1953) theorizes that interpersonal events can be interpreted as having much the same psychological meaning as catastrophic and other events over which the individual lacks control.

Marriage events clearly represent crucial changes in role for the individual and have important consequences for his life and for his self-esteem. Much of a person's identity is bound up with his work. A change in an individual's work status involves his status in the community and that of his family. A shift in jobs means altering a vast constellation of roles (Corwin et al., 1960) and values (Gersti, 1961), with possible mental health consequences (Breed, 1963).

Turning to changes in the social field, the finding that the exit of an individual from the immediate social field of the respondent is associated more strongly with changes in psychological distress than comparable entrance emphasizes the importance of object loss in the etiology of psychopathology in our culture, further suggesting a hierarchy of role transformations with respect to psychiatric symptomatology. American society with its secular, nontraditional attitudes has left the individual somewhat alone to cope with loss. Grief and mourning are denied to a larger extent in our society than in many others. Although we do have rituals to help the individual endure loss, much of this is in the form of denial. Owing to a pervasive skepticism of a world to come, once a loss occurs, the permanency of the loss is probably quite shattering to the individual. Ours is a society bent upon the pursuit of "happiness," and engagement, marriage, or birth are generally viewed as happy events. Moreover, although both gain and loss events involve challenges to an individual's role continuity and identity, more meaningful systems of social and interpersonal support may have developed around gain than around loss.

In this context, it is interesting that even changes in entrance-related events are related to changes in symptomatology, although only at the .10 level of significance. Apparently, the entrance of an individual into the social field of certain individuals is at times a sufficient threat to their psychological equilibrium to elicit symptoms associated with psychopathology. Perhaps such individuals have disturbances with libidinal cathexis which threaten identity maintenance. Or, perhaps there is a failure of immediately available support systems in the individual's social field. From a purely economic perspective, the addition of an individual to one's social milieu means parceling out vital necessities in ever-smaller portions.

As might be expected, undesirable events were found to be more highly related to changes in symptomatology than desirable ones. Clinicians have long observed the impact of frustrating experiences, or those perceived as such, upon the individual. This phenomenon has also been noted by theorists and researchers, and has been formulated in the classic frustration-aggression hypothesis of Dollard et al. (1939) and variations of it.

The results of this longitudinal study also help elucidate the meaning of symptoms and life events enumerated in the many cross-sectional community studies covering a single period of time. They emphasize clearly the importance of linking symptom prevalence and actual clinical phenomena to the overall matrix of the individual's recent life history. Psychiatric screening data are of value to the extent to which they are related to basic social and life event data. By themselves, symptom data are difficult to interpret. In interpreting these findings, we must note the possibility that the more impaired an individual, the more likely he is to report events because he feels they are stressful. However, the events we list are generally discrete and of such a factual nature that they are not likely to go unreported. For example, when the one-year time period is broken into two successive six-month periods, there is no significant difference in the number of events reported. Furthermore, what was recorded initially was the occurrence of an event, not the individual's perception of its stressfulness.

In summary, we have found a substantial and positive relationship between changes in life events and changes in psychological impairment over a two-year period. Both the quantity and quality of events have an impact upon symptoms. Certain cultural and social factors have been discussed as possibly helping to account for the relationships found. Finally, the importance of linking symptom prevalence and clinical phenomena to the matrix of the individual's recent life history has been noted.

COMMENTARY

WATT. For one type of change event, migration, you describe as one of your categorization principles that a move to a poorer area of residence is a negative change, and a move to a better area is an improvement or a positive change. Do you have any information about migration or even change of residence that does not mean a new community and its relationship to psychiatric or psychological status?

MYERS. Relocation, which is movement of any type, is the one area of social activity which is unrelated — a trend is there, but it is not statistically significant. We looked at our data almost case by case. You must recognize that we are dealing only with people who moved within metropolitan New Haven and around the state of Connecticut — if they went any great distance, we could not follow them. We found that most movement in lower-class areas was within a few blocks, and there was essentially no change in neighborhood or area. With middle-class people, there might be greater distances involved, but their moves were also to the same kind of neighborhood. For example, a young couple moved from a middle-class apartment area to a middle-class area of single family homes. Or people on the way up in their thirties and forties, who are established in the community, move one notch higher in the cost of housing, but the neighborhood is just five blocks away; even if it is five miles away, it is very much the same sort of neighborhood because the neighborhood they left was full of younger people of the same income group. So that in essence, the actual move within at least the New Haven community, which is of course a medium-sized metropolitan area, did not seem to entail the sort of change in equilibrium that our other categories did.

ROLF. One thing that differentiated our sample, at least the previous year, coinciding with maternal psychiatric treatment, was family mobility. The groups with disturbed mothers moved significantly more often than their matched controls. The year of the move was the year that the kids' grades fell apart. Should one interpret a move as stressful, or as simply associated with maternal breakdown, or what? Thus, in studying kids at risk, it's wise to match on mobility because it seems to be related to their other problems.

MYERS. Of course, we were studying persons 18 or over.

THOMAS. Was there any relationship in the group to involvement of the individuals with the community mental health centers?

MYERS. We are now studying the people in this sample who used mental health facilities, and I can't yet give you the results. We can check the Ss' reports of use of these facilities against actual records. We also have another population of people using not only the community health facilities but other kinds of facilities from this entire catchment area. We plan to get a much better picture of the use of facilities — what sort of problems bring people to a center, who comes and who doesn't, and so forth.

THOMAS. It would be of interest to learn whether some people come to the center for help when what's presumably a good event occurs in their lives.

MYERS. Oh yes.

THOMAS. This material emphasizes the dynamic importance of change, as such, in affecting intrapsychic equilibrium and level of adaptability. All the emphasis that is generally placed on the unfavorable event may miss this very issue of the stressfulness of change of any kind. On the social level, we see with all bureaucracies, and I think on the individual level, as well, that change itself is pertinent. I presume this is a major thrust of the further analyses that you are making.

MYERS. That is correct.

SCHOOLER. I have been intrigued that in the many discussions of precursors of schizophrenia at this meeting, social class really hasn't come up once except as a control. In the group that you have here, were there differences in social class and number of events? And even more intriguingly, were there differences in the effect of events within social class? In other words, did an event for somebody in a lower social class have more of an effect?

MYERS. Not much. We found the usual social class differences in the prevalence of impairment, twice as much at the bottom as at the top. We do find some social class differences in the ratio of desirable and undesirable events. That is, going down the class scale, there is a tendency for people to have more undesirable events. Also, undesirable events, or changes in them, are more strongly related to mental status than desirable events, although both are related. Clearly, some of the class differences in the prevalence is probably accounted for by this, but we do not know how much. There are no class differences in the total number of events, which surprised me. I had assumed that there would be. Also, when you control for class, by and large you get the same picture at all class levels. It may well be that class differences, if they exist, exist at different levels than this, or that a cumulative effect may be operating, but I can say that the differences by class were not nearly so striking as I had expected.

SCHOOLER. Given an event, or given a number of events looked at separately in different classes, would the number of events or the power of the event have a bigger effect on the illness level of individuals from one social class than from another?

MYERS. No, it doesn't.

VAILLANT. This paper shows the tremendous contribution that sociology is making to medicine, and I should like to try to return the favor by suggesting one kind of control that studies like this need from medicine. Doctors for a long time have learned to distinguish between signs of illness and symptoms of illness. Some people appear in general practitioners' offices who are fairly healthy and have no signs of medical illness, but who have symptoms. Also, people who have symptoms of emotional discomfort rather than signs of discomfort see psychiatrists — that is, people who are high in the Garrand score but on objective examination are pretty healthy tend to seek psychiatrists more than the stoic who may have objective emotional impairment but doesn't complain about it. I think that in studies of this kind, when you are looking at life events, you have to be sensitive to the fact that anybody who is depressed is going to be more responsive to questions such as "Has someone near to you died?" and "Do you sometimes have trouble sleeping?" In other words, if someone is depressed, and if he had pre-existing medical illness, it will be when he becomes depressed that the illness is most likely to come to his subjective impression. So that not only, as you suggested, is the emotionally ill person more sensitive, more likely to complain about life events, but it is also well to find some life events that you can check by a means other than self-report. In long-term follow-ups of individuals where I have considerable external information about their lives and also interview them, I am continually amazed at the important things that happen in someone's life which he doesn't mention in an interview. I don't think this casts any aspersion on your findings, but I think a control is to have some way, perhaps in a much smaller sample, of checking out the things that really happen.

MYERS. In a related study we're checking with family members as well, using the very same lists. Again, though, this is a very specific list in which Ss are cued, "Within the past year, did your wife die?" It is inconceivable that someone reports no when she did. But I don't know.

COMMENT. The opposite is more likely.

REFERENCES

Antonovsky, A., & Kats, R. The life crisis history as a tool in epidemiological research. *Journal of Health and Social Behavior*, 1967, 8, 15–21.

Breed, W. Occupational mobility and suicide among white males. *American Sociological Review*, 1963, 28, 179–188.

Brenner, M. H. Economic change and mental hospitalization: New York state, 1919–1960. *Social Psychiatry*, 1967, 2, 180–188.

————. Patterns of psychiatric hospitalization among different socioeconomic groups in response to economic stress. *Journal of Nervous and Mental Disease*, 1969, 148, 31–38.

Brown, G. W., & Birley, J. L. T. Crisis and life changes and the onset of schizophrenia. *Journal of Health and Social Behavior*, 1968, 9, 203–214.

Corwin, G., et al. Social requirements for occupational success: Internalized norms and friendships. *Social Forces*, 1960, 39, 135–140.

Dohrenwend, B. P., & Dohrenwend, B. S. The problem of validity in field studies of psychological disorder. *Journal of Abnormal Psychology*, 1965, 70, 52–69.

————. *Social status and psychological disorder: A casual inquiry.* New York: Wiley, 1969.

Dollard, J., Doob, L., Miller, N., & Sears, R. *Frustration and aggression.* New Haven: Yale University Press, 1939.

Duncan, O. D., & Hodge, R. W. Education and occupational mobility: A regression analysis. *American Journal of Sociology*, 1963, 68, 629–644.

Fischer, H. K., Dlin, B., Winters, W., et al. Time patterns and emotional factors related to the onset of coronary occlusion. *Psychosomatic Medicine*, 1962, 24, 516.

Gersti, J. E. Leisure, taste and occupational milieu. *Social Problems*, 1961, 9, 56–68.

Graham, D. T., & Stevenson, I. Disease as response to life stress. In H. I. Lief, V. F. Lief, and N. R. Lief (Eds.), *Psychological basis of medical practice.* New York: Harper, 1963.

Greene, W. A. Psychological factors and reticulo-endothelial disease. I. Preliminary observations on a group of males with lymphomas and leukemias. *Psychosomatic Medicine*, 1954, 16, 220.

———— & Miller, G. Psychological factors and reticulo-endothelial disease. IV. Observations on a group of children and adolescents with leukemia: an interpretation of disease development in terms of the mother-child unit. *Psychosomatic Medicine*, 1958, 20, 124.

————, Young, L. E., & Swisher, S. N. Psychological factors and reticulo-endothelial disease. II. Observations on a group of women with lymphomas and leukemias. *Psychosomatic Medicine,* 1956, 18, 284.

Gurin, G., Veroff, J., & Feld, S. *Americans view their mental health: A nation-wide survey.* New York: Basic Books, 1960.

Haberman, P. W. An analysis of retest scores for an index of psychophysiological disturbance. *Journal of Health and Human Behavior,* 1965, 6, 257–260.

Hawkins, N. G., Davie, R., & Holmes, T. H. Evidence of psychosocial factors in the development of pulmonary tuberculosis. *American Review of Tuberculosis and Pulmonary Diseases,* 1957, 75, 5.

Hinkle, L. E., Jr., & Wolff, H. G. Health and the social environment: Experimental investigations. In A. H. Leighton, J. A. Clausen, & R. N. Wilson (Eds.), *Explorations in social psychiatry.* New York: Basic Books, 1957. Pp. 105–137.

Hunt, W. A., Wittson, C. L., & Harris, H. I. The screen test in military selection. *Psychological Review,* 1944, 5, 37–46.

Jackson, E. F. Status consistency and symptoms of stress. *American Sociological Review,* 1962, 27, 469–480.

Kissen, D. K. Some psychosocial aspects of pulmonary tuberculosis. *International Journal of Social Psychiatry,* 1958, 3, 252.

Leighton, D. C., Harding, J. S., Macklin, D. B., MacMillan A. M., & Leighton, A. H. *The character of danger.* New York: Basic Books, 1963.

Lindenthal, J. J., Myers, J. K., Pepper, M. P., & Stern, M. S. Mental status and religious behavior. *Journal for the Scientific Study of Religion,* 1970, 9, 143–149.

———, Thomas, C. S., & Myers, J. K. Psychological status and the perception of primary and secondary support from the social milieu in time of crisis. *Journal of Nervous and Mental Disease,* 1971, 153, 92–98.

Lipset, S. M., & Bendix, R. *Social mobility in industrial society,* Ch. 7. Berkeley: University of California Press, 1957.

MacMillan, A. M. The health opinion survey: Technique for estimating prevalence of psychoneurotic and related types of disorder in communities. *Psychological Reports,* 1957, 3, 325–329.

Manis, J. G., Brawer, M. J., Hunt, C. L., & Kercher, L. C. Validating a mental health scale. *American Sociological Review,* 1964, 29, 84–89.

Myers, J. K., Lindenthal, J. J., & Pepper, M. P. Life events and psychiatric impairment. *Journal of Nervous and Mental Disease,* 1971, 152, 149–157.

——— & Ostrander, D. R. Life events and mental status: A longitudinal study. *Journal of Health and Social Behavior,* 1972, 13, 398–406.

Paykel, E. S., Myers, J. K., Dienelt, M. N., Klerman, G. L., Lindenthal, J. J., & Pepper, M. P. Life events and depression: A controlled study. *Archives of General Psychiatry,* 1969, 21, 753–760.

Phillips, D. L. The "true prevalence" of mental illness in a New England state. *Community Mental Health Journal,* 1966, 2, 35–40.

Rahe, R. H. Life crisis and health change. In P. R. A. May & J. R. Wittenborn (Eds.), *Psychotropic drug response: Advances in prediction.* Springfield, Ill.: Thomas, 1969, P. 92.

——— & Holmes, T. H. Social, psychologic and psychophysiologic aspects of inguinal hernia. *Journal of Psychosomatic Research,* 1965, 8, 487.

———, Mahan, J. L. Jr., Arthur, R. J., & Gunderson, E. K. E. The epidemiology of illness in naval environments. I. Illness types, distribution, severities, and relationship to life change. *Military Medicine,* 1970, 135, 443–452.

———, Meyer, M., Smith, M., Kjaer, G., & Holmes, T. H. Social stress and illness onset. *Journal of Psychosomatic Research,* 1964, 8, 35–44.

Rogler, L. H., & Hollingshead, A. B. *Trapped: Families and schizophrenia.* New York: Wiley, 1965.

Spilken, A. Z., & Jacobs, M. A. Prediction of illness behavior from measures of life crisis, manifest distress and maladaptive coping. *Psychosomatic Medicine,* 1971, 33, 251–264.

Srole, L., Langner, T. S., Michael, S. T., Opler, M. K., & Rennie, T. A. C. *Mental health in the metropolis,* New York: McGraw-Hill, 1962.

Stouffer, S. A., Guttman, L., Suchman, E. A., Lazarsfeld, P. F., Star, S. A., & Clausen, J. A. *Measurement and prediction.* Princeton: Princeton University Press, 1950.

————, Lumsdaine, A. A., Lumsdaine, M. H., Williams, R. M., Smith, M. B., Janis, I. L., Star, S. A., & Cottrell, L. S. *The American soldier: Combat and its aftermath.* Princeton: Princeton University Press, 1949.

Sullivan, H. S. The interpersonal theory of psychiatry. New York: Norton, 1953.

Tyhurst, J. S. The role of transition states — including disasters — in mental illness. In *Symposium on preventive and social psychiatry.* Washington, D.C.: GPO, 1957. Pp. 149–169.

Weber, M. *The Protestant ethic and the spirit of capitalism.* London: Allen & Unwin, 1948.

Weiss, E., Dlin, B., Rollin, H. R., et al. Emotional factors in coronary occlusion. *Archives of Internal Medicine,* 1957, 99, 628.

Wyler, A. R., Masuda, M., & Holmes, T. H. Magnitude of life events and seriousness of illness. *Psychosomatic Medicine,* 1971, 33, 115–122.

GEORGE E. VAILLANT

Antecedents of
Healthy Adult Male Adjustment

TWENTIETH-CENTURY man no longer perceives mental illness as bad luck that just happens. Nor is he content to believe that mental illness is retribution for immoral behavior. Unlike Sophocles, he does not believe that "when a house hath once been shaken from Heaven, there the curse falls evermore, passing from life to life of the race." Rather, in contemporary science, mental illness is perceived to have definite antecedents. Modern man believes that its etiology can be discovered by careful scrutiny of nature and nurture. However, the justification for even this belief system is anecdotal and retrospective. Adequate confirmation requires prospective examination of complete lifetimes.

Even when such studies are available, two further problems would arise to confound the quest for definitive etiology of mental illness. First, what do we really mean by this term? The definition of even the most obvious mental malady, schizophrenia, is hard enough. But what about depression, character disorder, and so forth? Then, even if we could identify mental illness with as much certainty as diabetes, there is ample evidence to suggest that complex socioeconomic factors play a major role in determining whether a given individual with given genes and a given childhood will ever be diagnosed mentally ill.

All these difficulties notwithstanding, the present paper seeks a still more elusive quarry: What are the antecedents of psychological health? The evidence will be drawn from a prospective study of 94 men from age 18 to 47. Before age 18, the data in the study are retrospective.

A twofold definition of mental health has been used. First, health has been rated for the degree to which evidence of known, labeled mental illness was *absent*. Second, mental health has been defined as the degree to which objective evidence of successful adjustment to middle life was present. The two ratings correlated with an *r* of 0.7 (Pearson's product-moment correlation).

In this study, socioeconomic differences proved fortuitously irrelevant. The sample was chosen from sophomores selected for healthy adjustment in a highly competitive college. The broad socioeconomic differences that existed at college entrance proved to have no significant correlation with any subsequent mental health or career success variable. Unfortunately, the childhood data before 18 were retrospective, but were gathered from both child and parent, and gathered not only by direct questioning but also by psychiatric interview. Although family history for mental illness also depended upon retrospective data, long-term follow-up often disclosed family skeletons that had been initially concealed.

METHODS

In the late 1930's, an interdisciplinary study was undertaken of a 7 per cent sample of several consecutive sophomore classes at a liberal arts college (Heath, 1945; Hooten, 1945). To be taken into the study, a student had to be considered by both the College Health Service and the Dean's Office to present no emotional or physical difficulties and to fall in the top half of the class academically (Vaillant & McArthur, 1972). Of 268 men originally selected in 1938–1942, 102 were chosen by chance in 1966 for reinterview. In college, 2 subjects had dropped out early from the subsample. Over the next 30 years, 6 died. Despite geographic dispersion, all of the 94 remaining members (aged 46–49) were interviewed.

In their sophomore year, all the men had been studied by a psychiatrist (8 interviews), an internist, a physiologist, an anthropologist, and a psychologist. A home visit was made to each subject's parents by a family worker who also interviewed each subject. Over the next 30 years, the men were followed both by a biennial questionnaire on many aspects of their lives and by a home interview at age 30.

Many independent, blind ratings were made:

I. The men were *somatotyped* (ie., rated 1–5 on endomorphy, mesomorphy, and ectomorphy).

II. On the basis of anthropometry, anthropologists rated each man on the strength of the *masculine component* of their physiques (strongly masculine, mild weakness, moderate weakness, strongly feminine).

III. *College Soundness:* At the end of a year of study, each sophomore was rated A, B, C, according to overall psychological soundness. An A rating implied research staff consensus that the subject was unusually well adjusted; B was an intermediate; and a C rating meant that the staff predicted future emotional difficulties for the subject. Only three subjects were thought overtly mentally ill.

IV. *Childhood Environment:* In 1971 a research associate who was blind to the fate of the men after their sophomore year, but who was not blind to more recent theories of child development, especially Erikson's, rated the men on the adequacy of their childhoods on a 20-point scale. The data made available to the blind rater were (a) the psychiatrist's and family worker's notes on the boy's reports of his home life, (b) the parents' description of their relationship with the boy, and (c) a developmental and medical history obtained by the family worker from the parents.

The 20-point scale was as follows:

a. Infant/Childhood Problems: Feeding problems, cried a great deal, dissocial, other noted problems (e.g., phobias) — no points. An average, not particularly problem-filled childhood — 1 point. No known problems age 0–10, normally social and "good-natured" — 2 points.

b. Childhood Health: Severe or prolonged illness, or physical disability — no points. A childhood with minor illnesses but no severe childhood diseases — 1 point. Consistent good health — 2 points.

c. Home Atmosphere: An uncongenial home with lack of family cohesiveness, with early maternal absences, separated parents, many moves or financial hardship which affected family life — no points. An average home or little information — 1 point. A warm, cohesive atmosphere where the parents did things together in a sharing atmosphere; few moves and financial stability — 2 points.

d. Mother-Child Relationship: A distant, hostile, or absent mother; one who blamed others (i.e., nurses, teachers, etc.) for her wrong methods of upbringing; a mother who seemed either overly punitive and demanding, or overprotective and/or seductive — no points. Lack of definite information or an apparently average relationship — 1 point. A warm mother who encouraged autonomy and esteem — 2 points.

e. Father-Child Relationship: An absent, distant, hostile, or overly punitive father; one with unrealistic expectations — no points. Lack of definite information or an apparently average relationship — 1 point. A warm father who encouraged positive autonomy, helped to develop his son's self-esteem, and who participated in activities of mutual interest — 2 points.

f. Sibling Relationships: Severe rivalry and destructive relationship where one sibling consistently undermined the other, or no siblings — no points. Lack of information — 1 point. Close enjoyable relationship with at least one sibling — 2 points.

g. High School Adjustment: Academic mediocrity, marked social problems, lack of competitive sports — no points. "Average" social adjustment but no competitive sports — 1 point. Academic and social success with participation in competitive sports — 2 points.

h. Global Impression (This was a subjective impression based on the available data): Impression of generally negative, non-nurturing environment — no points. Predominant impression neutral — 3 points. A positive, intact childhood which included good relationships with parents, siblings, and others of importance, and an environment conducive to good self-esteem — 6 points. Thus, each participant received a score from 0–20 points.

V. *Overall Adult Adjustment Score:* This was obtained by a research assistant who was blind to all the other assessments and had no information regarding childhood. She rated each surviving man on thirty-two relatively objective items (e.g., divorce, career advancement, length of vacation, days/year sick leave). These items are described in detail elsewhere (Vaillant, 1972b). Eight items reflected career adjustment, eight reflected social adjustment, eight medical adjustment, and eight psychological adjustment. On the Overall Adult Adjustment Score, scores ranged from 2–28.

VI. *Maturity of Defenses:* During his adult life, each man was rated on his use and nonuse of eighteen mechanisms of defense (Vaillant, 1971). Individual mechanisms of defense were identified by observing each man's style of adapting to crises and important life events. Mechanisms like projection, schizoid fantasy, and hypochrondriasis were called *immature.* Defenses like isolation, displacement, and repression were called *neurotic* (intermediate); and mechanisms like sublimation, suppression, and altruism were called *mature.* In 50 cases selected by chance, the ratings of these adaptive styles were made by two judges blind to all other ratings (Vaillant, 1972d). Each man then received a score (range 1–26) that numerically reflected the relative maturity of his defenses. Depending on the defense, rater reliability ranged from 60 to 90 per cent agreement. In this paper, only the defenses of the 50 blindly rated subjects will be discussed.

VII. *Social Class:* When each man was studied in college, his socioeconomic status was graded A–E on the basis of parents' education, father's occupation, family's social standing, and presence or absence of private education. At that time, 31 per cent were rated A or B (roughly corresponding to upper and upper-middle class); 49 per cent were rated C (middle class); and 20 per cent were rated D or E (lower-middle and lower class).

Rating I–VII were made by independent raters.

Four ratings were made by the author, who was *not* blind to the data from which the above ratings were made.

VIII. *Oral Dependence:* During their adult life, the men were also rated by the author on six traits: (a) pessimism, (b) passivity, (c) self-doubt, (d) fear of sex, (e) suggestibility, and (f) dependence. As a cluster, these traits characterize what clinicians call the oral-dependent character (Lazare et al., 1966). Depending upon the frequency with which behavior illustrating these traits was observed, the men received a score of 1–20.

IX. *Family History for Mental Illness:* The family worker specifically inquired about a history of mental illness in all known relatives. Over the years, the men often reported additional evidence of mental illness, especially in their parents and siblings. The author assigned tentative diagnoses to these relatives.

X. *Psychiatric Illness:* Each subject was rated 0–4 on overt evidence of mental illness. He received one point for each of the following items: (a) Hospitalization (usually in a general hospital) for an emotional problem (e.g., alcoholism, conversion reaction, depression). (b) Having been given a diagnostic psychiatric label by two observers other than the interviewer. (c) A clinical impression, after a recent two-hour interview, that the subject was schizoid, obviously neurotic, or clinically depressed. These clinical impressions were relative. (d) Frequent complaints over the years by the subject of excessive anxiety.

If two or more of the above items were noted, the subject was called "psychiatrically ill."

XI. On the basis of a two-hour interview and on his pattern of relationships over the past 30 years, each man was rated from 1–3 on his *object relations.* A rating of 1 reflected a man who was unusually warm, open, and candid toward others and who possessed obvious charm. A rating of 2 reflected an intermediate rating. A rating of 3 reflected a man with consistently ambivalent or distant object relations, and one who during the interview was often emotionally constricted, evasive, and avoided eye contact. These ratings correlated at an *r* of .64 with an independent rater's assessment of the more quantitative aspects of these men's social adjustment (Vaillant, 1972b).

RESULTS

Table A* presents the strong positive intercorrelation among the scores on the different variables which reflected different facets of mental health. These ratings were made by five individuals, each blind to the other ratings and often blind to all the information available to the other raters in the study. The significant, uniformly positive intercorrelations in Table A suggest that it may be just as legitimate to use the concept of positive psychological health as to speak of psychiatric illness. The quality of childhood was significantly associated with many mid-life parameters of psychological health — even in a sample preselected for health. Only maturity of defenses was not significantly correlated with childhood. In contrast, socioeconomic status in college correlated with none of the other variables. In adult life, oral-dependent traits showed strong negative correlations with variables reflecting psychological health.

	Correlation with Childhood Score
Career success	.01
Social class (age 19)	.10
Successful marriage	.10
Sexual adjustment	−.12
Mature ego mechanisms of defense	.21
Number of somatic symptoms with stress	.19
Recent objective health	.15

The accompanying tabulation, however, offers some real surprises. Career adjustment, marital success, and maturity of defenses were significantly correlated with all the other parameters of adult mental health in Table A and also with one another: the correlations ranged from 0.3 to 0.6 (Vaillant, 1972c). Yet, in this sample, these three variables were *not* significantly associated with childhood adjustment (Pearson's product-moment correlation coefficient). Similarly, at age 47, only 5 per cent of the men with the 20 best childhoods were in *Who's Who in America* or in *American Men of Science*, whereas 27 per cent of the remaining men were in one volume or the other. More astonishing still was the fact that the correlation between mature defense choice and childhood adjustment was

*For Tables A and B, order NAPS Document 02197 from ASIS/NAPS, c/o Microfiche Publications, 305 East 46th Street, New York, New York 10017, remitting $1.50 for microfiche or $5.00 for photocopies. Make checks payable to Microfiche Publications.

only .21 (not quite significant). A possible explanation is that marriage, job success, and choice of defense mechanism were ways in which these men — already selected in college for good adaptation — could compensate for having come from relatively inadequate childhoods. The tabulation also reflects the fact that objective physical health which was highly correlated with mature ego mechanisms and with absence of psychiatric illness, was only weakly related to the quality of childhood. Frank psychosomatic illness and multiple somatic symptoms with stress were not more common among men with relatively troubled childhoods (Vaillant, 1972c).

Many childhood variables, commonly cited in case histories as either causing or predicting future psychiatric illness, appeared to be unrelated to adult adjustment (Vaillant, 1972a). These items include difficult births, feeding problems, early or delayed toilet training, adolescent fingernail biting, loss of a parent, and below average mother/child relationships. In evaluating this finding, however, it must be borne in mind that the childhoods of these men were relatively good and that in 1940 they had already been selected for their capacity to adapt successfully to difficulties.

Table 1 compares the very best childhoods (scores of between 14 and 19) with the very worst childhoods (scores between 0 and 3). The trend seems clear. Thirteen of the worst childhoods and only one of the best childhoods had two or more items positive on the *psychiatric illness* scale. The less happy the childhood, the more visits the adult subject made to

Table 1. The Association of Some Adult Variables with Quality of Childhood as Assessed in Late Adolescence, in Percentages

Adult Variables	Worst Childhood[a]	Intermediate Childhood[b]	Best Childhood[c]
Psychiatrically ill	55	25	5**
Did visit psychiatrist	72	32	40
Does not visit family of origin	32	23	5*
No pastimes with non-relatives	59	38	15*
Poor object relations as adult	50	23	5**
Takes little vacation	41	45	10*
Too calm and unemotional	32	21	0*
Suppression *not* a major ego defense	41	25	15
Heavy use of drugs or alcohol	64	23	25**
Many oral-dependent traits	32	17	10*

[a]Scores of 0–3; $N = 22$.
[b]Scores of 4–13; $N = 53$.
[c]Scores of 14–19; $N = 20$.
*$p<.05$.   **$p<.01$.

a psychiatrist ($r = .23$, $p<.05$), and the fewer visits he made to his own next of kin.

In this population, if poor nurture has not severely impaired a man's capacity to marry happily and to excel on the job, it seems to have profoundly affected his capacity to play. Such men took briefer vacations, had more trouble expressing feelings, and seldom engaged in enjoyable relationships with friends and relatives.

The study also offered prospective confirmation of the retrospective assumption that heavy drug and alcohol use arises from the poor self-esteem and barren friendship patterns that, in turn, are the aftermath of an unsatisfactory childhood. Not only were drug use and poor object relations associated with such childhoods, but 41 per cent of the worst childhoods and only 10 per cent of the best resulted in adults rated high in oral-dependent character traits. Case histories showed that both poor human relations and oral-dependent traits preceded rather than resulted from heavy drug use (liberally defined as 6 ounces or more per day of alcohol or regular use of tranquilizers or sleeping pills by prescription).

Table 1 casts interesting light on the antecedents of emotional control. By a non-blind observer (GEV) the men were rated on their capacity to postpone gratification and to use optimistic stoicism (the ego mechanism of defense, *suppression*). In fifty cases, the correlation between the blind rating for *suppression* and the rating by GEV was .6. (In this study, *suppression* was differentiated from repression in that repression reflects a more complete pushing of conflict from consciousness and often the affect remains undiminished.) The men were also rated by GEV on whether or not they had appeared to go through life oblivious to any emotional upset — either pain or pleasure (*too calm and unemotional*). Suppression was the *only* ego mechanism that was associated with happy childhoods. In other words, men with poor childhoods either were unable to feel or autistically found comfort in drugs; men from the happiest childhoods could feel, but were good at controlling those feelings.

The accompanying tabulation illustrates some childhood antecedents associated with adults being classed as *psychiatrically ill* (total adds to 79, since one man had little information to classify). It was unusual for men from very happy childhoods or for those who in college had been judged psychologically sound to develop subsequent mental illness. If at 19 the subject perceived his father as his dominant parent, the subject was less likely to be later judged psychiatrically ill. Other work suggests this rela-

	Percentage Ill (N = 26)	Percentage Not Ill (N = 73)
Childhood among best in study	4	27**
College "soundness" rated A	12	42*
Father seen as dominant parent (age 18) ..	37	66*
Poor relationship with siblings	50	18**
Infant/childhood problems	69	44*
Relatively poor relationship with mother ...	58	48

*$p<.05$.   **$p<.01$.

tionship is as much due to the relative emotional maturity of the subject as it is due to the quality of the father per se (Vaillant & McArthur, 1972).

It was interesting that a good relationship with a sibling was not only associated with adult mental health, but that this was the only childhood variable statistically associated with mature defense mechanisms (Vaillant, 1972d). Unlike feeding problems and toilet training, other infant/childhood problems (for example, fears, tics, excessive shyness) were associated with adult mental illness. In their sophomore year, the subsequently mentally ill were statistically less likely to have been called friendly, practical, or well integrated by the research staff and were more likely to have been called asocial and thought to "lack purpose and values" and to show "mood fluctuations." However, 18-year-olds who were "introspective," "ideational," and "inhibited" were not more likely to develop mental illness than those who lacked these traits.

The mother-subject relationship did not appear statistically associated with later mental illness. Rather, other things being equal, during the course of 30 years there appeared to be intervening variables that mitigated the long-range effects of the early mother-child relationship. However, during their follow-up interview, the 14 middle-aged men who had had good relationships with *both* parents tended to appear warm, extroverted, energetic, and comfortable with intimacy. Only one was called psychiatrically ill. The 38 men who had had relatively poor relationships with both parents seemed distant, barren of warmth, and demonstrated relatively inflexible social behavior; 14 were called psychiatrically ill, and of these, 11 had three or four of the items supporting such a classification. It should be kept in mind, however, that in this study the term *psychiatric illness* is only relative. All of the men were functioning in the community at a relatively high level of occupational competence, and most were adequately meeting family responsibilities.

Turning from nurture to nature, the study examined the association of constitutional factors with positive mental health. Although mental illness in *parents* was associated with poor adult adjustment, this was not true of mental illness in the extended family (Vaillant, 1972a). There was no evidence that "tainted" heredity differentially affected the subsequent course of these men's lives. Except for the unsurprising fact that endomorphy in adolescence was associated with overweight in adult life, somatotype was uncorrelated with *any* of the many variables measured in adult life, including character type.

In general, native intelligence (as measured by the alpha tests of numerical and verbal aptitudes and as reflected by the Scholastic Achievement Test [SAT] and the Mathematical Attainments Test [MAT] was not correlated with either adult adjustment or psychopathology. The only outcome variable associated with relatively high intelligence was that 11 of the 33 brightest men and none of the 12 least intelligent men were in *Who's Who in America* or *American Men of Science* at age 47.

The one constitutional variable that did seem associated with adult psychological health was the masculine component of their physiques (Table B). If at eighteen the anthropologists had judged the subject's body build strongly masculine, the subject was more likely to have adjusted well both as a young child and in high school. He was more likely to have come from a home that a blind rater perceived as happy and cohesive. As adults, subjects high in androgyny were more likely to be viewed as extroverted, aggressive, and not orally dependent. In terms of global adult adjustment, such men had better mental and physical health, object relations, and greater career success. Conclusions about the cause and effect of a strongly masculine body build are confusing and will require extensive future work. Although specific somatotype was uncorrelated with outcome, men with feminine body builds were rated relatively higher in endomorphy, but not lower in mesomorphy or ectomorphy. Part of the confusion arises from the fact that strongly masculine body build in adolescence was correlated with social approval and with childhood variables that themselves predisposed the subject to a favorable midlife outcome.

DISCUSSION

The concept of positive mental health is not just a subjective will-o'-the-wisp. Although assessed by independent judges at different points in time, ratings of different facets of psychological health were strongly associated (Vaillant, 1972b). Poor adjustment to life (even in a sample relatively free of gross emotional impairment) at one age was statistically correlated with poor adjustment at other periods. Thus, the child with emotional problems in early life was more likely to get along poorly with his siblings and in adolescence to fail to shift from his mother to his father as a dominant parent. He would have trouble making a good college adjustment and, finally, his midlife adjustment would leave much to be desired. But the past did not inevitably predict the future. Over time, there also appeared to be many ways in which individuals could compensate for psychic insults in the distant past. The most dramatic examples were that career success and mature mechanisms of defense appeared relatively independent of childhood. Ingenious solutions to intrapsychic conflict were not just the province of the well-adjusted. The findings of Block (1971) on the subjects in the Berkeley Growth Study suggest that there are several personality subtypes in which individuals may appear impaired at one stage of life and not at another.

The accuracy of the childhood rating was undoubtedly blurred by subjective evaluation and by retrospective distortion. However, the ratings obtained predicted future object relations with sufficient power to suggest some specificity. Every subscale but those reflecting childhood physical health and sibling relationships were statistically associated with independently assessed adult object relations at age 47 (Vaillant, 1972a). The subjects of the Berkeley Growth Study, followed from birth to middle life, offer evidence that mother-child relationships — as reported in adolescence — are highly correlated with those actually observed in early childhood (Hunt & Eichorn, 1972). A necessary caveat is the possibility that human beings possess innate capacities for good or poor human relationships. If true, then an innately warm child might engender a warm childhood, and an innately schizoid child could poison the family atmosphere.

The present paper stimulates curiosity as to the significance of androgyny in mental health. Bayley (1951) observed that adolescent males with weakly masculine body builds had stronger masculine interest scores on Kuder Interest Scales than their peers with more masculine physiques. If true, then the relative failure of men with feminine body builds in career and social adjustments cannot be explained by a failure to cathect to masculine roles. But our study raises and does not answer the question, Does a stable, cohesive homelife facilitate endocrinological maturation or do endocrinological factors affect perception of past adjustment?

The most important conclusion of this paper is the clear association of troubled childhoods — as identified in late adolescence — with mental illness in adult life. However, longitudinal stress seemed far more important in effecting outcome than did isolated traumatic events. Thus, birth difficulties, feeding problems, early toilet training, and traumatic loss of a parent or sibling did not seem to occur more often in the poor outcomes than in the good outcomes. If a lost parent was relatively unimportant, a mentally ill but present parent was, indeed, statistically related to mental illness. Since there seemed an equal amount of mental illness in the rest of the families of both the best and worst outcomes, it seems fair to suppose that in this sample, mentally ill parents exerted their effect environmentally rather than genetically. Mother-child relationships were correlated with adolescent adjustment, but it was the quality of total childhood experience rather than the quality of any relationship with any one person that had the clearest association with psychopathology by the time the subjects reached 47.

COMMENTARY

WATT. In Table B, I think all but one of the variables listed on the left are also found to be more frequent in men at high risk for heart disorder. Rosenman and Friedman, in their huge collaborative study on the West Coast, found every one of those. Behaviorally, these are significant predictors of heart disorder and its accompanying kidney failure, cerebrovascular accidents, and hypertension. If these are really the healthiest men, is it possible that what you are finding from a psychiatric point of view is that the healthiest man is also going to have a shorter life?

VAILLANT. No, you're reversing it — the unhealthiest men have most of those variables. Also, those items correlate not only with heart disease, but also with psychosomatic illness in these men as a whole.

WATT. So what you find is that the worst outcome men took fewer vacations, were too calm and unemotional? Yes, that's consistent then with Rosenman and Friedman's findings; it means that these men also would be the most prone to heart disorder, peptic ulcer, and so on. Then you would expect that the least adapted in your psychiatric sense would have the shortest lives?

VAILLANT. Yes.

CHESS. I'm always a bit troubled with correlation studies that talk about the effect of disturbed childhoods on the outcome of adult health or pathology. Using the word *correlation* isn't just a matter of semantics — it means that you're looking at the data differently. Not only in our longitudinal study, but in all sorts of clinical situations where it has been possible to get another view of what happened in childhood from relatives or whoever, very often the question of the disturbed childhood adaptation, the relationship of child with mother or with father during childhood, is a reciprocal issue. What may be being tapped is not the nurturing of the child, but the childhood personality, which is then a continuum with the adult personality. So that when you talk about the effect of the disturbed childhood on the adult, I don't think we can be entirely sure that that is what you have described.

VAILLANT. Dr. Chess is completely right.

REFERENCES

Bayley, N. Some psychological correlates of somatic androgyny. *Child Development*, 1951, 22, 47–60.

Block, J. *Lives through time*. Berkeley: Bancroft Press, 1971.

Heath, C. W. *What people are*. Cambridge, Mass.: Harvard University Press, 1945.

Hooten, E. *Young man, you are normal*. New York: Putnam, 1945.

Hunt, J. V., & Eichorn, D. H. Maternal and child behaviors: A review of data from the Berkeley Growth Study. *Seminars in Psychiatry*, 1972, 4, 367–382.

Lazare, A., Klerman, G. L., & Armor, D. J. Oral, obsessive, and hysterical personality patterns. *Archives of General Psychiatry*, 1966, 14, 624–630.

Vaillant, G. E. Theoretical hierarchy of adult ego mechanisms of defense. *Archives of General Psychiatry*, 1971, 24, 107–118.

———. Natural history of male psychological health, II: Some antecedents of good adult adjustment. Submitted for publication, 1972. (a)

———. Natural history of male psychological health, III: Empirical dimensions of positive mental health. Paper presented at the meeting of the American Psychiatric Association, Dallas, May 1–5, 1972. (b)

———. Natural history of male psychological health, IV: What kinds of men do not get psychosomatic illness. Paper presented at the meeting of the American Psychosomatic Society, April 25, 1972. Submitted for publication, 1972. (c)

———. Natural history of male psychological health, V.: The relation of choice of defense mechanisms to good adult adjustment. Paper presented at Psychiatric Grand Rounds, Boston University School of Medicine, October 25, 1972. (d)

——— & McArthur, C. C. Natural history of male psychological health, I: The life cycle from 18–50. *Seminars in Psychiatry*, 1972, 4, 417–429.

DANIEL J. LEVINSON
CHARLOTTE M. DARROW
EDWARD B. KLEIN
MARIA H. LEVINSON
BRAXTON MC KEE *The Psychosocial
Development of Men in Early Adulthood
and the Mid-Life Transition*

THIS IS NOT a formal research report, but a statement of thinking and progress, as of May 1972. We are in the third year of a projected four-year study. We have obtained interview and TAT material on a sample of 40 men, all of whom are currently aged 35–45. There are 10 men in each of four occupational groups: blue- and white-collar workers in industry; business executives; academic biologists; and novelists. Each man was seen 6–10 times for a total of 10–20 hours over a period of 2–3 months. We had a single follow-up interview with most of the men about two years after the initial interviews. The focus is on the current status of our efforts to construct a theory of adult male development over the age span of about 20–45. We hope in further study to get beyond that, but that's where we are now. In view of the comments that have been made during the discussions of the previous papers, which have dealt heavily with problems of research design, measurement, and statistical analysis, let me say in advance that I shall not talk about methodology or data.

DEVELOPMENTAL PERIODS IN THE ADULT LIFE COURSE

We have found it convenient to distinguish several gross chronological periods in the adult life course: early adulthood, roughly ages 20–40; middle adulthood, ages 40–60; and late adulthood, age 60+. We are

NOTE: The project is carried out by the Research Unit for Social Psychology and Psychiatry, at the Connecticut Mental Health Center and the Department of Psychiatry, Yale University.

studying early adulthood and the "mid-life transition" — that is, the several years on either side of 40 that constitute a transitional period between early and middle adulthood.

These are descriptive time units that we use to begin making developmental distinctions within adult life. Something even as simple as this is necessary because of the tremendous neglect of development and socialization in the main adult years, roughly 20–65, in psychology, psychiatry, sociology, and so on. We speak as though development goes on to age 6, or perhaps to age 18; then there is a long plateau in which random things occur; and then at around 60 or 65 "aging" begins.

There is little work in sociology on adult socialization. In psychology there are the concepts and "psychohistorical" approach of Erikson and the extensive work of Jungian depth psychology, which is almost totally ignored by the academic disciplines. Like Jung and Erikson, we assume that there is something we can call adult development, that there is a psychosocial evolution just as in pre-adult life, and that we won't understand adults and the changes they go through in their lives if we don't have a conception of what is intrinsic to adulthood. We can then see how derivatives of childhood operate to facilitate or hinder certain kinds of development.

One of our chief theoretical aims is to formulate a sociopsychological conception of the life course and the various developmental periods, tasks, structures, and processes within it. There are, of course, wide individual and group differences in the concrete life course, as our findings show. At a more conceptual level, however, we are interested in generating and working with hypotheses concerning *relatively universal, genotypic, age-linked, adult developmental periods* within which variations occur. As we conceive of these periods, their origins lie both in the nature of man as a biosocial and biopsychological organism, and in the nature of society as an enduring multigenerational form of collective life. The periods do not represent simply an unfolding of maturational potentials from within; they are thus different from the Freudian or Piagetan stages of childhood development, which are seen largely as an internal unfolding. Nor do they simply represent stages in a career sequence as shaped by an occupational, educational, or familial system. In other words, the periods are not simply a function of adult socializing systems, although these systems play an important part in defining timetables and in shaping one's course through them.

We are trying to develop an embracing sociopsychological conception of male adult developmental periods, within which a variety of biological, psychodynamic, cultural, social-structural, and other timetables operate in only partial synchronization. (It could be an important further step to do similar studies of women and to learn about similarities and differences between the sexes under various social conditions.) The remaining sections of this paper set forth our theoretical conception of these periods from roughly age 20 to 45. Within the framework of this overall theory we shall note some illustrative concepts, findings, and areas of exploration. Again, we emphasize that this is a report of work in progress and by no means a final statement.*

LEAVING THE FAMILY (LF)

We conceive of Leaving the Family (LF) as a period of transition between adolescent life, centered in the family of origin, and entry into the adult world. In our sample, LF ordinarily occupies a span of some 3–5 years, starting at age 16–18 and ending at 20–24. It is a transitional period in the sense that the person is half in and half out of the family: he is making an effort to separate himself from the family, to develop a new home base, to reduce his dependence on familial support and authority, and to regard himself as an adult making his way in the adult world.

The separation from the family proceeds along many lines. In its external aspects, it involves changes such as moving out of the familial home, becoming financially less dependent, and getting into new roles and living arrangements in which one is more autonomous and responsible. In its internal aspects, it involves an increase in self-parent differentiation and in psychological distance from the family. Of course, these processes start earlier and continue well beyond the LF period. We say that someone is in this period when there is a roughly equal balance between "being in" the family and "moving out." From the point of view of ego development, the young man is in the stage that Erikson has identified as Identity versus Role Diffusion.

LF ordinarily begins around the end of high school (graduation or dropping out). Those who enter college or the military have a new, institutional life situation that is in many respects intermediate between the family and fully adult life in the community. The institution constitutes a home base providing some degree of structure, control, support, and

*In May 1973, as we do the final editing of this manuscript for publication, we wish to note that the theory has been elaborated and modified in certain respects but the general framework continues to hold.

maintenance. It also provides spheres of autonomy and privacy in which the young person is largely responsible for himself and can strike out in new paths. He has increasing opportunities to form relationships, as a compeer, with adults of various ages and thus to begin experiencing himself as an adult who is part of that world (rather than an adolescent standing reluctantly at the edge of it).

Those who move directly from high school into the labor force — and this is most often the case within the working-class population — have no institutional matrix to shape the transition into adult life. These young men do, nonetheless, go through the LF transition. They may continue to live at home for several years on a semi-boarder status, "leading their own lives" and yet remaining in some ways subject to parental authority and integrated within the family network. This is a common pattern among ethnic groups with strong communal and extended family bonds. Often the young man works with his father or relatives during this period. If he marries during LF, the couple may live for some time with one spouse's parents or relatives. The initial work history has the same transitional character. For several years (in some cases, permanently) the young man has no genuine occupation. He works at various jobs and acquires a variety of skills. But, lacking seniority, influence, and broader competence, he tends to be given the worst jobs on the worst shifts and to have the least job security. Even though a young man in this position may be economically self-sufficient and living on his own, he is still on the boundary between the family and the fully adult world; and getting across this boundary is his major developmental task.

The LF period ends when the balance shifts — when one has for the most part separated from the family (though further work on separation-connectedness in relation to family continues for many years, if not forever) and has begun to make a place for himself in the adult world.

GETTING INTO THE ADULT WORLD (GIAW)

The period we call Getting into the Adult World (GIAW) begins when the center of gravity of one's life shifts from the family of origin (or an equivalent authoritative-protective social matrix) to a new home base and an effort to form an adult life of one's own. This period ordinarily starts in the early 20's and extends until roughly age 27–29. It is a time of exploration and provisional commitment to adult roles, memberships, responsibilities, and relationships. The young man tries to establish an occupation, or an occupational direction, consistent with his interests, values, and sense of self. He begins to engage in more adult friendships and sexual relationships, and to work on what Erikson has termed the ego stage of Intimacy versus Aloneness.

The overall developmental task of the GIAW period is to explore the available possibilities of the adult world, to arrive at an initial definition of oneself as an adult, and *to fashion an initial life structure* that provides a viable link between the valued self and the wider adult world.

The concept of life structure is of central importance in our thinking. In its external aspects it refers to the individual's overall pattern of roles, memberships, interests, condition, and style of living, long-term goals, and the like — the particular ways in which he is plugged into society. In its internal aspects, life structure includes the personal meanings these have for the individual, as well as the inner identities, core values, fantasies, and psychodynamic qualities that shape and infuse one's engagement in the world and are to some degree fulfilled and changed by it. Traditional behavioristic and sociological approaches tend to emphasize the external aspects and to ignore the internal. Conversely, depth psychological approaches tend to emphasize the internal dynamics without taking sufficiently into account the nature of the sociocultural world and the individual's actual engagement in it. Our approach is to use concepts such as life structure to provide an initial focus on the *boundary between individual and society*; from this base, we can then move outward to a fuller examination of the social world and inward to a fuller examination of the personality.

GIAW is, like all entry periods, a time of exploration and initial choice. It involves, to varying degrees and in varying sequences, the processes of exploratory searching, of making provisional choices, of further exploratory testing through which the rightness of an initial choice is assessed and alternatives are considered, of increasing commitment to certain choices and the construction of a more integrated, stable life structure.

There are wide variations in the course, duration, and outcome of this period. These are a few of the patterned sequences we have found:

a. Perhaps the most frequent pattern we find is that of the man who makes a provisional commitment to an occupation and goes through the initial stages of a career. That is, during the 20's he is establishing a tentative structure, including an occupational choice and the beginnings of commitment to an occupational identity. Then, somewhere in the interval between age 28 and 32, he enters a transitional period in which he works on the questions: Shall I make a deeper commitment to this occupation and build a stable life structure around it? or I still have a chance to change; shall I take it? There is a kind of bet that's being made here, at around age 30. Many of our subjects remain in the occupation initially chosen in their 20's; they get married or reaffirm the existing marriage, and they enter a new period, Settling Down.

b. In some cases, the man at around 30 decides that his initial occupational choice was not the right one — that it is too constraining, or that it is a violation or betrayal of an early dream which now has to be pursued, or that he does not have the talent to succeed in it — and he makes a major shift in occupation and in life structure, sometimes including marriage. In this pattern the man makes a provisional structure in his 20's and then makes a moderate or drastic change at about 30.

c. Still another variant is that of the man who during his 20's lives a rather transient, unsettled life. He then feels a desperate need at around 30 to get more order and stability into his life. It is our tentative hypothesis that if a man does not reach a significant start toward settling down by about age 34, his chances of forming a reasonably satisfying life structure, and one that can evolve in his further development, are quite small. A number of movies in the last few years have depicted this particular kind of age 30 crisis. One is *Five Easy Pieces*. Another is *Getting Straight*, which is about an ex-college radical who has been in a transient, wandering stage during his 20's. Around 30 his tentative occupational choice is to become a high school teacher, and he makes an effort which he and the educational establishment collude to destroy.

A concept of great value in the analysis of the GIAW period is the *dream*. Many men, though certainly not all, enter adulthood with a dream or vision of their own future. This dream is usually articulated within an occupational context — for example, becoming a great novelist, winning the Nobel Prize (a common dream of our biologists), contributing in some way to human welfare, and so on. Where such a dream exists, we are exploring its nature and vicissitudes over the life course. Major shifts in life direction at subsequent ages are often occasioned by a reactivation of the sense of betrayal or compromise of the dream. That is, very often in the crises that occur at age 30, 40, or later a major issue is the reactivation of a guiding dream, frequently one that goes back to adolescence or the early 20's, and the concern with its failure. We are also interested in the antecedents and consequences of not having a dream, because the dream can be such a vitalizing force for adult development.

A second, crucial concept is that of the *transitional period*. The time around 28–32 seems to be a transitional period, a link between the termination of GIAW and the onset of the next period. We are trying to be very specific about age-linkages in order to counteract the strong tendency to assume that in adulthood very little is age-linked because development isn't occurring. We pursue tenaciously the possibility that the age-linkages are stronger than has been recognized. The Age 30 Transition, and others like it at different points in the life course, may occasion considerable turmoil, confusion, and struggle with the environment and within oneself; or it may involve a more quiet reassessment and intensification of effort. But it is marked by important changes in life structure and internal commitments, and presages the next stage in development.

SETTLING DOWN

The next period is Settling Down (SD). As noted above, this period ordinarily begins in the early 30's. The individual now makes deeper commitments; invests more of himself in his work, family, and valued interests; and within the framework of this life structure, makes and pursues more long-range plans and goals.

The imagery and meaning of Settling Down are multifaceted. One aspect of this period involves *order*, stability, security, control. The man establishes his niche in society, digs in, builds a nest, and pursues his interests within the defined pattern. This aspect may be stronger or weaker in a given case. A second, contrasting aspect has more the quality of *making it*. This involves planning, striving, moving onward and upward, having an inner timetable that contains major goals and way stations and ages by which they must be reached. The executive has to get into the corporate structure by age 40 or has to be earning at least $50,000 by 40; the assistant professor has to get tenure by 40; and so on.

So these are two aspects of SD. One has more to do with *down, in, order*; the other has more to do with *up, mobility, ambition*. Antithetical to both of these is the disposition to be free, unfettered, not tied to any structure no matter how great its current satisfaction nor how alluring its future promise, always open to new possibilities, ready to soar, wander, quest in all directions as the spirit moves one. We see the surgence of this disposition in the present state of society. This disposition is usually not predominant during the early SD period, but this does not mean it is necessarily absent nor that it may not in time reassert itself. Indeed, it frequently reappears toward the end of SD.

The SD period lasts until the late 30's or early 40's, when various internal and external changes bring on new developments. We shall note just a few major characteristics of this period. In creating an integrated life structure, one can utilize only parts of one's self, and this means that important parts of the self are left out. A myth supported by most theories of pre-adult development is that at the end of adolescence you get yourself together and, as a normal, mature adult, you enter into a relatively stable, integrated life pattern that can continue more or less indefinitely. This is a rather cruel illusion since it leads people in early adulthood to believe that they are, or should be, fully adult and settled, and that there are no major crises or developmental changes ahead. The structure one creates in SD cannot fulfill or reflect all of oneself. Parts of the self are repressed or simply left dormant. At some point the life structure must be enlarged, reformed, or radically restructured in order to express more of the self.

One reason the SD structure must change is that it is based to some degree upon illusions — illusions about the importance and meaning of achieving one's occupational goals, about one's relationships with significant others, about what it is one truly wants in life, and so on. A *de-illusioning* process — by which we mean the reduction or removal of illusions and not a cynical disillusionment — is an important aspect of post-SD development. For example, the man in the early SD period tends to regard himself as highly autonomous. He is making his own way, he is not a child anymore, his parents are not telling him what to do, he is on his own. One of his illusions is that he is, in fact, freed of what we would call tribal influences. In actuality, however, the ambitions and the goal-seeking of the 30's are very much tied in with tribal influences. We seek to a large extent what the institutions and reference groups important to us are helping us define. We may be more free of our parents, but we find or invent others who guide us, protect us, tell us what to do. Toward the end of SD, a new step is taken.

BECOMING ONE'S OWN MAN

The next step is Becoming One's Own Man, BOOM. Calling this the BOOM time has a certain metaphorical rightness. We are now inclined to regard BOOM not as a separate period but as a time of peaking and culmination of the Settling Down period and a connecting link to the Mid-Life Transition.

BOOM tends to occur in the middle to late 30's, typically in our sample around 35–39. It represents the high point of early adulthood and the beginning of what lies beyond. A key element in this period is the man's feeling that, no matter what he has accomplished to date, he is not sufficiently his own man. He feels overly dependent upon and constrained by persons or groups who have authority over him or who, for various reasons, exert great influence upon him. The writer comes to recognize that he is unduly intimidated by his publisher or too vulnerable to the evaluations of certain critics. The man who has successfully risen through the managerial ranks with the support and encouragement of his superiors now finds that they control too much and delegate too little, and he impatiently awaits the time when he will have the authority to make his own decisions and to get the enterprise really going. The untenured faculty member imagines that once he has tenure he will be free of all the restraints and demands he's been acquiescing to since graduate school days. (The illusions die hard!)

The sense of constraint and oppression may occur not only in work but also in marriage and other relationships. We have been greatly impressed by the role of the mentor, and by developmental changes in relationships with mentors and in the capability to be a mentor. The word *mentor* is sometimes used in a primarily external sense — an adviser, teacher, protector — but we use the term in a more complex psychosocial sense. The presence or absence of mentors is, we find, an important component of the life course during the 20's and 30's. The absence of mentors is associated with various kinds of developmental impairments and with problems of individuation in mid-life.

The mentor is ordinarily 8 to 15 years older than the mentee. He is enough older to represent greater wisdom, authority, and paternal qualities, but near enough in age or attitudes to be in some respects a peer or older brother rather than in the image of the wise old man or distant father. He may be a teacher, boss, editor, or experienced co-worker. He takes the younger man under his wing, invites him into a new occupational world, shows him around, imparts his wisdom, cares, sponsors, criticizes, and bestows his blessing. The teaching and the sponsoring have their value, but the blessing is the crucial element.

The younger man, in turn, feels appreciation, admiration, respect, gratitude, love, and identification. The relationship is lovely for a time, then ends in separation arising from a quarrel, or death, or a change in circumstances. Following the separation, the processes of internalization are enhanced, since internalization is increased by loss, and the personality of the mentee is enriched as he makes the valued qualities of the mentor more fully a part of himself. In some respects the main value of the relationship is created after it ends, but only if there was something there when it was happening. This is probably true of psychotherapy as well.

The number of mentor relationships in an individual's life does not vary widely. Few men have more than three or four, and perhaps the modal numbers are none and one. The duration of the intense mentor relationship is also not extremely variable, perhaps 3–4 years as an average and 10–12 years as the upper limit. When this relationship ends, the pair may form a more modest friendship after a cooling-off period. The ending of the mentor relationship may take a rather peaceful form, with gradual loss of involvement. More often, however, and especially during the 30's, termination is brought about by increasing conflict or by forced separation, and brings in its wake intense feelings of bitterness, rancor, grief, abandonment, and rejuvenation in the mentee.

The final giving up of all mentors by those who have had them tends to occur in the middle or late 30's. One does not have mentors after 40. One may have friendships or significant working relationships after this, but the mentor relationship in its more developed form is rare, at least in our sample and in our life experience. It is given up as part of Becoming One's Own Man. The person who was formerly so loved and admired, and who was experienced as giving so much, comes now to be seen as hypercritical, oppressively controlling, seeking to make one over in his own image rather than fostering one's independence and individuality; in short, as a tyrannical and egocentric father rather than a loving, enabling mentor. Among the more dramatic examples of this are Freud's relationships with Breuer and Fliess, and Jung's with Freud.

There are clearly irrational elements in this process, such as the reactivation and reworking of Oedipal conflicts, which have their origins in childhood. To focus solely on these, however, is to restrict our vision and to miss the adult developmental functions of the relationship and its termination. Whatever its Oedipal or early childhood–derived meanings, the relationship with the mentor has crucial adult meanings as well. It enables the young man to relate *as an adult* with another man who regards him as an adult and who welcomes him into the adult world on a relatively (but not completely) mutual and equal basis.

The young man must in time reject this relationship, but this is largely because it has served its purpose. He is ready to take a further step in becoming his own man: to give up being a son in the little boy sense and a young man in the apprentice-disciple-mentee sense, and to move toward assuming more fully the functions of mentor, father, and peer in relation to other adults. This kind of developmental achievement is of the essence of adulthood and needs to be studied. It is probably impossible to become a mentor without first having been a mentee.

Relationships of this kind are probably also of crucial importance in initiating and working on the ego stage of *generativity versus stagnation* and its attendant virtue, *caring* (for adults). Erikson has identified this stage as beginning at around 40 and as involving one's relationship to future generations in general and to the next generation of adults in particular. This goes beyond caring about one's small children, which one ordinarily has to learn in the 20's. The issue now is caring about adults, being generative in relation to adults, taking responsibility in the adult world, and getting over being a boy in the adult world. We are saying that one can't get very far with this before age 40 and that the BOOM time of the late 30's is the beginning of work on it.

During BOOM a man wants desperately to be affirmed by society in the roles that he values most. He is trying for that crucial promotion or other recognition. At about age 40 — we would now say within the range of about 39 to 42 — most of our subjects fix on some key event in their careers as carrying the ultimate message or their affirmation or devaluation by society. This event may be a promotion or new job — it's of crucial importance whether one gets to be vice-president of a company, or full professor in a department, or foreman or union steward. It may involve a particular form of symbolic success: writing a best seller or a prize-winning novel, being recognized as a scientist or executive or craftsman of the first rank, and so on. This event is given a magical quality. If the outcome is favorable, one imagines, then all is well and the future is assured. If it is unfavorable, the man feels that not only his work but he as a person has been found wanting and without value.

Since the course and outcome of this key event take several (perhaps 3–6) years to unfold, many men at around 40 seem to be living, as one of our subjects put it, in a state of suspended animation. During the course of the waiting, the next period gets under way.

The next period we call the Mid-Life Transition. A *developmental transition*, as we use the term, is a turning point or boundary region between two periods of greater stability. A transition may go relatively smoothly or may involve considerable turmoil. The Mid-Life Transition occurs whether the individual succeeds or fails in his search for affirmation by society. At 38 he thinks that if he gains the deserved success, he'll be all set. The answer is, he will not. He is going to have a transition whether he is affirmed or not; it is only the form that varies.

The central issue is not whether he succeeds or fails in achieving his goals. The issue, rather, is what to do with the *experience of disparity* between what he has gained in an inner sense from living within a particular structure and what he wants for himself. The sense of disparity between "what I've reached at this point" and "what it is I really want" instigates a soul-searching for "what it is I really want."

To put it differently, it is not a matter of how many rewards one has obtained; it is a matter of the *goodness of fit between the life structure and the self*. A man may do extremely well in achieving his goals and yet find his success hollow or bittersweet. If, after failing in an important respect, he comes primarily to castigate himself for not being able to "make it," then he is having a rough time but he is not having a mid-life crisis. He just regrets failure. He is having a crisis to the extent that he questions his life structure and feels the stirrings of powerful forces within himself that lead him to modify or drastically to change the structure.

In making the choices out of which the Settling Down structure was built, he drew upon and lived out certain aspects of himself: fantasies, values, identities, conflicts, internal "object relationships," character traits, and the like. At the same time, other essential aspects of the self were consciously rejected, repressed, or left dormant. These excluded components of the self — "other voices in other rooms," in Capote's vivid image — now seek expression and clamor to be heard.

We shall note briefly some of the major issues within the Mid-Life Transition: (a) The sense of *bodily decline* and the more vivid recognition of one's *mortality*. This brings the necessity to confront one's mortality and to deal in a new way with wounds to one's omnipotence fantasies, to overcome illusions and self-deceptions which relate to one's sense of omnipotence. It also brings greater freedom in experiencing and thinking about one's own and others' deaths, and greater compassion in responding to another's distress about decline, deformity, death, loss and bereavement. (b) The sense of *aging*, which means to be old rather than young. The Jungian concepts of puer and senex as archetypes that play a significant part in the mid-life individuation process are important here.

(c) The polarity of *masculine and feminine*. Ordinarily in man's Settling Down structure masculinity is predominant; the emergence and integration of the more feminine aspects of the self are more possible at mid-life. During the mid-life period there is often a flowering of fantasies about various kinds of women, especially the maternal (nurturing and/or destructive) figures and the younger, erotic figures. These fantasies do not represent simply a belated adolescence, a final surge of lasciviousness, or self-indulgence or dependence (though they may have these qualities in part). The changing relationships to women may also involve the beginnings of a developmental effort. The aim of this effort is to free oneself more completely from the hold of the boy-mother relationship and to utilize one's internal relationships with the erotic transformative feminine as a means of healing old psychic wounds and of learning to love formerly devalued aspects of the self. It is the changing relation to the self that is the crucial issue at mid-life.

RESTABILIZATION AND THE BEGINNING
OF MIDDLE ADULTHOOD

For most men the Mid-Life Transition reaches its peak sometime in the early 40's, and in the middle 40's there is a period of Restabilization. There seems to be a 3–4-year period at around age 45 in which the Mid-Life Transition comes to an end and a new life structure begins to take shape and to provide a basis for living in middle adulthood.

We are not presenting this as the last developmental change or the one in which everything will be resolved. For many men little is resolved, and the chickens come home to roost later. But it is a time both of possibility for developmental advance and of great threat to the self. Men such as Freud, Jung, Eugene O'Neill, Frank Lloyd Wright, Goya, and Gandhi went through a profound crisis at around 40 and made tremendous creative gains through it. There are also men like Dylan Thomas, F. Scott Fitzgerald, and Sinclair Lewis, who could not manage this crisis and who destroyed themselves in it. Many men who don't have a crisis at 40 become terribly weighted down and lose the vitality that one needs to continue developing through adulthood. Arthur Miller's play *The Price* tells something of the crisis of a man at 50: the sense of stagnation he has because of what he didn't do earlier, especially at 40 when he considered changing his life structure and didn't; he is now sinking in it.

We regard the Restabilization, then, as an initial outcome of the

Mid-Life Transition. We are examining various forms of Restabilization and considering their implications for an understanding of the possibilities and problems of middle adulthood.

COMMENTARY

ZUBIN. After such a literary and poetic description of life stages, a hard-bitten differential psychologist like me shouldn't really say anything. However, I have to give a testimonial, I believe he's been reading my autobiography. It is so true! Yet I have enough egocentricity to wonder whether all people are like me — aren't there any individual differences left? I mean, are there not some differences, even within his own group, which could be documented? As Levinson was talking, I began to ask myself, What other classification of stages of man would I have adopted in trying to make sense out of these data? Of course, one can go back to Ethics of the Fathers who had about thirteen stages of man, Shakespeare who had several, Freud who had at least three, and Erik Erikson, Jean Piaget, etc. Mightn't you take a crack at showing what other options are open and what similarities and differences you would have got if you had tried different frameworks?

STIERLIN. Levinson has beautifully shown the complexity of a badly neglected life phase. I would like to add a few comments from my own research, which is a study of underachievers who were high risks for schizophrenia and other serious psychopathology. We conducted family therapy from three months to two years. We followed up the *Ss'* parents, becoming increasingly interested in how these parents tried to solve their life crises, and how their life crises affected the separation of their children from the home. For example, we found that parents can get so bogged down with resolving aspects of their middle-age-specific tasks or crises that children are experienced as nuisances and are expelled, or at least insidiously neglected. Many of these children in our sample ran away in a casual, drifting manner (in contrast to other runaways who gave more evidence of inner turmoil [Stierlin, in press]). But other children appeared "delegated" to fulfill aspects of the parents' unresolved life crises. The word *delegate* very nicely conveys two aspects. It conveys, first, "to send out," and, second, to bestow with a mission. Thus, the delegate, while sent out, is also held back, as he remains beholden to the sender. His mission can be to experiment on behalf of the parent. For example, a father who is constantly preoccupied with breaking away from his job or breaking away from a stifling marriage, now encourages his son to experiment with things he is afraid to do himself but is completely preoccupied with. The boy will have a sort of scout function. He runs away, but he comes back and feeds the parent the needed information or enacts some aspect of his (the father's) developmental task. At the other extreme, there are parents who try to solve various aspects of the middle-aged crises you have outlined, holding onto the adolescent in an extremely tight manner. I call these the binding parents. Binding parents maintain on various levels a symbiotically clinging, sucking type of relationship, as salvation for their life crises. They hold on for dear life to what the adolescent offers them. This accounts for a very different kind of separation from the home — a dynamic dilemma which I have outlined in its various ramifications (Stierlin, 1972; Stierlin, Levi, & Savard, 1971; Stierlin & Ravenscroft, 1972).

JESSICA SCHAIRER. As you spoke, I could see that many of the people around me felt that your paper struck very close to home. While not affecting me in the same way, something in what you said is relevant to my situation, which I would like you to think about. Epstein (1970), in a paper on the participation of women in the professions, found that the lack of a mentor is what holds so many women back in professional development. Your whole paper seems to show, almost categorically, that it should be theoretically impossible for a woman to have a mentor in a professional field. This is a sociological problem which people here should think of as professionals and as life historians — even though your paper, like so many others, specifically addresses itself only to men.

LEVINSON. I endorse that. Having more women in senior positions in professional life in the university would have a number of functions. It would give female students female mentor figures. It would give male students female mentor figures, which might help them. I'm greatly indebted to the female mentors that I was lucky enough to have. And it would help to overcome that whole polarization of masculine and feminine with which we struggle so.

SCHAIRER. Was I correct in thinking that your paper says that theoretically it should be impossible because of the psychodynamics of the mentor relationship?

LEVINSON. Well, a man can be a genuine mentor to younger women. I must say that I have worked fairly hard at that myself, and I'm sure Harry Murray could tell stories of his functioning as a mentor. But it's a challenge because the older man who is in that position with, say, female graduate students or students in professional school has to be careful that his conscious or unconscious sexism doesn't lead him to make the female student into a little girl, rather than welcoming her into the peer relationship.

SELECTED REFERENCES

Brim, O. G., & Wheeler, S. *Socialization after childhood.* New York: Wiley, 1966.
Buhler, C. The curve of life as studied in biographies. *Journal of Applied Psychology*, 1955, 19, 405–409.
Cain, L. Life course and social structure. In R. E. L. Faris (Ed.), *Handbook of modern sociology.* Chicago: Rand-McNally, 1964.
Campbell, J. (Ed.) *The portable Jung.* New York: Viking, 1971.

Epstein, C. F. Encountering the male establishment: Sex-status limits on women's careers in the professions. *American Journal of Sociology*, 1970, 75, 965–982.

Erikson, E. H. Identity and the life cycle. *Psychological Issues*, 1959, 1 (1).

————. *Gandhi's truth.* New York: Norton, 1969.

Jaques, E. Death and the mid-life crisis. *International Journal of Psycho-Analysis*, 1965, 46, 502–514.

Jung, C. G. *Memories, dreams, reflections.* New York: Pantheon, 1963.

Neugarten, B. L. (Ed.) *Middle age and aging: A reader in social psychology.* Chicago: University of Chicago Press, 1968.

Stierlin, H. Family dynamics and separation patterns of potential schizophrenics. In Y. Alanen (Ed.), *Proceedings of fourth international symposium on psychotherapy of schizophrenia.* Amsterdam: Excerpta Medica, 1972. Pp. 169–179.

————. A family perspective on adolescent runaways. *Archives of General Psychiatry*, in press.

————, Levi, L. D., & Savard, R. J. Parental perceptions of separating children. *Family Process*, 1971, 10, 411–427.

Stierlin, H., & Ravenscroft, K., Jr. Varieties of adolescent "separation conflicts." *British Journal of Medical Psychology*, 1972, 45, 299–313.

NOTE: There are excellent biographies and autobiographies of persons such as Sigmund Freud, Eugene O'Neill, Bertrand Russell, Henry James, James Joyce, and F. Scott Fitzgerald. There are also novels and plays about men in the mid-life transition, often written by men during or just following their own mid-life transition — for example, *The Iceman Cometh* (O'Neill), *Who's Afraid of Virginia Woolf?* (Albee), *The Tempest* (Shakespeare), *The Man Who Cried I Am* (Williams), *Chimera* (Barth), and *Herzog* (Bellow). Works of this kind are of great value, both in forming a theory of adult development and in testing and extending our present theory.

BENEDICT J. GROESCHEL ⫼ *Social Adjustment*
after Residential Treatment

THIS PAPER evaluates the family background, case history, and later adjustment of 124 boys discharged from Children's Village between July 1, 1965, and September 1, 1966. The practical goals of the study reported here were identifying variables which predict successful or poor adjustment and suggesting procedures for minimizing the effect of negative factors after discharge from treatment. Children's Village is a residential treatment center for emotionally disturbed boys located in Dobbs Ferry, New York. The boys studied had been referred to it by family court and other social agencies for a wide variety of behavioral and emotional problems. They all came from the northeastern United States and 80 per cent came from New York City. Independent evaluations were made of the background and case history of each boy and of his later adjustment. The mean age of the boys on admission to Children's Village was 11 years, 11 months, and the mean age at discharge from the in-care program was 14 years, 6 months, with the average stay being 2 years, 7 months. The mean age at the time of this study was 17 years, 8 months. Of the 137 boys discharged from Children's Village during the period studied, 10 were not located, and 3 had died. Those who were not located or who had died were not significantly different from those who were studied in terms of the variables considered in this study.

Two trained staff members independently recorded information about the family background and the treatment history of the boy while he was at Children's Village. Thirty-five different variables were considered.* Variables related to family background included ethnocultural group, religion, family composition, home management and support,

*All instruments used in these evaluations, including questionnaires, rating scales, and structural interview forms, are available on request from Reverend Benedict J. Groeschel, O.F.M., Children's Village, Dobbs Ferry, New York 10522.

number of siblings, social disorganization of home neighborhood, quality of parental relationships, psychopathology of parents, and social behavior of parents. Variables related to treatment history included age at admission and discharge, length of stay, reason for referral, behavioral classification or diagnosis at admission and discharge, child's performance in various areas of the Children's Village program, and prognosis.

The evaluation of adjustment was made by the author, who, as chaplain of the agency, knew each boy personally. Two to three years after the boys had been discharged from Children's Village, I interviewed 110 boys and their parents, wives, employers, teachers, and other significant persons. In 14 cases, boys had to be evaluated on the basis of information from secondary sources such as relatives, former employers, and police officials. Evaluation of adjustment was based on ten variables, including data related to vocational, educational and home adjustment, criminal record, and narcotics use.

Since ethnocultural group emerged as important in this study, an explanation of this term is necessary. The three ethnocultural groups represented in this study — Caucasians (60), Blacks (4), and Puerto Ricans (20) — are sociocultural groups and not races in the strict sense of the term. They are social groupings of persons who have been exposed to similar familial, economic, educational, and environmental influences. This is particularly true of the Black and Puerto Rican boys in this study. Almost without exception, they came from and returned to homes in high or medium crime areas with inferior educational services, severe economic handicaps, and multiple, chronic social problems. Within each of these groups, particular familial patterns exist, sometimes reflecting the effects of centuries of deprivation. Ethnocultural groups were found to be significantly related to all important variables in this study. It is not implied that the ethnocultural group was itself a causative factor. The term does, however, serve as a means of social identification and was found to be related to a wide variety of environment factors, including parental relationship and behavioral classification.

It is important to take note of features of the ethnocultural groups in this study. It was observed that the Puerto Ricans in the sample were least likely to experience parental rejection, but were the most vulnerable to it when it occurred. I have noted that in selected populations of rejected Puerto Rican children, such as an orphanage, there is a high level of alienation which was not observed among the Puerto Rican boys at Children's Village.

The Caucasian boys were less homogeneous than the Black and Puerto Rican boys and their adjustments presented a bimodal pattern. However, the same variables (for example, quality of parental relationship) which significantly discriminated between and within the other two ethnocultural groups with respect to adjustment, also discriminated between Caucasian boys who succeeded and those who failed.

FINDINGS

Background. Significant relationships were found between a number of variables in the case histories of the boys, and between those variables and adjustment. A relationship was found between ethnocultural group and social level of the neighborhood. Because of the need for an objective and uniform evaluation of the social level of neighborhoods, only boys from New York City were considered in terms of this variable. The evaluation was based on statistics of the New York City Police Department for 1968. It was found that 38 per cent (11) of the Caucasians, 91 per cent (31) of the Blacks, and 100 per cent (20) of the Puerto Ricans came from and returned to high crime areas.

Table 1 indicates that ethnocultural group was also related to certain diagnostic categories, with Blacks more likely to have been seen as passive-aggressive, and Puerto Ricans and Caucasians more likely to have been diagnosed as neurotic or inadequate ($p<.05$). These diagnostic categories were drawn mainly from the American Psychiatric Association classification (1952) and from Cameron (1963). Specific indicators of behavior which the evaluators used as guides were drawn from *Psychological Disorders in Childhood* (GAP, 1966) and from McCord and McCord, *The Psychopath* (1964).

Ethnocultural grouping was significantly related to a diagnosis of

Table 1. Behavior Classification at Discharge from Children's Village by Ethnocultural Group

Behavior Classification at Discharge	Caucasian		Black		Puerto Rican		Total	
	N	%	N	%	N	%	N	%
Inadequate	5	8	7	15	2	10	14	11
Neurotic	20	33	5	11	5	25	30	24
Passive-aggressive ..	18	30	25	57	6	30	49	40
Active-aggressive ..	9	15	4	9	3	15	16	13
Prepsychotic	6	9	3	7	3	15	12	10
Psychotic	2	4			1	5	3	2
Total	60	100	44	100	20	100	124	100

neurosis. Boys diagnosed as passive-aggressive had a poorer rate of adjustment than neurotics, prepsychotics, or inadequates. In terms of parental relationships, boys were divided into those who experienced unambiguous relationships with mother and father figures, ranging from acceptance to total rejection, and those with missing parents.

Ethnocultural group was found to relate significantly with maternal acceptance ($p<.05$): 35 per cent of the Puerto Ricans (7) had accepting mothers whereas only 19 per cent of the Caucasians (11) and 17 per cent of the Blacks (8) experienced maternal acceptance.

Because of the disproportionately large percentage of boys with missing fathers in the Black and Puerto Rican groups, it was not possible to compare accurately the different effects of paternal acceptance. Whereas only 21 per cent (13) of the Caucasians had missing fathers, 35 per cent (7) of the Puerto Ricans and 39 per cent (17) of the Blacks had no father present in the house. However, it should be noted that 29 per cent (17) of the Caucasians but only 14 per cent (6) of the Blacks and 10 per cent (2) of the Puerto Ricans had totally rejecting fathers at home. This suggests that social pressures are more likely to keep a rejecting Caucasian father in the home than fathers from other ethnocultural groups.

Boys were also divided into those who had mothers or fathers engaged in antisocial behavior, ranging from chronic and overt alcoholism to felonies, and those who were law-abiding. Although there were no significant group differences in fathers engaged in antisocial behavior, 32 per cent (13) of the Black youngsters, 13 per cent (3) of the Puerto Rican youngsters, and 18 per cent (11) of the Caucasian youngsters had mothers engaged in antisocial behavior.

Treatment History. The case records of the boys were evaluated. Because of the nature of the information available, simple 10-point rating scales were employed to measure the quality of involvement in various therapeutic programs, including clinical services, child care, school, recreation program, and the religious program. Information on the therapeutic involvement of the boy was gathered from departmental reports, case conference minutes, caseworkers' notes, and discharge summaries. For clinical services, the evaluation was made on the basis of the use the boy made of casework services and of psychological and psychiatric services. A boy who was seen as having become seriously involved in a psychotherapeutic relationship for at least the last third of his stay was given a rating from 1 to 3. A boy with moderate to superficial involvement was rated 4–7. A boy who refused to use these services or who resisted them throughout his stay was rated 8–10. In the milieu areas of child care (social adjustment in the cottage), school, recreation, and religious programs, the child was evaluated on performance. Since children generally perform much better in these areas toward the end of their stay, performance ratings were based on the final case conference reports and the discharge summary. The evaluation of school performance was based on the quality of the boy's application to schoolwork and his attempts to make educational gains, rather than on any actual assessment of improvement. Case conference reports from the school contain information on both performance and educational advancement.

In all areas the mean performance scores were between 3.0 and 3.5 on a 10-point scale with 1 as the highest positive score. Performance scores in clinical services correlated highly with performance in child care (.63), in school (.62), in religious services (.50), and in the recreation program (.35).

In summary, background information and treatment histories suggested that Caucasians were likely to come from more favorable social environments and Puerto Ricans were more likely to enjoy more favorable parental relationships. The Black youngsters in this study were significantly disadvantaged as regards neighborhood, parental relationships, and social behavior of their mothers. They had more diagnoses in which aggression was the dominant symptom, and fewer in which neurotic or psychotic defenses predominated.

Follow-Up Adjustment. At the time of evaluation, Black youngsters were found to have favorable vocational patterns (in school or at least part-time employment) in 43 per cent (21) of the cases, whereas 57 per cent (34) of the Caucasians and 65 per cent (13) of the Puerto Ricans presented favorable patterns of vocational adjustment.

Caucasians were less likely to be involved in extensive use of narcotics (70 per cent [42] were non-users) than either of the other groups. The number of Blacks (40 per cent [18]) who had not used narcotics at all was significantly smaller ($p<.05$) than the number of non-users in the other groups.

To get one single index of adjustment level, all of the information gathered during the evaluation phase, including data from questionnaires, and the results of open-ended interviews with the boys and significant persons in their lives were reduced to a single composite four-point scale, from very good to very poor. The following descriptions indicate the specific qualities in each category.

1. *Very good adjustment.* Boys were rated as having made a very good adjustment if they were employed or going to school full time and were doing well in these pursuits, if they were getting along with others where they lived, and if they were avoiding narcotics and crime. Apart from a few minor problems which they were coping with successfully, these boys were apparently functioning better than most people in their social environment. No boy who had been in any serious legal difficulty since leaving the Village was judged to have made a very good adjustment, even if at the time of follow-up he seemed to be doing very well.

2. *Fairly good adjustment.* Boys were rated as making fairly good adjustments if they were doing reasonably well in school or at work, and either (a) had one identifiable life problem which, though not threatening their basic adjustment, was limiting their potential in some way; or (b) they were doing well at present but had been in some legal difficulty in the past. In this second category were two boys who were actually in training schools, but who were considered to be making an excellent adjustment and were expected to do well when they returned home by the school officials who rated them.

3. *Fairly poor adjustment.* Boys were judged to be doing fairly poorly if they were not self-supporting or going to school, but were at least avoiding serious difficulties. This included school dropouts who are not yet working, partially unemployed boys, or boys whose employers and families complained about their failure to contribute positively on the job or at home. Also included in this group are most of the boys in training schools, who were seen as just conforming but not really making permanent gains in adjustment.

4. *Very poor adjustment.* Boys were judged to be doing very poorly if they were in prison for serious crimes. This category also included boys still in the community who were involved in criminal careers, who were using hard narcotics, or who were fugitives from the law. Also included were psychotic boys who were totally incapable of coping with life and were either hospitalized or totally withdrawn from society.

Data on the adjustment of the subjects are given in Table 2. More Puerto Ricans made good adjustments ($p < .10$) or very good adjustments than Blacks ($p < .05$). More Blacks made very poor adjustments than did boys in other groups ($p < .10$).

After examining relationships between other background variables (besides ethnocultural group), the relationship of these to adjustment was explored. A number of background variables were not significantly related to adjustment. These included religion, IQ, educational level of parents, pathology of parents, economic support of home, and number of siblings. No significant relationships were found between adjustment and the following measures derived from treatment histories: age at

Table 2. Composite Index of Adjustment and Ethnocultural Group

Boys According to Index of Adjustment	Caucasian		Black		Puerto Rican		Total	
	N	%	N	%	N	%	N	%
Very good	21	35	5	11	8	40	34	28
Fairly good	17	29	16	37	6	30	39	31
Total	38	64	21	48	14	70	73	59
Fairly poor	11	18	10	23	4	20	25	20
Very poor	11	18	13	29	2	10	26	21
Total	22	36	23	52	6	30	51	41
Total	60	100	44	100	20	100	124	100

admission and at discharge, length of stay, and performance in the religion and recreation programs.

Three variables reflecting the boys' performance in treatment were significantly and positively correlated to adjustment: performance in school (.21), performance in child care (.22), and involvement in casework services (.27). These correlations, though small, suggest that the children who had better emotional control and less severe pathology were likely to relate to authority figures more positively during residential treatment than other boys, and to make better adjustments after discharge.

The prognosis given by staff members at the time of discharge did significantly relate to later adjustment (.35). However, it is interesting to note that staff ratings were often guarded or pessimistic in the cases of boys whose adjustments at follow-up were very good.

Of equal or greater importance were the relationships discovered between adjustment and ethnocultural groups on the one hand and the four background variables of parental relationships, behavioral classification, social behavior of mothers, and social disorganization of neighborhood. For the most part, these variables tended to be related to one another and to be, in turn, associated with the ethnocultural identity of the boys.

In terms of positive acceptance, the relationships of boys with their mothers were divided into accepting, confusing, and totally rejecting. These were found to be significantly related to outcome in that 73 per cent (19) of boys with accepting maternal relationships and 60 per cent (45) of those with confusing relationships made good adjustments, whereas only 34 per cent (7) of those who experienced total rejection made such adjustments. It has already been noted that 35 per cent of the Puerto Rican boys had accepting relationships with their mothers while only 19 per cent of the Caucasians and 17 per cent of Blacks had such a relationship. The importance of the ethnocultural factor becomes even clearer when it is noted that of the 7 boys who had accepting maternal relationships but who made poor adjustments, 5 were Black, 1 was Puerto Rican, and 1 was Caucasian. This suggests that having an accepting mother may not be able to mitigate social factors leading to poor adjustment in the case of a Black youngster, whereas such a maternal relationship might help a Puerto Rican boy who comes from the same socially disadvantaged environment.

There were no statistically significant differences in the adjustment of boys with differing paternal relationships, but while only 10 per cent (6) of the Caucasians and 19 per cent (8) of the Blacks had accepting fathers, no less than 45 per cent (9) of the Puerto Rican boys had such fathers. In the group of 9 boys who had accepting fathers but who made poor adjustments, there were 7 Blacks but only 1 Puerto Rican and 1 Caucasian. This suggests, again, that even an accepting paternal relationship may not be able to moderate the social disabilities which the Black youngster faces.

The ability to adjust in spite of rejection or confusing parental relationships appeared also to be related to predischarge diagnosis. Among boys who had confusing parental relationships, the 15 neurotic boys had the highest rate of adjustment (86 per cent) as compared with the 30 passive-aggressive boys, whose rate of good adjustment was only 50 per cent. The neurotic boys were overwhelmingly Caucasian and Puerto Rican.

The possibility of obtaining the help of intervening persons or agencies from outside the family also appeared to be associated with ethnocultural group. The Puerto Ricans who had favorable maternal and/or paternal relationships were most likely to make good adjustments, but they were unlikely to find or accept help from outside their own homes. The Blacks were most likely to have experienced rejecting parental relationships and also to have the more unfavorable diagnoses, and they lived in areas which offered few sources of assistance outside their homes. Caucasians were most likely to be able to find social assistance. Both Black and Caucasian boys who made good adjustments, despite parental rejection, seemed to have been able to find, and to respond to, positive intervention from non-parental figures.

A comparison between behavioral classification before discharge from the Village and adjustment yielded significant results ($p<.05$). These results are found in Table 3. A striking finding was the rate of good

Table 3. Behavior Classification at Discharge versus Adjustment ($N = 124$)[a]

Behavior Classi-fication at Discharge	Very good		Fairly Poor		Fairly Good		Very good		Total	Percentage Making Good
	N	%	N	%	N	%	N	%	N	Adjustment
Inadequate	3	21.5	2	14	5	37	4	28.5	14	64
Neurotic	2	7	4	13	11	37	13	43	30	80
Passive-aggressive	8	16	13	27	20	41	8	16	49	57
Active-aggressive	10	63	4	25			2	12	16	13
Prepsychotic	2	16.6	2	16.6	2	16.6	6	50	12	67
Psychotic	1	33	1	33			1	33	3	33

[a] $\chi^2 = 40.77$, $p < .05$.

adjustment of the 30 neurotics (80 per cent) and the low rate of good adjustment of the 16 active-aggressive boys (12 per cent). The second highest record of good adjustment (67 per cent) was made by the 12 prepsychotic boys, who seemed to be able to continue to function as they had in the Village, despite severe personality problems.

Thus, a pattern emerges: consistent positive prognostic signs for Puerto Ricans, fairly positive prognostic signs or the possibility of outside ameliorating factors for Caucasians, and overriding social, psychological, and personal disadvantages for the Black youngsters.

A significant difference ($p<.05$) was found to exist between the number (65) of successful boys who had law-abiding mothers (68 per cent) and the number of successful boys (12) who had mothers involved in antisocial behavior (43 per cent). It has already been noted that 13 per cent of the Puerto Rican, 18 per cent of the Caucasian, and 32 per cent of the Black mothers were so involved. Thus, in this sample, the social behavior of mothers is yet another variable related to the poor adjustment of the Black boys and the good adjustment of the Puerto Rican boys. Considering only boys who returned to New York City, the 6 boys from low crime neighborhoods (all Caucasians) made good adjustments. The 12 Caucasian boys from medium crime areas had a lower frequency of good adjustment (50 per cent) than the overall sample (59 per cent). Although 100 per cent of the Puerto Ricans came from high crime areas, 70 per cent (14) made at least fairly good adjustments, a record well above the 59 per cent base rate for the entire group. The 31 Black youngsters from high crime neighborhoods had a poorer rate of good adjustment (45 per cent).

From the data available, the most plausible explanation of the high adjustment rate of the Puerto Rican boys despite their poor social environment is the quality of parental relationships — in which, as has been noted, the Puerto Ricans had significantly higher ratings than the other ethnocultural groups.

Apparently, boys from high crime areas reacted differently to their social situation according to their ethnocultural group. Boys from low crime areas tended to be diagnosed as neurotic or prepsychotic, to be able to seek help effectively, and to disentangle themselves from rejecting families. Boys from medium crime areas also tended to be neurotic, but included a number of passive and active aggressives. Examination of individual case histories suggests that these boys' successful adjustment may be related to positive changes in their parents' attitude toward them.

Summary of Findings. A significant relationship has been observed throughout this study between ethnocultural group and adjustment. With the sole exception of neighborhood social disorganization, the Puerto Rican boys have had the most positive prognostic signs and they have tended to make good adjustments most frequently. Black youngsters have the greatest handicaps and the poorest rate of adjustment (good adjustment of 48 per cent compared with a rate of 59 per cent for the whole sample); one quarter of the Black youngsters made very poor adjustments. Among the Blacks in this sample who made favorable adjustments, there were none who had left home and cut themselves off from their families, as was the case with successful Caucasians. The Black youngster who succeeded found support and encouragement from his family and friends. A number succeeded after one arrest and probation, but very few succeeded after sentence and detention.

The difference between the Puerto Ricans and the other groups becomes apparent particularly in the quality of parental relationships: 3 Puerto Ricans, 1 Black, and no Caucasian experienced complete maternal acceptance; 9 Puerto Ricans out of 20 experienced full or limited paternal acceptance, whereas only 6 Caucasians out of 60 had such an experience; and whereas 28 per cent of the Caucasians experienced total paternal rejection, only 10 per cent of the Puerto Ricans had this experience. When combined maternal and paternal relationships are considered, 55 per cent of the Puerto Ricans can be said to have experienced at least one accepting relationship, as compared with 21 per cent of the Caucasians and 30 per cent of the Black youngsters. Even Puerto Rican boys who had some negative feelings toward their parents remained emotionally close to their families. Puerto Ricans who had lost their families through death or mishap sought out another family and were often "adopted." The 2 Puerto Ricans who made very poor adjustments were the only boys in this ethnocultural group who were actually without close emotional ties to some family group.

The Caucasian boys were socially and psychologically the most varied of the three ethnocultural groups. The Caucasians included the largest proportion of neurotics, active-aggressive antisocial personalities, and psychotics, thereby encompassing both extremes of the psychological spectrum. Despite this bimodal distribution, their rate of adjustment (63 per cent) is closest to the base rate (59 per cent) for good adjustment of the entire sample.

Examination of individual case histories suggests that the Caucasians who got into difficulties more often found help and rehabilitation than did similarly troubled boys from minority groups. The Caucasians who failed were frequently the most disturbed (active-aggressives and psychotics) or boys with extremely rejecting home situations where the rejecting parents, apparently responding to middle-class social pressure, maintained a hostile and destructive relationship with the boy rather than abandoning him. This kind of destructive relationship was observed in a quarter of the Caucasians who failed. Even though the Caucasians have the highest percentage of rejecting and confusing parental relationships, moderating and ameliorating factors were frequently found in the individual case histories of Caucasian boys. In fact, all 6 Caucasians from low crime areas cut themselves off from their pathological families, found help, and made successful adjustments.

Boys from different ethnocultural backgrounds who made good adjustments usually faced different obstacles and found different solutions. Black youngsters who made good adjustments tended to remain in their own communities and found either in their own family or in some other person a source of emotional support, recognition, and counsel. In many cases, however, there simply was no supporting person available to help them deal with the challenges of adjustment. The Puerto Rican boys also remained at home and usually found parental acceptance and care; those who lacked accepting families usually adopted another family. The Caucasian boys who adjusted well tended to look outside their homes to individuals or social agencies for help and emotional support.

The trend of successful boys to look for acceptance and relationships at home or elsewhere was also noted in the treatment histories at the Village of boys who eventually made good adjustments. There were significant correlations between adjustment at follow-up and a child's use of clinical services and his performance in the child life and educational programs of Children's Village. The boys who were able to relate to caseworkers and to staff and peers in the treatment program eventually made the best adjustments. The observed association of "relatedness" and adjustment led to a search for a single common factor of adjustment which might conceptualize personal qualities predicting good adjustment after residential treatment.

CONCLUSIONS

The need for positive recognition as an individual and the need for a place in one's social group has been conceptualized as the need for social integration by a number of social scientists, including Parsons (1951) and Srole (1956). Expanding Durkheim's concept of anomie or alienation, Srole applied the concept to societies and individuals. Minority groups or subcultures experience anomia when they feel that they are not part of the society in which they live. Individuals experience anomie when they lack integration into the "total action fields of their interpersonal relationships and reference groups"(Srole, 1956).

It appears likely that anomia and anomie apply differently to the three ethnocultural groups represented in this project. Without experiencing anomia, a Caucasian boy might experience personal alienation (anomie) to a fairly high degree. The Caucasian boys tended to have rejecting parents, fathers who were involved in antisocial behavior, and emotionally confusing home environments. However, since they were members of the dominant social group, the Caucasians did not experience anomia or alienation from society. Put quite simply, a place in society could be found if they looked for one.

The Puerto Ricans, on the other hand, had little experience with anomie at home, although they experienced anomia or alienation from the dominant society in which they lived. Puerto Rican boys experienced social integration in their own family and were able to transfer this experience to their extended families of surrogate parents and siblings. The Puerto Ricans were also protected from the alienating hostility of the majority by the fact that they usually lived in Spanish-speaking ghettos of thousands who shared the same Latin American cultural heritage. Puerto Ricans, encountering the Caucasian world with its social pressures, were aware that if they did not win acceptance in it they might at least return to their families and neighborhoods and experience the sense of belonging that these gave them.

In terms of alienation on a familial and social level, the Black youngster had the most obstacles to overcome. Black youngsters in this study frequently had rejecting or socially rejected antisocial mothers, absent fathers, and parental relationship patterns marked by ambiguity. Two Blacks who made good had been helped by strong parental substitutes even when the child had been involved in delinquency and his parents were socially maladjusted. He might still experience the anomia common among American Blacks in a northern city, but he had a better chance of dealing with it because of the experience of social integration in the Black community.

A number of practical conclusions arising from this study apply to residential treatment centers like Children's Village. Space does not permit a review of these, but they relate to intake procedures, the application of some insights into ethnocultural needs drawn from social psychology, and continued care and after-care needs of children. The author hopes to be able to re-evaluate the adjustment of the same boys about ten years after discharge and is attempting to remain in touch with the young men in the sample. He is also conducting a pilot project in providing emotional support and acceptance for a number of representative boys in the sample who are now in their late teens. This project includes a self-supporting residence which the young men operate under the author's direction.

COMMENTARY

GITTELMAN-KLEIN. Robins (1966) has emphasized the importance of antisocial fathers. I wonder what you found along that line?

GROESCHEL. I used Robins's study as a model for this study. Many of the boys in this study had missing fathers, and so our statistics were incomplete: 30 per cent of the Puerto Ricans and 35 per cent of the Blacks had no fathers. Many of the Caucasians had fathers who might have departed but social pressures kept them at home. Only 13 per cent of the Caucasians had absent fathers. This made it impossible to obtain statistically significant data. We did observe the following trend. Of Black fathers present in the home, 45 per cent were involved in antisocial behavior, and of the Puerto Rican fathers 15 per cent were engaged in antisocial behavior, but 45 per cent of the Caucasian fathers were also so engaged. These are interesting data, but they were not statistically significant.

ZUBIN. I think your description is very interesting and certainly very humanistic. However, you pointed out that this was a residential home of a special kind and that the people that you dealt with were highly special. What made the residential home unique? Secondly, how much can you generalize from a situation where you have a special residential home and some specialized types of Puerto Ricans?

GROESCHEL. I am cautious about generalizing from these data. Perhaps the only generalization that would be completely valid is that those boys who had accepting mothers did well and those who did not, did poorly. That is hardly unexpected. Perhaps one might be able to generalize further by comparing residential treatment centers in the Northeast. They tend to have similar problems and populations. One might compare populations of Puerto Rican children who are mostly foundlings with our population and discover some interesting trends. People who work among Puerto Ricans hold an adage that the unloved Puerto Rican dies. This was certainly true in this study. The two rejected Puerto Ricans adjusted very poorly, and the rest seemed to do well.

Another fact that makes this population specialized is that a tremendous number of children coming into placement from the New York area are Black and Puerto Rican. A residential treatment center may be tempted to select children who need treatment, but might tend to take those who appear more treatable. This would mean that, generally, a Black and Puerto Rican population should be a little healthier than a Caucasian population.

THOMAS. One advantage of letting Zubin speak first is that he always asks the question that you have in mind. The question, of course, is of generalization from this population. As you indicate, there is such a pressure of cases being referred to these specialized residential centers that in a study of this kind, it would be extremely important to get a base line of what the population was like at the time of entry, and then comparisons could be made thereafter. It may very well be that the white, Black, and Puerto Rican children are very different — your caution that there may be special selection of these children by the agencies is a gentle warning. As some of you know, one of the great hidden scandals in the New York area, which I am sure is duplicated in other major metropolitan centers, is that voluntary residential agencies and institutions treating children accept populations heavily weighted in the direction of the white middle-class child. This kind of selection is accomplished in many ways, such as by setting a floor on IQ. Thus, a child will not be accepted if he has an IQ below 70, 75, or whatever, although it is known that IQ scores attained by many Black and Puerto Rican children are entirely unreliable. Also, a number of institutions will not take the aggressive, acting-out child. So I think any conclusion that such a child cannot be treated or is, perhaps, not a good risk for putting money into has to be made very carefully because of the way such findings are utilized by agencies in this kind of biased selection process.

GROESCHEL. Thomas's observations are to the point, although perhaps oversimplified. It should be noted that the ethnic balance of Children's Village is very different now than in the past, with a smaller Caucasian population. I notice this on Sunday, because the Black youngsters tend to be Protestant and Caucasians referred in New York tend to be Catholic. I have been telling our Protestant chaplain for years that the Catholics in Children's Village are much sicker than the Protestants, because I end up with more of the Caucasians in my congregation. On the point of active-aggressive children, though, I must add that I am convinced that an open residential setting with an easy, nondirective structure cannot even contain them. They burn the buildings down, go over the wall, and quickly end up in the state hospital. A lot of creative thinking should go into what kind of private residential facility is necessary for these children.

GITTELMAN-KLEIN. Your single best predictor of outcome is diagnosis. Of the neurotics, 80 per cent make a good adjustment. I am puzzled about what sort of child is diagnosed as neurotic and referred for inpatient treatment.

GROESCHEL. Generally, these are children driven by fear or guilt, who have nightmares and tics, but no overt psychotic symptoms. These boys haunt their caseworker, want to be in therapy, and are verbal. Of course, these are also the kids who know how to get help when they leave.

GITTELMAN-KLEIN. But why are they there? How do they get there?

GROESCHEL. Ordinarily, they have been totally impossible to control in school. They often have serious learning disabilities. Almost all were referred for severe school problems. They often steal or act out to get sent away from home. One of the best neurotics in the study picked the pocket of a bookie in Harlem and stole five thousand dollars to get to Children's Village. He has made a wonderful adjustment.

REFERENCES

Cameron, N. *Personality development and psychopathology.* New Haven: Yale University Press, 1963.

Diagnostic and statistical manual of mental disorders. Washington, D.C.: American Psychiatric Association, 1952.

Group for the Advancement of Psychiatry. *Psychopathological disorders in childhood.* Vol. 6. Report No. 62. New York: Group for the Advancement of Psychiatry, June 1966.

McCord, W., & McCord, J. *The psychopath.* Princeton, N.J.: Van Nostrand, 1964.

Parsons, T. *The social system.* Glencoe, Ill.: Free Press, 1951.

Robins, L. N. *Deviant children grown up: A psychiatric and sociological study of sociopathic personality.* Baltimore: Williams & Wilkins, 1966.

Srole, L. Social integration and certain correlaries. *American Sociological Review,* 1956, 21, 6, 709–716.

DAVID F. RICKS *Supershrink: Methods of a Therapist Judged Successful on the Basis of Adult Outcomes of Adolescent Patients*

Dᴜʀɪɴɢ ᴛʜᴇ last decade, three growing beliefs have begun to reorient therapeutic practice. The first, developing from observations in mental hospitals, is that hospitalization itself can produce social deterioration so severe that prevention of hospitalization through early identification and treatment must become one of the main strategies of mental health work (Goffman, 1961; Mednick & Schulsinger, 1970).

The second grows out of experience and research in psychotherapy. Like hospitalization, psychotherapy can both help and hinder those who experience it (Bergin, 1966, 1971). In examining the implications of deterioration effects for therapeutic practice, Bergin argued that therapists "should find out who they are making better or worse, and how . . . They should find out if some therapists make people better and some make them worse, or if individual therapists do both."

The third is the growth of a life history perspective on disturbance. This viewpoint is coming to be widely shared. Even Eysenck (1966) has realized that improvement and deterioration both require demonstration of lasting effects that have real, long-term, life significance.

This paper is a beginning attempt to describe some therapeutic methods that may be effective in preventing hospitalization. The observations concern methods employed by a therapist who was unusually helpful in early psychotherapeutic intervention with severely disturbed boys. At some points contrasting results obtained by an apparently harmful therapist, together with the methods that seemed to produce them, are described. The criterion of effectiveness is adult outcome, that is, whether each patient in a set seen by a particular therapist was chronically hospitalized, briefly hospitalized, or not hospitalized in adult life, and for those not hospitalized, the level of adjustment, whether inadequate or socially adequate.

This report, based largely on notes kept by different therapists, can cover only a few aspects of the therapeutic relationship. No comparisons will be made of the therapists' experience levels, training, or professions, since we do not want to identify individuals. Personal qualities such as warmth, adequacy of adjustment, or empathy will not be described, since therapy notes provide inadequate data for judging these. Even the methods used by the therapists, which can be described in some detail, may be considerably distorted by the process of recording and the judgments made by researchers some years later. But the importance of the problem justifies an attempt to describe these methods, and a start now may lead to more adequate research.

No claim is made here that psychotherapy was the only, or even the most powerful, influence on the adult adjustment levels of the children with whom the report is concerned. But if the adult outcomes of children seen by different therapists differ reliably, and if the differences seem related to specific therapeutic methods, a beginning description of therapeutic methods that further growth or hasten deterioration can be made. Since methods of helping people are more interesting to clinicians than methods of harming them, the focus of this article will be on useful methods of intervention, with description of apparently destructive types of intervention described for background and contrast.

METHODS

Sample. Cross checking the records of a major child guidance center with lists of patients kept by the local state department of mental health revealed that of approximately 15,000 patients seen at the center and grown to adulthood, 196 had been hospitalized in the state and given either a final diagnosis of schizophrenia with no history of repeated conflicting diagnoses, or had repeated diagnoses of schizophrenia. Of this sample 84 were still hospitalized in 1965, at the time of the study, while 112 were released and back in the community.

A comparison sample was gathered by selecting for each child in the schizophrenic sample another child seen during the same era in the center's history, and matched to the pre-schizophrenic child on age when seen, IQ, ethnic background, sex, social class, and when possible, on presenting symptoms.

Comparison children were followed up by telephone calls to the patient or to immediate family members, and a few were visited or came back to the center to report on their adult lives. Like the children and adolescents who were later schizophrenic, those in the comparison sample proved to have a wide range of adult adjustments. Those who met only the minimal criteria of never having been hospitalized or jailed were classified in a *socially inadequate* group. Those who met rather stringent criteria of responsible social participation (if over 25, married, or if single, head of own household, not living with or supported by parents, and evidence of heterosexual dating) and an adequate work history (if 25 or older, steady employment at a level consistent with early IQ and school achievement; if under 25, active in school, armed forces, or work) were considered to be in a *socially adequate* group.

The adolescents whose adult lives are the standard for our comparisons, then, could be grouped into four levels of adult adjustment, ranging from (1) chronic schizophrenia, to (2) life patterns marked by one or more episodes of schizophrenia followed by release from hospitalization, to (3) socially inadequate life patterns, and (4) patterns of adjustment with clear evidence for social adequacy.

Preliminary study of a sample with mixed sets of diagnoses, and hence not usable for our final samples, indicated that records containing at least six therapy hours were necessary to provide evidence of the methods of the therapist. The study was accordingly limited to the records of children and adolescents who had been seen for six or more hours by at least one therapist. The composition of the sample is shown in the accompanying tabulation.

	Male	Female	Total
Chronic schizophrenic ...	15	8	23
Released schizophrenic ...	32	6	38
Socially inadequate	18	6	24
Socially adequate	21	15	36
Total	86	35	121

The records of this set of 121 children were inspected to find which therapists had treated them. Nine of the cases had been seen by therapists who were represented by only one or two cases. Most of these therapists had been in training. Since none of them were represented by enough children or enough therapy hours to permit a thorough study of their therapy methods, these records were put aside.

The other 112 children had been seen by therapists who had worked with at least 3 children for a minimum of 6 hours. They averaged about 12 hours per child, so that the methods of each were represented by about 36 descriptions of therapy hours. These descriptions appeared to provide at least preliminary suggestions of helpful, neutral, and harmful methods of intervention.

Close study of the therapy protocols, however, indicated that the case loads seen by different therapists were not generally comparable. Two of the therapists had worked in the early, court-connected days of the clinic, when study of the child and recommendations to the court and other agencies were the method of choice. Their methods could not be considered those of therapeutic intervention, by current standards. Two other therapists worked predominantly with sets of diagnostically diverse young children. Another therapist appeared to establish little relationship with the children he treated, so that any effect he achieved would appear to be only chance. And still another therapist, with a national reputation, had been presented with a sample of children biased toward higher levels of social class and intelligence.

Elimination of these therapists left the study with two therapists whose effects appeared open to comparison. Each had seen a large number of boys, more than any other therapists. They had worked over the same period in the history of the clinic, and, as shown below, their case samples were rather closely matched at the time of clinic contact.

The children in the residence operated by the center have given therapist A the title Supershrink. The other therapist will be called Therapist B. Both men worked only with boys, and predominantly with boys in late childhood and early adolescence. The contrasting trajectories of boys who had seen Therapist A and Therapist B are shown in the accompanying tabulation.

	Therapist A	*Therapist B*
Chronic schizophrenic	0	3
Released schizophrenic	4	8
Socially inadequate	5	2
Socially adequate	6	0

Ricks and Berry (1970) have argued that the main determinants of chronicity in schizophrenia are poor neurological and personality integration. Other determinants have to do with the family atmosphere and with the hospital into which a person is placed. On the assumptions that therapy in adolescence might influence whether one has a young adult schizophrenic episode, but is not likely to be the major determinant of whether that episode develops into chronic schizophrenia, we might combine the two schizophrenic groups seen by each therapist. If we also combine the two groups who were never hospitalized, we have the simple four-fold tabulation below.

	Therapist A	Therapist B
Schizophrenic outcome	4	11
Non-schizophrenic outcome ..	11	2

A χ^2 test of significance produces a value of 7.21, indicating that the probability of a difference this great is less than .01; it seems reasonable to conclude that this difference is not likely to be owing to chance.

It remains to be shown, however, that the difference is not due to some difference in the samples seen by the two therapists. The development of schizophrenia is related to a number of variables, among them low IQ (Lane & Albee, 1970; Pollack, Woerner, & Klein, 1970), low social class (Faris & Dunham, 1939; Hollingshead & Redlich, 1958), and ethnic background. It has also been shown that parental personalities, family relationships, and the milieus these create for the developing child must be taken into account (Waring & Ricks, 1965). An effort had been made to match each adolescent who was later schizophrenic to a control who was not, but since the sample seen by the two therapists considered here was a much reduced selection from the original set, it seemed possible that biases had crept in during the reduction process. Our task, then, was to find whether the two samples were matched on all variables other than the two crucial ones of adult outcome and therapist seen in adolescence. The following variables were considered:

a. Sex. There were no differences, since all were boys.
b. IQ. The mean IQ for both samples was near the usually expected population mean, 103 for those seen by Supershrink, 97 for those seen by Therapist B. One child in each sample was in the 70–80 range, the level at which low IQ begins to be a severe handicap to social adjustment.
c. Class. Both samples were predominantly working class, with only one boy in each sample coming from a background above Hollingshead's Class III.
d. Age. The mean age of both groups was early adolescence, 13 and a few months for Supershrink, slightly above 14 for Therapist B.
e. Ethnic status. Both samples contained a mix of ethnic backgrounds representing the complex elements of a large city, and neither contained an unusual representation of children from any particular ethnic background.
f. Period seen. All were seen between 1938 and 1948, and both groups were spread fairly evenly over that period.

g. Frequency of psychotic or schizoid parents. All parents had been studied before investigation of the therapeutic intervention. The classification of the parents is described in detail by Waring and Ricks (1965). No differences were found with regard to the frequency of any type of parent between the samples seen by the two therapists.

Probably the most crucial comparison, however, is between the syndromes the boys demonstrated at the time they were seen at the center. In earlier work on this project each boy had been classified by a team of an experienced psychologist and an experienced social worker into one of four groups, in decreasing order of severity.

1. Schizophrenic, either diagnosed by clinic or by other agencies, or evident in the record in a few cases, though no diagnosis given.
2. Definite psychotic symptoms, but not clearly schizophrenic. Bizarre acting out, depression, suicidal gestures, extreme obsessions and compulsions, extreme object-directed hostility.
3. Schizoid or withdrawn, extremely passive and/or acting out. Evidence of predominantly asocial or antisocial orientation.
4. No psychotic symptoms, only neurotic or mild acting out, and some evidence of personality integration in patterns of work, play with other children, etc.

The distribution of the samples seen by Supershrink and Therapist B are shown in the accompanying tabulation. The two distributions are

	Therapist A	*Therapist B*
1	4	4
2	7	5
3	3	2
4	1	2

virtually identical, with the majority of the boys seen by both therapists falling in the more disturbed two categories. Three of the boys seen by Supershrink, and none of those seen by Therapist B, had definite symptoms of brain damage. On the other hand, five of the boys seen by Therapist B, and none of those seen by Supershrink, were over 17, which may be a late age for intervention with boys as severely disturbed as these. This is also a convenient place to point out that the sample being discussed, for both therapists, is quite a disturbed one. Both had seen many boys who had less severe symptoms, and so did not fall into either the schizophrenic group or the comparison group of this study. A complete follow-up for both of these therapists, therefore, would find many more boys who turned out well, and the findings of extreme difference in outcome apply only to their work with quite disturbed boys.

DIFFERENCES IN PSYCHOTHERAPEUTIC METHODS

The nature of the present sample does not permit any interpretation of the two therapists' effectiveness with children or with adults unlike the small set of unusually disturbed boys considered here. Inspection of their therapy protocols suggests that both were intelligent, sensitive, articulate men with impressive insight into psychopathology in general and male adolescent problems in particular.

There seem to be four major ways in which the methods of the two therapists differed. Compared with Therapist B, Supershrink appeared to allocate his efforts more appropriately, to make more frequent and better planned use of community resources, to handle families with more firmness and directness, and to set up deeper and more lasting therapy relationships. The main elements in these relationships, in turn, seemed to be help to the boys in achieving autonomy and in developing competence in school and work.

Appropriate Allocation of Effort. Both therapists spent an average of 12 hours with children in the two least disturbed categories. With children in the most disturbed two groups, on the other hand, Therapist B averaged 20 hours, and Supershrink averaged 28. With children in the most disturbed group, already schizophrenic, Therapist B spent an average of 11 hours, Supershrink an average of 18. Since each hour typically represents a week in the life of the boy, this means that the most disturbed boys stayed in therapy with Supershrink about two months more than such boys stayed with Therapist B.

The differences are also apparent when the mean hours spent are classified according to the boys' adult outcome, as in the accompanying tabulation. One can conclude from this that Supershrink spent the most

	Therapist A	*Therapist B*
Chronic schizophrenic	—	9
Released schizophrenic	38	19
Socially inadequate	25	24
Socially adequate	13	—

time with the children who needed his help most, judged by the long-term criterion of their later outcomes. If therapy were the only influence on the lives of these children, one could draw a cynical conclusion — the more time spent with Supershrink, the worse the outcome. But it is abundantly clear that therapy is an intervention into an ongoing life, and one with limited effects compared with the effects of biological endowment and family environment. The fairest interpretation of these data seems to be that Supershrink gave his time in proportion to the degree of potential disturbance in the boy, while Therapist B gave more time to those who were easier to reach.

The decision to terminate or to maintain therapy with an adolescent boy of course involves not just the therapist, but also the boy and the family. Inspection of the final therapy hours of Supershrink and Therapist B suggests that Therapist B lost some of these vulnerable boys (Fleming & Ricks, 1970) by overloading an already tenuous relationship with too much anxiety- or depression-arousing interpretation.

Is very disinclined to talk. I tell him that there is a contradiction in his behavior, that he won't tell me anything about himself now, that he complains that he is losing his mind and suffering so, and yet he tells me that at work he fools around with the other fellows, tells dirty stories with them.

After the hour summarized by this comment and others like it, the boy decided not to come back, arguing that all of his troubles were due to his difficulty in breathing; Therapist B allowed the case to be closed.

Another premature conclusion came about after a boy, in his sixth session, contrasted how active he used to be and how many friends he used to have, with his present state — two strikes against him, no brains, no chance to do anything, and so on. Ignoring the implicit argument he was offering for possibly being again what he had been before, Therapist B emphasized the depressed feelings.

I tell him my impression is that his spirit has been broken. . . . At the present time it is certainly impossible to get him interested in any occupation, and there doesn't seem to be anything else to do but have him come in for psychotherapy and perhaps if his condition is ameliorated we might get him to do something later on.

Later, after he had missed two appointments before coming again, Therapist B noted: "He is still very depressed and hardly said anything to me at all. The case certainly has an ominous aspect." In this case, as in several others, Therapist B seemed to get caught up in the child's own depressed and hopeless feelings. This seemed to confirm the boy's own views of himself as worthless or beyond help, and effectively robbed further therapy of any value. The child therefore stopped coming.

Use of Resources outside the Immediate Therapy Situation. Under this heading we may group a number of resources used by both therapists at various times: foster homes, summer camps, boarding school placements, or jobs that provided a place to live or a refuge from conflicts at home. Supershrink more frequently used outside resources, particularly camps and other temporary group placements. The main difference in this regard, however, is the thoroughness and care with which he helped the boy work out, in the therapy hours, the meaning of placement and what to expect from it (see the case of James, p. 288).

Firmness and Directness in Relationship with Parents. Although both Supershrink and Therapist B were psychoanalytically trained, Supershrink was less inclined to work problems through in terms of intrapsychic dynamics (though he did this at times with admirable skill) and more inclined to coordinate changes in the child with changes in the way he was treated by his parents. For example, Tobe, a 13-year-old, had had his bicycle and his allowance denied for misbehavior. Later his bicycle was allowed him again, but his parents did not reinstate his allowance. Supershrink and the mother's social worker insisted on the child's right to some definite expectation from the parents, helped the mother to see that Tobe seldom knew what to expect, and then helped her work through her feelings of envy and resentment growing out of her own desperately deprived childhood.*

Supershrink met with parents fairly often to reinforce a point he had made with a boy. Two boys, for instance, had been told by their fathers that masturbation led to insanity. Supershrink met with each father and attempted to change his attitudes enough to prevent further advice of this sort. Several parents seemed to see perfectly ordinary adolescent behavior — such as masturbation, reading pornography, experimenting with smoking, or hiding things in one's room — as evidence of craziness. His meetings were devoted to reassuring them about the usualness of their sons' behavior and to persuading them to stop threatening their sons and interfering with their development.

Support for Autonomy. Many of these children were locked in an extreme symbiotic attachment with a parent (Ricks & Nameche, 1966; Waring & Ricks, 1965). Supershrink seemed particularly competent in helping children and their parents to recognize the ways in which overprotection stunted the child's emotional growth and in helping both to free themselves from destructive ties.

A quotation from Supershrink's notes after his first hour with Harry, a neurologically impaired child, aged 10, indicates his early recognition of symbiosis and his immediate support for efforts toward autonomy.

*Unfortunately, the sample considered here is not large enough to permit a comparative study of social workers and social work methods. Waring's (1966) related research suggests that the difference in impact of these is at least comparable with the difference in the impact of therapists.

My suspicions of his being a closely supervised child were confirmed when he talked about the fact that he always came right home after school and either stayed in the house or did errands for his mother. He never went to the movies with any of the other children. In fact, he usually went to the theater "because we like it better." In referring to all of his activities he usually said "we" because there is hardly anything he does without his mother except going to school. I asked about the possibility of coming to the clinic alone, and he was horrified by the idea. He said that his mother always went with him and he would probably get lost if he came alone. [He lived about five blocks from the clinic, and would have walked through a pleasant residential neighborhood.]

Supershrink summed up his impressions after this first hour as follows:

The patient presents the picture of an overprotected child. There is no indication of his resenting his being tied so closely to his mother. He seemed to think that everything he did was all right and actively verbalized his desire to be with his mother rather than with other boys, whom he doesn't get along with too well. I do not believe that this is the type of problem we can handle unless the mother is able to accept her responsibility. If a strong relationship should be obtained with the boy, and he began to resent being treated like a baby, the mother, unless she had some insight into the situation, would withdraw him from the clinic very quickly.

Harry's mother was given a great deal of support by her social worker in letting go of Harry. The social worker's notes some time later indicate something of the nature of her conflict, and of the ways in which she was supported in resolving it.

Mother continues to complain of Harry in each interview, listing the things he has done which have been upsetting and repeatedly stressing the fact that anyone as low in intelligence as Harry is cannot be expected to do too much. . . . During one interview mother brings in the camp report, which is very brief, but does state that Harry did fairly well at camp. Mother immediately becomes derogatory, saying she is sure that he didn't make as good progress as this sounds. But during the same interview Mother wonders about the possibility of private school, since he got along fairly well at camp and the home situation is impossible. I agree with mother that the home situation is pretty bad for all concerned, and that, even though I realize she has been making a very good effort, it is hard on her. She says that she has been thinking that if he goes away to school she could again go to work. She has been restless for a long time and has been searching for things to fill up her life.

By the fourth hour of his therapy Harry "mentioned with a great deal of pleasure that he is coming to the clinic alone." Later, camp experiences supported his growing independence and helped him in overcoming some of the handicaps produced by his neurological impairments and the impact of his disturbed parents.

Supershrink's notes from an hour with Tobe illustrate the ways in which this passive, compliant 13-year-old who was still being bathed by his mother was encouraged to develop some small seeds of autonomy:

> We continued the previous week's theme. I am trying to get him to see the situation he is in — on the one hand trying to conform to the parent's wishes and on the other hand trying to grow up. He says that the other boys never *call* him a sissy, but that at times he thinks he might be one, "I never go out with the other kids." I tried to help him clarify in his own mind whether he believes there is any advantage to him to come to the clinic, other than (1) getting excused from school early, and (2) coming because his mother wants him to and it is easier to comply with her wishes than to resist. I tried to show him how this conflict between conformity and growing up is tied up with his lack of school and social success. I also tried to get him to think about the question of whether he wants to take the path of least resistance and remain a small boy with the possibility of future unhappiness, or take the more difficult path leading to growing up, with the possibility of a more satisfactory future life.

The next hour Tobe decided that he really wanted to come, because he did want to grow up. A note two years later indicates the changes he made, with an exaggerated adolescent rebellion under way at 15:

> Quite in contrast to the last years, he seems to have many boys to pal around with. A group of them have been building a clubhouse. He has been invited to numerous parties and also has a girl friend about whom he talks quite freely. He seems to have achieved considerable freedom in doing what he wishes after supper and is becoming more defiant of his parents. In this connection he is smoking and doing some minor stealing from local stores.

Having succeeded in his rebellion, Tobe later became a devout young candidate for the ministry.

Development of some sense of autonomy seems crucial to recognition of oneself as a person in one's own right, with the opportunity to make decisions, learn from mistakes, and test beliefs in the laboratory of one's own experience. Failing to develop autonomy, many children go through the path described by Laing (1960, 1962), from compliant unemotional "goodness" to genuine but unsocialized "badness," and when this badness alienates people or is too strikingly confirmed, to "madness" that ends in schizophrenia.

The Therapy Relationship as an Anchor in Reality. A fourth contrast between Supershrink and Therapist B begins in a seemingly trivial observation and ends in a mystery. The first thing apparent on inspection of the records of children seen by the two men was that Supershrink's files contained many letters, some written years after therapy ended, keeping him up to date on how the boy's life had progressed and some-times asking for advice about adult problems. Superficial inspection also revealed many spontaneous visits to the clinic, so that more than half of Supershrink's case folders contain notes, often several years after the ter-mination of therapy, beginning, "Patient dropped in today without an ap-pointment," "George was in the neighborhood today, so he came in," etc. Like the many hours that disturbed, withdrawn, angry boys were able to maintain in therapy with him, these letters and visits suggest that Supershrink became a supportive factor in the real life of the patient and a resource to be turned to when problems arose. But he was also a friend to whom good things could be reported, and more than half of the spon-taneous visits seem to be just that — renewal of old remembrances and bringing a valued relationship up to date. He was also, in contrast with most therapists, remembered vividly in our follow-up interviews.

The factors in Supershrink's own personality that contributed to this depth of impact cannot be gauged on the basis of the materials in his case files. Their existence is confirmed by his later nickname, but what his special personal qualities might be remains hidden in the unseen process of therapy.

The specific methods that produced this impact, on the other hand, may be judged in part from therapy notes. The first thing apparent in his discussions with children is that he expected every therapy hour to be used, and if it was not being useful to the child, he wanted to know why. There is a direct contrast here between his methods and those of Thera-pist B, who often seemed to be drifting without clear focus from hour to hour, and at other times following up sidelines that interested him (and were sometimes fascinating to the reader interested in the intricacies of psychopathology) but were of no use to the child in solving his day-to-day problems. Supershrink expected the boy to take responsibility for coming to therapy, and make a clear decision not to stay if it failed to help him.

Supershrink's comments also mirror an unusual openness to the boy's feelings and unusual freedom from threat in the presence of extreme love or extreme hostility. His equilibrium is suggested in some of the notes he kept:

When Tim first started coming to the clinic he thought it was some form of punishment or that he would be put away. He was very protective of him-self, as would be expected. Now, however, he is very happy about his ap-pointments here. Sometimes it is extremely difficult to get him out of the office when his time is up. He wants to stay on indefinitely. He has sug-gested that it would be nice if I adopted him. [A few weeks later] . . . Tim got very silly, as he has before, got on the couch and refused to leave when the time was up. He hunted around the room for something he could take with him, alternating between swearing at the therapist and demanding to know when his next appointment was.

Dan opened the interview by saying that he thinks it is a waste of time to come in here, but was very much taken aback when I agreed with him. He likes to say things that start arguments or create concern. When he found that I agreed with him, he immediately began to assure me that he didn't mean that. I insisted that I felt that it was a waste of time unless he was more active in helping work out his own problems. . . . [A few weeks later, when the therapist had required that they talk over a negative evaluation from a foster home,] he was not interested, but did say that he was sorry that I had failed, the whole idea being that I hadn't been able to get him to get along better in the foster home or to get along better in school. He was apparently trying to provoke me, since he several times asked if I had ever had any success with anyone, and he wondered a number of times whether I had any standing in this field.

Supershrink seemed to be the first person, in contrast with a long series of unfortunate adults that Dan had known, who could tolerate his provocativeness without retaliation or rejection. Two years after his therapy had ended, when he was well over the age range of the clinic, he again approached Supershrink, still full of sarcasm and explanations of why the therapist's personality did not encourage confidence and his technique was faulty, but asking for further help. Supershrink worked with him long enough to find a therapist at another agency. Follow-up reports indicate that Dan went on to a successful career after a few turbulent years that included brief hospitalization. It seems reasonable to speculate that Supershrink's acceptance and help may have enabled him to emerge from his later troubles by again reaching out for therapy in later years. Several of the other boys seen by Supershrink sought further psychotherapy, either through him or independently, after their adolescent contact. One of the values of early work with a helping therapist may have been its role in preparing the boys to seek further therapy later, and to use it effectively in avoiding extremes of regression.

Therapist B tended to take a distant, cognitive attitude toward expressions of feeling. He also seemed selective in the feelings he did respond to. Unless there were expressions of depressions or anxiety, he seemed to believe that nothing was happening in therapy.

It is still very difficult to know just how much to do with this boy. He seems so dull and lacking in ability to converse. He denies any other worries, any other need for advice, yet at the same time he gives me the impression of enjoying his visits here.

When this same boy expressed feelings not of liking to come, but of the depressed type that Therapist B tended to tune in to, the therapy notes contained long, detailed comments:

. . . the essential points that come out of all this are that he feels terribly insecure, very much discouraged, and seems completely blocked from putting forth his best efforts. His insecurity comes from various sources, *all of which I discuss with him* — the broken home, the abusive father, the peculiar mother, the inferior siblings, poverty . . .

It was difficult for Therapist B not to share depressive feelings, and even to reinforce them.

Promoting Competence. Unlike those therapists who feel that it is best to avoid giving direct advice, Supershrink often expressed opinions on how problems might be handled and sought to work out with the boy the consequences of different courses of action.

I tried to help James think about the problem of whether he really wants to stay there or not, and to show him that if he really wants to stay there, then that means a certain amount of conformity. I am not suggesting that he stay there — maybe that is not the place for him. But since he is always saying how much he likes the farm, he really must decide to accept their ways of doing things if he wants to remain. Of course I don't expect him to go too far in this change of behavior, but perhaps a slight improvement may make all of the difference in his remaining on the farm and leaving. I also tried to help him see that even if he were living with his own parents they would not always consult him, and he would still have to do many things that displeased him.

Supershrink's interest in helping boys reach solutions to problems in real life was most evident in his work toward realistic understanding of vocational ambitions and possibilities. Even more than other adolescents, those with a high risk for schizophrenia go through role diffusions and turmoil as they seek vocational roles and try to relate present schoolwork to future possibilities. Some of the elements in Supershrink's approach may have reflected the background he brought to psychotherapy, in which teaching and camp work had developed some unusual skills in fostering ego growth and reality testing. He seemed unusually able to bring these skills to bear on highly charged issues of how to reconcile the realities of school and work with fantasies and fears that fed unrealistic ambitions.

Therapist B appeared to be caught between his own tendencies to give advice, be helpful, and so forth, and his desire to bring out a great deal of material of deeper psychodynamic interest. For example, whenever he referred to material from an hour as "interesting," it proved to be fantasy, early childhood memories, and the like. Such an attitude often made these adolescents reticent, so that his records contained a number of comments on how hard it was to get each child to talk. With younger children this approach proved more successful, so that the liveliest hours Therapist B recorded were those spent bringing out fantasy through play and drawing and working it through with preadolescents. With those few adolescents who responded to Therapist B's interest in ordinarily repressed material with pressured compliance, the initial effects seemed to be promotion of regression, immersion in depressed feelings with which neither boy nor therapist could cope, and quick withdrawal from further therapy.

DISCUSSION

To the observer looking over the course of therapy with each of these boys, and now gifted with the hindsight that a 20-year follow-up makes available, it seems that Supershrink was both working actively with each boy toward the solution of immediate problems and, probably much less consciously, setting an example, through his own realistic effectiveness, of how problems could be approached and solved (Shonbar, 1967). Therapist B, on the other hand, was often sophisticated enough to know how to bring out a great deal of anxiety, depression, and pathological fantasy, without having yet the sophistication or the resilience to know what to do with it once it was out in the open.

Inspection of the therapy notes made by the other successful therapists suggests that the methods Supershrink used are not the only successful ones. Two successful therapists, for example, saw younger children, mostly girls, and both used play therapy more than the conversational methods used with adolescent boys. The active methods used by Supershrink may require modification for younger children — one lively little girl who is now a chronic schizophrenic was quickly withdrawn from therapy by her mother when a strong female therapist seemed too successful in supporting the child's autonomy without supporting the mother through her fears of losing her baby. The small numbers of young children and of girls studied here make discussion of successful therapy with these groups outside the scope of this paper. Until such groups have been studied, the conclusions reached here have to be understood as applying only to therapy with adolescent boys, and within that group, to those whose disturbances are severe enough to produce a high risk of schizophrenia in adult life.

The thrust of child guidance methods toward early intervention and work with the disturbed child and his family has provided an opportunity to increase our understanding of how psychopathology develops and how intervention might affect its development. As the child guidance movement came into full maturity, we have become able to study childhood development of all types, not just through adult recall, but also through the eyes of skilled observers in childhood. The research reported in these volumes indicates how fruitful this approach may be in tracing the natural history of different mental and emotional disorders.

The work reported here indicates that these materials can also be used in the study of early childhood intervention, basing the comparison of therapists on the pragmatic ground of how children seen by them turn out in adult life. In this study, a long-term follow-up comparison of the outcome of children who saw two different therapists suggests consistent differences in therapeutic effectiveness. Those children who saw Supershrink were likely to go on to lives free from schizophrenia, often containing much evidence of social adequacy. Those who saw Therapist B were more likely to be schizophrenic in adult life. Although there were some small differences between the samples seen by the two men, they were well matched in most ways, with the only strong differences the therapist seen and the adult outcome.

The methods of the more effective therapist were characterized by more appropriate allocation of effort, more effective use of resources outside the immediate therapy situation, firmness and directness in dealing with parents, support of efforts toward autonomy (and stimulation of these when they were latent), anchoring the children in reality through setting up strong therapeutic relationships on which the boys tended to rely even after formal termination of therapy, and the promotion of competence in handling everyday problems in real life.

This list is not necessarily exhaustive. There are probably subtle ways in which the two therapists differed that could not be detected in their therapy notes. But the list does seem complete enough to have implications for planning therapy with children who have a high risk for schizophrenia.

Boys who later become schizophrenic seem to have all of the usual problems of adolescence (Gardner, 1959), but they come to these problems handicapped with many developmental lags and deficiencies, and often they face them with minimal parental support or have to overcome interference with their development (Stierlin, Levi, & Savard, 1971). The therapist who is most helpful in working with such boys would seem to be one who approximates (and modifies also, to fit his own personality and style), the methods used by Supershrink. Given the precarious hold on socialized living that these children bring to therapy, it is not surprising that supportive ego strengthening methods produced much more helpful changes than the methods of Therapist B, who moved too precipitously into presumably deep material. Successful therapy with adolescents requires a continuous process of diagnosis, with modification of "opening up" methods whenever the child, or the therapist, becomes unable to cope with the material brought out.

If the results achieved by successful therapists argue against the pessimistic belief that therapy never helps, the apparently destructive effect of some interventions by Therapist B also suggest that the potential harmfulness of therapeutic efforts can hardly be ignored. The children considered here were already experiencing nearly intolerable degrees of anxiety, vulnerability, feelings of unreality, and isolated alienation (Fleming & Ricks, 1970). When the therapist increased those feelings, without being at the same time able to help the boy develop ways of living with them, he may have played a part in the subsequent psychotic developments. Therapy may lead one into health, but it may also be a part of the complex process that ends up driving one crazy (Searles, 1959).

More speculatively, we may look at what Supershrink seemed to provide for children, see that his patients generally did not become schizophrenic, and suggest that children whose earlier lives have failed to provide these characteristics are especially prone to schizophrenia in adult life. On this basis we could say that the prodromal stage of schizophrenia is characterized by lack of autonomy, inability to find anchors in social reality, and incompetence in finding solutions to the social and vocational problems of adolescence. The early stages of schizophrenia are still interpersonal affairs, with the family, school, and community doing much to stunt the emotional growth of the child and offering him little inducement to grow up. The developing schizophrenic process is at this stage still fluid, and the evidence presented above suggests that like many deficiency "diseases," it is still open to deflection, and perhaps even reversal, if therapy can offer what the earlier environment failed to provide.

A MODEST PROPOSAL

The strongest reaction of students and colleagues who have read earlier versions of this paper has been concern for how to prevent long-term therapeutic practice by therapists known to be harmful. The second strongest reaction is an attempt to examine the methods of Supershrink and adapt them to their own personalities and ways of work.

I believe that all major hospitals, faced with the need to protect their patients against incompetence, have developed "tissue boards" who examine the results of surgery and decide on its necessity and the competence of its execution. No such boards exist for psychotherapy, and there is no evidence that traditional examinations in any of the groups trained to do psychotherapy provide for this kind of evaluation of the outcomes of a therapist's work. Life history research suggests a possible model for such evaluation. If a major clinic were to set up an "outcomes board" to look over the long-term outcomes of therapy conducted by staff psychotherapists, it would be possible to determine, within a few years, whether particular therapists were unusually harmful or helpful. The difficulties in the way of establishing such a board are not small, nor is its method of operation clearly foreseeable on the basis of current clinical and research experience. But given the voluminous evidence already assembled on deterioration effects (Bergin, 1971), to which this study adds yet another bit of evidence, it would seem clinically and scientifically irresponsible not to begin making the effort.

[This paper was not read at the conference, but copies of it were distributed to participants. The discussion is drawn from subsequent correspondence with individuals who read the paper.]

COMMENTARY

STRAUSS. One of the major problems is determining whether the patients seen by the two therapists would have had different prognoses, just in terms of their clinical characteristics, irrespective of treatment. Stephens and Astrup (1965) describe how the results of Therapist A and Therapist B types could have been predicted by prognostic variables, regardless of therapist characteristics.

Since you are talking about patients treated when they were children, the Stephens-Astrup prognostic variables might not apply. But you might want to have some clinicians review the records of all the patients treated by Supershrink and by Therapist B and make prognostic judgments based on the data available from the original course of treatment. Or, to avoid the predictors being contaminated by the therapist's notes, it might be possible to have judgments made on the data available in intake conference summaries.

RICKS. I would certainly plan to do this in any replication of this kind of study. The prognostic variables that we would use for children and adolescents could be based on Roff's work on peer relations, Albee and

Lane's work on IQ, Watt's work on teacher perceptions of the kids, and so on.

BERGENN. Is it possible that you mis-diagnosed the cases seen by Supershrink, giving them too pessimistic a prognosis, and were more accurate about those seen by Therapist B?

RICKS. I doubt it. We did the diagnostic judgments well before we planned a comparison of these two therapists, and we used the same criteria on all cases. When Supershrink read the paper, he did comment that he didn't think he had seen any preschizophrenic boys, but that is perhaps a reflection of his approach, not of the diagnoses of the boys.

QUESTION. I disagree with your belief that to be socially adequate a man must be heterosexual. My experience with homosexuals has led me to believe that many of them are socially adequate, far more so than many unhappily married men or men whose heterosexual life is with prostitutes.

RICKS. We are dealing with a general social bias here. It may be wrong, but society generally considers a heterosexual adjustment preferable to a homosexual one. In some of our other papers we have argued that any kind of relatedness to others is preferable to no relationships, and so a homosexual adjustment would be a positive factor in quite a few lives.

R. KLEIN. I don't think you can separate the personality of the therapist from his methods and techniques. The fact that Supershrink utilized community resources effectively, that he gave the parents firm direction, that he maintained relationships with his patients long after therapy was formally discontinued — these certainly tell us something about his personality as well as his methods. He had enough confidence in himself to take firm stands, and his ability to utilize the community to help the boys is an indication that he did not need the boys to depend on him.

RICKS. What I had in mind is the sort of study that can report measures of the threapist's MMPI scales or his judged warmth from therapy protocols. Here we can't do that.

ROFF. But you are dealing with personality all the way through. You credit Supershrink with equilibrium, which is not unrelated to personality. I have asked a reader to judge if there was any difference in "warmth" between Supershrink and Therapist B. She said that there was no question that Supershrink was far ahead in warmth and empathy, just like the TV laundry commercials. So you may not have thought that you were describing these qualities, but they surely become inescapably obvious by the end of the paper. Therapist B didn't even get a nickname from the kids.

RICKS. I had two hopes here. First, I wanted to abstract out of the records some methods that I thought would be learnable, so that other people might try them. I suspect that only people with strong psychopathic trends can learn a new personality in order to do a job, but anybody can learn methods. Second, I didn't want to get into personalities, because that gets you into persons, and this paper is sensitive enough as it is.

ROFF. Your separation may be too sharp, though. I became aware of this problem many years ago, when dealing with the problem of parent practices. Psychologists like to think in terms of disembodied practices unattached to any person. Thus, if a mother should occasionally dribble a baby's head like a basketball, this would surely be classified as an undesirable practice. It might also suggest something about the mother who was doing this.

RICKS. I have one bit of evidence that I can add to the paper on separating Supershrink's methods and his personality. Soon after doing the first draft of this paper I selected from our own clinic a boy who had all of the familial and personality characteristics, other than low IQ, that we have found to predict later schizophrenia. He was extremely obsessive, could eat no food cooked by anyone other than his mother, had no friends, and had some ideas that most people would classify as paranoid. I tried to use Supershrink's methods with him, and after two years of therapy, on a once a week basis, he had a few friends, was no longer suspicious and hostile about peers, had tried his aunt's food, and had had a sleep-over with another boy that included breakfast at his home. Near the end of his therapy he several times asked me to give half of the hour to his mother "because she needs it more than I do now." My own personality is very different from that of Supershrink, but apparently I can use his methods.

WATT. Karon and Vandenbos (1970) have shown that experience is an extremely crucial variable in determining the effectiveness of treatment. Could you comment on the extent of previous clinical experience of the two therapists?

RICKS. I believe that they were about the same age, and both were in psychoanalytic training at the same time. So in formal clinical experience they would not differ. But Supershrink did have the advantage of a lot of school and camp experience with normal kids in a variety of settings.

ROFF. I am deeply skeptical of the generality of the preschizophrenic sequence you attribute to Laing. From all that I can find out, he has never heard of the concept of validity.

WATT. I agree with this description of the evolution of madness in schizophrenia. One of the hardest things for me to communicate about the results of the school records study concerns what I consider a rather serious misunderstanding of the evolution of "schizophrenic withdrawal." The early studies of the child guidance clinic records from the thirties and forties lead to the conclusion that the withdrawn schizophrenic in young adulthood was withdrawn since birth. I am much more impressed with the evidence that such withdrawal is in fact merely the last phase of an extended psychological struggle in adolescence, which is often manifested in anything but shyness, withdrawal, introversion, or passivity. It is true that a substantial minority of schizophrenics appear to be congenitally shy or introverted, but this is not true of the majority.

R. KLEIN. The various things that Supershrink did, e.g., supporting autonomy and promoting competence, are also good child-rearing practices for normal children. Perhaps looking at good child-rearing practices would help therapists work more effectively with their patients.

FREMOUW. Therapist B sounds to me like more than just an ineffective therapist — he is typical of traditional training for psychotherapy. His emphasis on fantasy and negative emotions, avoiding the real problems of these children's lives such as the mother's need of her son's dependence in crossing the street, is typical of the traditional intra-psychic orientation of psychotherapy. I wonder what kind of training, if any, can produce a therapist able to form strong relationships with disturbed children and to proceed to the real questions of their lives like allowances and privileges without therapeutically meaningless forays into the psyche. The high grades and college boards required for graduate training probably eliminate a lot of potential Supershrinks and yield too many Therapist Bs.

RICKS. A lot of graduate training programs in clinical psychology are looking into the life history of the applicant to see if he has worked in camps, has done some teaching, and has shown in his life that he has a concern with people. That ought to counterbalance the concern with grades.

ROFF. In relation to your "tissue boards," the Food and Drug Administration insists that a drug have demonstrable positive effects before it can obtain approval. I wonder what such an approach would do to psychotherapy.

RICKS. It seems to me that a concern with systematic evaluation is coming in several parts of our society. I have recently read some proposals for evaluating welfare services that in design, sampling, and evaluation of data are superior to almost all of the published psychotherapy research. I doubt that the public will buy psychotherapy without evaluation much longer. Milgram (1972) has made this point very strongly.

STRAUSS. I think that the model you suggest for a board to evaluate the work of actual psychotherapists would be extremely valuable. There is a lot of understandable resistance to any such move in any center, but the merits of the plan in terms of teaching, delivery of care, and research are probably strong enough to convince people of its utility.

STIERLIN. I am sure that such boards would find many Supershrinks. The hospital where I worked for many years certainly had one.

WATT. I wonder if you are missing the boat in recommending *psycho*therapy for adolescent preschizophrenics, rather than some form of sociotherapy that would focus on the deficiencies in our social system for the last phases of socialization in youth. The most notable deficiency is that our society provides few forms of vocational apprenticeship, especially outside of academic pursuits. We offer virtually no sympathetic introduction to the complex social and sexual roles of adulthood. Very few appropriate role models are available for children who have been deprived of them. We have virtually no provision in our educational system that enables troubled youngsters to explore their feelings in a sympathetic atmosphere. It seems to me that Supershrink was providing many of these things for the youngsters he treated in adolescence. Only one of these areas, exploration of feelings, fits with my understanding of individual psychotherapy. It makes me wonder if the interventions recommended for such youngsters ought not to be cast in a somewhat broader perspective.

RICKS. What you say fits with Rosalea Shonbar's view of therapy as offering a new developmental opportunity, a chance to make up a deficit in identity formation. It may be that some communes, some schools of the Summerhill type, and some residential colleges do this in a better way than therapy can. Supershrink would probably agree with you — he runs a fine summer camp for disturbed boys, and he must have designed it to do some things that individual therapy could not do.

REFERENCES

Bergin, A. E. Some implications of psychotherapy research for therapeutic practice. *Journal of Abnormal Psychology*, 1966, 71, 235–246.

————. The evaluation of therapeutic outcomes. In A. E. Bergin & S. L. Garfield (Eds.), *Handbook of psychotherapy and behavior change.* New York: Wiley, 1971.

Eysenck, H. J. *The effects of psychotherapy.* New York: International Science Press, 1966.

Faris, R. E. L., & Dunham, H. W. *Mental disorders in urban areas: An ecological study of schizophrenia and other psychosis.* Chicago: University of Chicago Press, 1939.

Fleming, P., & Ricks, D. F. Emotions of children before schizophrenia and before character disorder. In M. Roff & D. F. Ricks (Eds.), *Life history research in psychopathology.* Vol. 1. Minneapolis: University of Minnesota Press, 1970. Pp. 240–264.

Gardner, G. E. Psychiatric problems in adolescence. In S. Arieti, *American handbook of psychiatry.* New York: Basic Books, 1959.

Goffman, E. *Asylums.* Garden City, N.Y.: Doubleday (Anchor), 1961.

Hollingshead, A., & Redlich, F. C. *Social class and mental disease.* New York: Wiley, 1958.

Karon, B. P., and Vandenbos, G. R. Experience, medication, and the effectiveness of psychotherapy with schizophrenics. *British Journal of Psychiatry*, 1970, 116, 427–428.

Laing, R. D. *The divided self.* Chicago: Quadrangle Books, 1960.

————. *The self and others.* Chicago: Quadrangle Books, 1962.

Lane, E. A., & Albee, G. W. Intellectual antecedents of schizophrenia. In M. Roff & D. F. Ricks (Eds.), *Life history research in psychopathology.* Vol. 1. Minneapolis: University of Minnesota Press, 1970. Pp. 189–207.

Mednick, S. A., & Schulsinger, F. Factors related to breakdown in children at high risk for schizophrenia. In M. Roff & D. Ricks (Eds.), *Life history research in psychopathology.* Vol. 1. Minneapolis: University of Minnesota Press, 1970. Pp. 51–93.

Milgram, N. A. The examination of clinical fallout: The iatrogenic medical model. *The Clinical Psychologist*, 1972, 25 (2), 2.

Pollack, M., Woerner, M. G., & Klein, D. F. A comparison of childhood characteristics of schizophrenics, personality disorders, and their siblings. In M. Roff & D. F. Ricks (Eds.), *Life history research in psychopathology.* Vol. 1. Minneapolis: University of Minnesota Press, 1970. Pp. 208–225.

Ricks, D. F., & Berry, J. C. Family and symptom patterns that precede schizophrenia. In M. Roff & D. F. Ricks (Eds.), *Life history research in psychopathology*. Vol. 1. Minneapolis: University of Minnesota Press, 1970. Pp. 31–50.

Ricks, D. F., & Nameche, G. F. Symbiosis, sacrifice, and schizophrenia. *Mental Hygiene*, 1966, 50, 541–551.

Searles, H. F. The effort to drive the other person crazy — an element in the aetiology and psychotherapy of schizophrenia. *British Journal of Medical Psychology*, 1959, 32, 1–18.

Shonbar, R. A. Identification and the search for identity. *Contemporary Psychoanalysis*, 1967, 2, 75–95.

Stephens, J. H., and Astrup, C. Treatment outcome in process and non-process schizophrenics treated by A and B types of therapists. *Journal of Nervous and Mental Disease*, 1965, 140, 449–465.

Stierlin, H., Levi, L. D., & Savard, R. J. Parental perceptions of separating children. *Family Process*, 1971, 10, 411–427.

Waring, M. A search for possible saving events in averting hospitalization for adult schizophrenia. *Journal of the National Association of Social Workers*, October 1966.

——— & Ricks, D. F. Family patterns of children who became adult schizophrenics. *Journal of Nervous and Mental Disease*, 1965, 40, 351–364.

JOSEPH BALKIN *Once More with Feeling:*
Moods Before and After Psychotherapy

THE UNDERSTANDING and amelioration of human suffering is among the central concerns of psychology. Psychotherapy, as the chief tool of this trade, has been widely studied and evaluated. The reviews have been mixed. Among the less favorable appraisals is that of Eysenck (1961), who claims that one has a slightly better chance of improving if he stays away from a therapist. Other studies have shown beneficial effects.

Many criteria have been used to assess therapeutic outcome. One of the more popular is the therapist's rating of the degree of improvement of his patients (Ellis, 1957; Garfield & Kurz, 1952; Myers & Auld, 1955; Zubin, 1953). Specialized populations have sometimes suggested particular criteria. Work with hospitalized patients has been evaluated in terms of discharge rate (Zubin, 1953). With students, changes in grade-point average have been used (Kircheimer, Axelrod, & Hickerson, 1949). For juvenile delinquents the criterion has been the incidence of criminal behavior (Bronner, 1944).

Outcome studies of less specialized groups have utilized changes in maturity of behavior, as rated by therapist, patient, and/or peers (Cartwright & Roth, 1957; Hoffman, 1949; Rogers & Dymond, 1954); social effectiveness (Stone, Frank, Nash, & Imber, 1961); self-consistency (Cartwright, 1961); and discrepancy between actual and ideal self (Rogers & Dymond, 1954).

A different approach was taken by Strupp, Wallach, and Wogan (1962), who surveyed 44 people who had completed therapy. They were asked in rather open-ended fashion to describe the reasons they had sought therapy and the changes they experienced by the end. The most prominent initial problems mentioned were feelings of depression, anxiety, unhappiness and guilt, and physiological symptoms. The major changes reported included decreased anxiety, increased enjoyment, satisfaction, well-being, and self-esteem, greater awareness of feelings and improved ability to deal with problems.

It was striking that when people were asked to evaluate their need for and benefit from therapy in their own terms, there was a noteworthy absence of the old familiar phrases like maturity of behavior, self-ideal discrepancy, and so on. They seemed instead to be talking about how badly they felt before and how much better they felt afterward. They also talked about unhappiness, enjoyment, satisfaction, and well-being, words not so common in the psychiatric lexicon. I felt that a more thorough study of the relationship of feelings to the seeking and termination of therapy was needed. This was the purpose of the work to be reported here.

WHEN TO ASSESS AND WHOM TO ASSESS

In many outcome studies the amounts of treatment have been quite limited. In one, for example (Garfield & Kurz, 1952), of 142 patients, 104 had fewer than fifteen interviews. In two others (Stone et al., 1961; Myers & Auld, 1955), therapy was limited to six months and a year, respectively. Some studies made their evaluations at the end of treatment, but did not specify the amounts involved or the conditions of termination — whether by therapist or patient, or for what reasons. I felt that therapy could be meaningfully assessed only after voluntary termination. Understandably, one might not want to wait five years for the data to come in; within a limited amount of time, the best solution seemed to be comparing a group awaiting treatment with a group already treated.

Bergin (1966) has shown that although some people may improve in various ways as a result of therapy, others may not change or may become worse. He demonstrated that several outcome studies had included all of these types in their assessments, thereby obtaining overall effects of no changes in treatment, and obscuring the fact that some people had indeed improved. His analysis implied that cases of therapeutic success and the nature of such success could be disclosed if cases of failure were acknowledged, distinguished, and excluded at the outset. I therefore decided that in this study the group already treated should be limited to "successful" cases.

A third group was also studied: people who had never had nor felt the need for therapy. Bergin observed that "there are no studies in which treated neurotics had improved to a level of functioning which is similar to that of control normals . . ." (1966). The question arose whether a similar relationship would obtain in terms of feelings.

METHOD

The study examined and compared the feelings of three groups of people: those seeking psychotherapy, those having completed therapy, and those who had never had nor felt the need for therapy.

Subjects. The three groups were defined as follows:

a. Post-therapy group: people who have completed a course of psychotherapy, terminated with the agreement of therapist and patient that there was no need for further treatment, for reasons other than the feeling that therapy had been of little or no help. A period of at least one year must have elapsed since termination, and the patient must at no time since then have sought further therapy.

b. Pre-therapy group: people voluntarily seeking psychotherapy for the first time.

c. Non-therapy group: people who, while aware of the existence and availability of therapy, have never felt the need for, nor sought it, for reasons other than a belief that therapy is in general of little or no effectiveness.

The post-therapy group was drawn from the closed cases of the New Rochelle Guidance Center, a county-subsidized clinic serving New Rochelle, New York, and several surrounding communities. At the time of the study the Guidance Center had been in operation for over fifteen years and had a relatively stable staff; as such, it provided a substantial number of closed cases, in relatively few of which termination occurred because of the therapist's departure.

Included in the case files was a closing form giving the reason for termination. Those marked terminated on the basis of "no need for further treatment" were taken as providing the therapist's assessment. The case material provided the patient's reasons. Typically, the patient talked about ending treatment in conjunction with things going better, feeling better, problems being resolved, and not feeling the need to come anymore. Such cases were accepted as suitable for the study. About 85 per cent of these were married women, so the entire sample for this and the other groups was restricted to this category, eliminating several sources of demographic variability. Starting with cases closed a year previously and going back to the ten-year mark, a total of 52 cases was obtained.

Some aspects of the treatment of this group can be summarized as follows: The number of interviews ranged from 30 to 218, with a mean of 77. The duration of therapy varied from 1.0 years to 5.8 years, with a mean of 2.5. The mean time since termination of therapy was 3.7 years, with a range of 1.0 to 8.8 years.

Of their former therapists, eight were still at the clinic at the time of the study, and accounted for 21 of the patients who ultimately responded. Four of the eight were psychologists, two were psychiatrists, and two were psychiatric social workers. Their amounts of experience, at the times they saw their patients, varied from four to nineteen years. All described their orientations to treatment as within the analytic spectrum; five mentioned Sullivan's ideas as most influential in their work.

Subjects in the pre-therapy group came from the adult outpatient clinics of Jacobi Hospital and the Sound View — Throggs Neck Community Mental Health Center, both in New York City. All had been seen for an initial evaluation of two to five interviews, and then told they had been accepted for treatment, which would begin as soon as a doctor had time available — usually within a month or two at most. The selection of this group was restricted to provide demographic and initial diagnostic characteristics comparable with those of the post-therapy group. Forty cases were chosen for the pre-therapy group.

The members of the non-therapy group came through the efforts of the New Rochelle Volunteer Bureau, which had in the past provided volunteer help to the New Rochelle Guidance Center. Subjects in this group were told that a study was under way comparing the feelings of people before and after psychotherapy, and that similar information on people who had never sought therapy was desired. After it was determined that a person had never had nor sought therapy, she was asked why. Typically, the reply was to the effect of not having felt the need for it, which was taken as acceptable for this group. Thirty-five women appropriate for this group agreed to participate in the study. Their selection was also governed by the need for demographic similarity to the other two groups.

For the pre- and post-therapy groups, clinic records provided information about presenting problems and psychiatric diagnoses. The two groups did not differ appreciably in these respects. For both, the problems mentioned most frequently were depression, anxiety, problems with husband, and problems with children. These were mentioned by roughly half the women in each group. The most common diagnoses were, in descending order of frequency, passive-aggressive personality, character disorders (other types), depressive reaction, and anxiety reaction.

All three groups were similar demographically. Most were high school graduates, Jewish, married, working part time. The mean age was 44, number of children 2.3, and total family income $8,600 per year.

Measures. All subjects recorded their feelings every day for 28 days, using the Personal Feeling Scales of Wessman and Ricks (1966). There are sixteen unidimensional scales, dealing with various kinds of feelings and moods. Each scale consists of ten numbered statements, defining particular affective states relating to the mood or feeling involved. The ten statements provide a continuum ranging from extremely negative through more neutral to extremely positive states. For example, Scale I is entitled *Fullness versus Emptiness of Life* (How emotionally satisfying, abundant or empty, your life felt today). The ten scale points, in descending order, are:

9 Consummate fulfillment and abundance.
8 Replete with life's abundant goodness.
7 Filled with warm feelings of contentment and satisfaction.
6 My life is ample and satisfying.
5 Life seems fairly adequate and relatively satisfying.
4 Some slight sense of lack, vague and mildly troubling.
3 My life seems deficient, dissatisfying.
2 Life is pretty empty and barren.
1 Desolate, drained dry, impoverished.
0 Gnawing sense of emptiness, hollowness, void.

The other scales are:

II. *Receptivity Toward and Stimulation by the World* (How interested and responsive you felt to what was going on around you.)

III. *Social Respect versus Social Contempt* (How you felt other people regarded you, or felt about you, today.)

IV. *Personal Freedom versus External Constraint* (How much you felt you were free or not free to do as you wanted.)

V. *Harmony versus Anger* (How well you got along with, or how angry you felt toward, other people.)

VI. *Own Sociability versus Withdrawal* (How socially outgoing or withdrawn you felt today.)

VII. *Companionship versus Being Isolated* (The extent to which you felt emotionally accepted by, or isolated from, other people.)

VIII. *Love and Sex* (The extent to which you felt loving and tender, or sexually frustrated and unloving.)

IX. *Present Work* (How satisfied or dissatisfied you were with your work.)

X. *Thought Processes* (How readily your ideas came and how valuable they seemed.)

XI. *Tranquility versus Anxiety* (How calm or troubled you felt.)

XII. *Impulse Expression versus Self-Restraint* (How expressive and impulsive, or internally restrained and controlled, you felt.)

XIII.   *Personal Moral Judgment* (How self-approving, or how guilty, you felt.)

XIV.   *Self-Confidence versus Feeling of Inadequacy* (How self-assured and adequate, or helpless and inadequate, you felt.)

XV.   *Energy versus Fatigue* (How energetic, or tired and weary, you felt.)

XVI.   *Elation versus Depression* (How elated or depressed, happy or unhappy, you felt today.)

The ten scale points for each scale, and a description of their development and validation, can be found in *Mood and Personality* by Wessman and Ricks (1966).

Procedures. All subjects were sent a set of the Personal Feeling Scales and 28 Daily Record sheets, along with a letter introducing the study. The letters to the women in the post-therapy group came from the New Rochelle Guidance Center, and said that the clinic was doing some research and would appreciate their supplying some information by filling out the enclosed material. The letter was signed, where possible, by the patient's former therapist. The covering letters to the pre-therapy women originated from the clinic where therapy was being sought, and explained in like manner that the clinic was doing some research and would like the enclosed material filled out. Each letter was signed by the psychiatrist who had seen the particular patient for the intake evaluation. The women in the non-therapy group had already agreed to participate in the study; the letters to these people thanked them and were signed by the experimenter.

In all cases, the letters went on to say that the enclosed material was for keeping a record of day-to-day feelings and moods. The subjects were asked to begin on it right away, and told that I would call in a few days to answer any questions that might arise. It was pointed out that the subject's name was not to appear on any of the material. A sheet requesting basic demographic information and an envelope for mailing back the completed material were included.

A set of instructions described the scales and asked the women to fill out one of the Daily Record sheets at the end of each day by entering, for each scale, the number of the statement best describing how they felt, on the average, for the day, and also the highest and lowest they felt during the day. They were asked to do this for 28 consecutive days.

One week after the material had been sent, I called the subjects. Typically they had begun filling out the scales and had no questions. Those that did arise most commonly had to do with the meaning of a word or phrase, or whether it was acceptable for the daily high not to exceed the average. Only one woman asked to know more about the purpose of the study, and she turned out to be unable to participate, being about to move out of the state.

Ten women in the post-therapy group refused at the outset to participate. Their reasons included moving, recent deaths in the family, and illness; some claimed not to have enough time for it. After an appropriate interval, all but 7 of the remaining records had been returned. These 7 were called, and said they had been delayed in starting but would do so. None of these records, however, ever arrived. It was felt that these people were unable or unwilling to refuse openly, and their tacit refusals were accepted. For this group, 35 returns were ultimately received.

There were 2 initial refusals in the pre-therapy group, and 6 tacit refusals. The final returns here totaled 32. There were but 2 refusals in the non-therapy group, both tacit; 33 records were returned.

RESULTS

For each subject, each of the Personal Feeling Scales yielded three measures of level: the means over the 28 days of the daily average, high, and low. Group means were then obtained for these three variables on all sixteen scales.

The results were first analyzed to determine whether the members of each group experienced predominantly positive or negative feelings. Each scale midpoint (4.5 in all cases) divides the positive and negative feeling states; those numbered from 4 to 0 are increasingly negative, while those numbered 5 through 9 are increasingly positive. The analysis involved examining the difference between each group mean daily average and the scale midpoint with a *t* test. Table A* shows the mean daily averages together with the results of the *t* tests. The mean daily averages of the pre-therapy group were significantly less than 4.5 for all sixteen scales. The averages of the post- and non-therapy groups were in all cases significantly greater than 4.5.

The qualities of the feelings of these people are sharply illustrated by the descriptive statements most closely corresponding to the scale means. Thus, in the domains represented by the sixteen scales, the feelings most characteristic of the people seeking therapy were as follows:

   I.   Some slight sense of lack, vague and mildly troubling.
  II.   Slightly disinterested and unresponsive.

*For Tables A–C, order NAPS Document 02197 from ASIS/NAPS, c/o Microfiche Publications, 305 East 46th Street, New York, New York 10017, remitting $1.50 for microfiche or $5.00 for photocopies. Make checks payable to Microfiche Publications.

III. Some people don't seem to see much value in me.
IV. Somewhat constrained and hampered. Not free to do things my own way.
V. A little bit annoyed, somewhat "put out." Minor irritations.
VI. Not particularly outgoing. Feel a little bit unsociable.
VII. Feel a little bit left out.
VIII. Not much feeling of mutual understanding. Some lack of interest.
IX. Somewhat dissatisfied with my work. Not much enjoyment doing it.
X. Not particularly alert. My ideas trivial and commonplace.
XI. Somewhat concerned with minor worries or problems. Slightly ill at ease, a bit troubled.
XII. Keep a check on most whims and impulses.
XIII. Somewhat short of what I ought to be.
XIV. Feel my performance and capabilities somewhat limited.
XV. Slightly tired. Indolent. Somewhat lacking in energy.
XVI. Feeling a little bit low. Just so-so.

In contrast, the people who had completed therapy, and the people who had never sought therapy, most commonly felt:

I. My life is ample and satisfying.
II. Open and responsive to my world and its happenings.
III. Confident that some people think well of me.
IV. Free, within broad limits, to act much as I want to.
V. Get along well and rather smoothly.
VI. Companionable. Ready to mix with others.
VII. Feel accepted and liked.
VIII. Pleasant companionship and some affection. Sharing interests and good times.
IX. Satisfied with my work. Encouraged to go on with it.
X. Quite alert. Thoughts fairly quick and clear.
XI. Nothing particularly troubling me. More or less at ease. Pretty generally secure and free from care.
XII. Moderate acceptance and expression of my own needs and desires.
XIII. Consider myself pretty close to my own best self.
XIV. Feel my abilities sufficient and my prospects good.
XV. Fairly fresh. Adequate energy.
XVI. Feeling very good and cheerful.

The people seeking therapy experienced predominantly negative feelings, while those who had completed therapy and those who had never sought it experienced predominantly positive feelings, in all the areas covered by the scales.

The groups were next compared for differences in levels of feelings. For each scale, differences among the three group mean daily averages were examined with an analysis of variance. Wherever significant results appeared, particular differences between the groups taken two at a time were explored with *t* tests. The same procedure was carried out for the other two measures of level, mean daily highs and lows.

Given the findings that the mean daily averages of the pre-therapy group were significantly less than 4.5 while those of the other two groups were significantly greater than 4.5, it would be expected that the means of the post- and non-therapy groups would be greater, for each scale, than those of the pre-therapy group. Direct analysis showed that this was indeed the case, with all differences significant at the .001 level; it also showed no significant differences in mean daily average between the post- and non-therapy groups on any of the scales. So, in their most characteristic daily feelings, the people who had finished therapy felt better in every way than those seeking it, and as good as those who had never needed it.

The mean daily highs of the three groups formed a pattern identical to that of the daily averages (Table B). All the means of the post- and non-therapy groups were significantly greater than those of the pre-therapy group, and there were no significant differences between the post- and non-therapy groups.

As an example, in terms of Elation versus Depression (Scale XVI), the people in the pre-therapy group at their best were "feeling pretty good, OK," while those in the post- and non-therapy groups were "feeling very good and cheerful" or "elated and in high spirits." In every case, the best feelings of the people who had finished therapy reached levels higher than those of the people seeking it, and as high as those of the people who had never needed it.

When the mean daily lows of the three groups were compared, in every respect, the same relationships were maintained (Table C). For all scales, corresponding means of the post- and non-therapy groups were significantly greater than those of the pre-therapy group; there were no differences between the post- and non-therapy groups.

In terms of Elation versus Depression, for example, the people in the post- and non-therapy groups at their worst felt "pretty good, OK"; those in the pre-therapy group felt "spirits low and somewhat blue." In all ways, in their worst feelings, the people who had completed therapy did not feel so bad as those seeking it, and no worse than those who had never needed it.

DISCUSSION

The results form a clear, consistent, and meaningful pattern. They demonstrate the importance of feelings in the seeking and termination of psychotherapy and their usefulness in assessing its effects, and suggest that therapy can result in marked changes in feelings.

All conclusions are limited by the special nature of the post-therapy group. Only those people were studied who regarded their treatment as satisfactory; cases of little or no change were acknowledged and excluded at the outset. It cannot be asserted that everyone feels good after therapy. But it cannot be said that the selection of this group guaranteed these results. All that was ensured was that some changes important to the patients and their therapists had taken place. It can be concluded that when people have undergone therapy they regard as satisfactory, they feel good in a variety of ways.

A second qualification concerns the particular demographic character of the subjects. All were women, predominantly married, mostly in their forties, of high school education and lower-middle-income families. The question arises whether the results have more general relevance. Wilson (1967) summarized previous findings on correlates of avowed happiness, the bulk of which indicated little relationship to age, sex, education, intelligence, or economic level. Happiness is closely related to the dimension of Elation versus Depression (Scale XVI), but not necessarily to the other feelings assessed. Wessman and Ricks (1966) found no differences in level between men and women on any of twelve scales used.

It is noteworthy that several studies (Constantinople, 1965; Reinhardt, 1968; Wessman & Ricks, 1966) using the Personal Feeling Scales, primarily with college students, obtained mean daily averages about one scale point lower than those of the post- and non-therapy groups studied here. This is probably accounted for by the fact that most of the students were unmarried, whereas practically all the women in this study were married; Wessman (1956) found that married people tend to avow more happiness. That levels of feelings may vary with some demographic characteristics does not necessarily mean, however, that studies like this with different demographic groups would yield different relationships. The levels might all be shifted up or down the scales, while the relationships were maintained. The evidence available is not conclusive, but tends more to support than to deny the generality of the results.

The question of bias in reporting feelings should be considered. It might appear, for example, that the women seeking help would tend to represent themselves as feeling worse than they actually did in order to secure treatment. But they had already been guaranteed treatment, and participated voluntarily and anonymously. Similarly, it might be questioned whether the post-therapy women represented themselves as happier than they were. Their anonymity precluded misrepresentation to anyone but themselves. The possibility that they might need to see themselves as happier to justify their investment in therapy seems slight; clinic costs were low, and over half the women had fewer than 65 interviews and had been out of treatment for more than three years. In general, there appears little ground for assuming response biases that significantly affected the results.

The Case for Feelings. That the women seeking treatment felt relatively bad, while those who had completed it felt relatively good, underlines the importance of feelings in the seeking and termination of therapy. The results affirm the usefulness and validity of feelings, in particular as measured by the Personal Feeling Scales, as a criterion in the evaluation of psychotherapy. The Scales could also be profitably used in process studies, examining changes in feelings during the course of therapy. Clinically, they might serve as a kind of barometer, indicating periodic progress or the lack of it.

It should be noted that the observed differences encompassed a wide range of feelings. Not only anxiety and depression, but also feelings about work, fullness of life, sociability, and the others assessed seem important in the seeking and termination of therapy. It may be that traditional psychological thinking about affective dysfunction has been too narrow.

The use of bipolar scales assumed that feelings could be meaningfully conceptualized in this way; the present findings cannot be taken as establishing the truth or falsity of this approach. But the ability of the scales to differentiate meaningfully among the three groups provides empirical justification for their continued use. It appears that people can be studied in terms of the degree of unhappiness or happiness they have; not just the absence of depression, but the amount of elation, is important. A psychology that focuses solely upon the manifestations of unhappiness may miss half the range of human feeling.

The absence of differences between the post- and non-therapy groups would make this study, according to Bergin's report (1966), the first showing treated patients functioning at the same level as control normals. This finding no doubt rests heavily on the exclusion of failures and the assessment after voluntary termination. But perhaps also responsible was the use of feelings as the criterion.

The results of this study, together with the reports of the people questioned by Strupp et al. (1962), could be taken as support for the contention that feelings are fundamental in the seeking and termination of therapy. That is, people come for help not because of symptoms or inter-personal conflicts per se, but out of unpleasant feelings engendered by them. Similarly, therapy will be regarded as satisfactory, and terminated, when people have shifted toward experiencing more positive feelings. Although the evidence is consistent with this view, the point does not appear logically susceptible to proof. Such proof would require the performance of successful therapy, demonstrating improvements in feelings, with all other factors held constant. Such manipulation is not possible in the therapeutic process. Feelings might in fact underlie all cases of the seeking and termination of therapy, but to the extent that they are concomitants of other factors, the latter will change as feelings change. At best, repeated results like those obtained here can establish that positive feelings are a necessary, but perhaps not sufficient, condition of successful therapy.

The Effects of Psychotherapy. Since the groups differed only in their status with respect to therapy, it might appear that the observed differences between the pre- and post-therapy groups could be taken as representing the effects of psychotherapy for the latter group. This conclusion would rest on the inference that the pre-therapy group at the time of assessment was similar to the post-therapy group at the time the latter sought help. The two groups were carefully matched, not only demographically, but also in problems and initial diagnoses; apart from the treatment variable, there are no apparent ways in which the groups differed systematically that might have been responsible for the observed differences in feelings. Nonetheless, it cannot be assumed that all relevant factors were controlled. It will be recalled, for example, that only successful cases were used, and these comprised a minority of the people seen at the Guidance Center. It is possible that these people were better off when they started therapy than the pre-therapy group examined here. So the effects of therapy must be demonstrated by before-and-after measures on the same people. In the process of identifying successful cases, it might be possible additionally to study some of the conditions of success — qualities of therapist, patient, and process that contribute to it. A before-and-after study shows promise of providing meaningful information.

COMMENTARY

QUESTION. You are not dealing with all of the cases seen at this clinic, are you? Could this just be a sample of 50 out of 500 cases?

BALKIN. I didn't count it up at the time, but that would be my estimation. I was busy looking for the successful ones. It could be even 50 out of 1,000.

GITTELMAN-KLEIN. I would like to take strong exception to the conclusions you come to on the basis of your study. You say that 50 out of perhaps 500 are successful in psychotherapy, and that when psychotherapy works it works very well. But even if the patients had been identical with your pre-therapy patients, you can't come to that conclusion. It is not even plausible because, assuming that patients seek treatment because they are slightly depressed — as we know, and Ricks has demonstrated (Wessman & Ricks, 1966) — these feelings fluctuate over time. It may be that after a period of spontaneous remission and feeling well, the patients leave treatment; the decrease in depression may have nothing to do with treatment effectiveness. I would like to caution that control groups are essential before you draw conclusions as to the efficacy of any treatment.

BALKIN. Are you suggesting that the people who ended up feeling better might have ended up feeling better anyway, without therapy?

GITTELMAN-KLEIN. It is something that you should contemplate.

BALKIN. It is possible. I am not claiming that therapy made them feel better. What I am saying is that different levels of feeling go along with therapy felt to be successful. That is all I am saying.

GITTELMAN-KLEIN. I disagree, and I don't think that is all you say.

KNIGHT. I would like to take issue with your conclusion that good feelings were necessary but not sufficient for improvement in psychotherapy. I would like to have you talk to the point raised by Gordon Paul (1966). Paul was dealing with a problem of interpersonal anxiety as defined by talking in front of people. He found that there were no differences between treatment groups in subjects' self-ratings. But when blind judges rated the behavior of subjects talking before a group, the behavior modification group was significantly improved over the insight therapy and other control groups. Other studies using behavior modification techniques have found that self-reports were unrelated to behavioral improvement. It would seem that the subjects' good feelings might not be necessary for improvement.

BALKIN. So you are assailing the validity of the self-reports?

KNIGHT. No, but you are saying that better feelings are necessary for improvement in psychotherapy, and I think that might not be true.

BALKIN. Well, if you demonstrated that this kind of change took place before and after, on the same group, that would show that changes in feelings were necessary, but maybe not sufficient. But I don't think that I've demonstrated that.

KNIGHT. I would say that even the statement that changes in feelings are necessary is false.

BALKIN. If you assessed people before therapy and after therapy, and always found that their feelings had changed significantly, then that would not show that changes in feelings are a necessary condition of successful psychotherapy ?

KNIGHT. I think one should have some objective measure of improvement, a behavioral measure, in addition to the subjective feelings. These two measures might be independent, as they were in Paul's study.

BALKIN. Well, my measure would be success, as I defined it. Why do you think something other than that is necessary?

KNIGHT. Because someone might feel improvement, feel better after his therapy, without his behavior having objectively changed. Someone rating him might say, indeed, that he was as nervous as he was before. Another person might feel the same as before, but show improvement in his behavior.

BALKIN. So that his own report might not be valid?

KNIGHT. It might be valid in terms of his feeling better, but I don't think that should be considered a necessary criterion for success in psychotherapy.

BERGIN. What were the criteria for success that you used?

BALKIN. Terminated with mutual agreement that there was no need for further therapy.

BERGIN. But you picked out 50 case histories. Was that the only way that they were selected?

BALKIN. As I recall, there would be a note by the therapist in the files, giving the reasons for termination. The category selected would be "no need for further treatment." And in the patient material, the patient would be talking about wanting to terminate because she felt better and didn't feel the need for it any more.

BERGIN. So there were no behavioral criteria?

BALKIN. No. Except patients' reports of their feelings.

HUNT. Not all kinds of psychopathology will necessarily be the same in this regard. Many "basket cases" being treated behaviorally feel a lot worse as they are getting better. Sometimes they feel worse just before they get better. I wouldn't necessarily assume that because one study finds one thing and another finds something else, with widely differing kinds of patients, one of the indicators is wrong.

KNIGHT. I am taking issue with the idea that one could say, "For successful change in psychotherapy, good feelings are necessary."

BALKIN. But I am not saying that in order for it to be successful there have to be changes in feelings. I am saying that when therapy is felt to be successful, this may be a characteristic of success.

RICKS. I want to raise a question. I don't have an answer, but I think it is a curious and interesting thing. These women who had been through psychotherapy, and the other women who matched them very well, in terms of age and so on, are the very women that Women's Liberation would say are caught in the household trap. They are the happiest groups we have yet studied, in comparison with male and female college students, to people in mental hospitals, and so on. These trapped women are the happiest people we have found. It makes me wonder about some of our current rhetoric.

BERGIN. I think Ricks succeeded in provoking a good deal of feeling with that, and we ought to move on before those feelings lock us into an endless discussion.

REFERENCES

Bergin, A. E. Some implications of psychotherapy research for therapeutic practice. *Journal of Abnormal Psychology*, 1966, 71, 235–246.

Bronner, A. F. Treatment and what happened afterward. *American Journal of Orthopsychiatry*, 1944, 14, 28–35.

Cartwright, D. W., & Roth, I. Success and satisfaction in psychotherapy. *Journal of Clinical Psychology*, 1957, 13, 20–26.

Cartwright, R. D. The effects of psychotherapy on self-consistency: A replication and extension. *Journal of Consulting Psychology*, 1961, 25, 376–382.

Constantinople, A. P. Some correlates of happiness and unhappiness in college students. Ph.D. thesis, University of Rochester, 1965.

Ellis, A. Outcome of employing three techniques of psychotherapy. *Journal of Clinical Psychology*, 1957, 13, 344–350.

Eysenck, H. J. The effects of psychotherapy. In H. J. Eysenck (Ed.), *Handbook of abnormal psychology*. New York: Basic Books, 1961. Pp. 697–725.

Garfield, S. L., & Kurz, M. Evaluation of treatment and related procedures in 1,216 cases referred to a mental hygiene clinic. *Psychiatric Quarterly*, 1952, 26, 414–424.

Hoffman, A. E. Reported behavior changes in counseling. *Journal of Consulting Psychology*, 1949, 13, 190–195.

Kircheimer, B. A., Axelrod, D. W., & Hickerson, G. X., Jr. An objective evaluation of counseling. *Journal of Applied Psychology*, 1949, 33, 249–257.

Myers, J. K., & Auld, F. R. Some variables related to outcome of psychotherapy. *Journal of Clinical Psychology*, 1955, 11, 51–54.

Paul, G. L. *Insight versus desensitization in psychotherapy: An experiment in anxiety reduction*. Stanford: Stanford University Press, 1966.

Reinhardt, S. Studies of mood in women. Ph.D. thesis, Teachers College, Columbia University, 1968.

Rogers, C. R., & Dymond, R. F. *Psychotherapy and personality change*. Chicago: University of Chicago Press, 1954.

Stone, A. R., Frank, J. D., Nash, E. H., & Imber, S. D. An intensive five-year follow-up study of treated psychiatric patients. *Journal of Nervous and Mental Disease*, 1961, 133, 410–421.

Strupp, H. H., Wallach, M. S., & Wogan, M. Psychotherapeutic experience in retrospect: Questionnaire survey of former patients and their therapists. *Psychological Monographs*, 1962, 76 (43).

Wessman, A. E. A psychological inquiry into satisfaction and happiness. Ph.D. thesis, Princeton University, 1956.

——— & Ricks, D. F. *Mood and personality*. New York: Holt, 1966.

Wilson, W. Correlates of avowed happiness. *Psychological Bulletin*, 1967, 67, 294–306.

Zubin, J. Evaluation of therapeutic outcome in mental disorders. *Journal of Nervous and Mental Disease*, 1953, 117, 95–111.

JOHN S. STRAUSS
WILLIAM T. CARPENTER, JR.] *Evaluation of
Outcome in Schizophrenia*

UNDERSTANDING outcome in schizophrenia is important in clarifying
the nature of this disorder and in evaluating treatment methods. Conceptu-
ally, there is much disagreement and confusion regarding the characteristics of outcome in schizophrenia. At one extreme are those who hold that
poor outcome is an integral part of the concept. Kraepelin (1919) used
poor outcome as a validating criterion of dementia praecox. Although
Bleuler (1950) modified the concept somewhat and gave it the name
schizophrenia, he was even more adamant than Kraepelin that there was
never total remission in this disorder. Kleist (1960) and Leonhard (1961)
claim that if the patient recovers, he cannot have been schizophrenic. Also
linking poor outcome to "true" schizophrenia, Langfeldt (1969), Faergeman (1963), and Vaillant (1964) define a separate group of schizo-
phrenia-like disorders with good outcome (schizophreniform psychoses,
psychogenic psychoses, or acute schizoaffective psychoses) that presumably have a different etiology and pathogenesis.

In contrast to the poor outcome concept of schizophrenia, Wittman
(1941), Phillips (1966), and others have used outcome as one basis for
defining benign (reactive) and malignant (process) subtypes within
schizophrenia.

Adolf Meyer's (1922) view that schizophrenia is not linked to any
particular outcome has been influential in American psychiatry. Besides
its conceptual importance, this view has served as a counterforce to the
fatalism that often accompanies a schizophrenic diagnosis.

In addition to contributing to the resolution of these important conceptual differences, understanding outcome in schizophrenia can provide
the basis for evaluating treatment methods and specifying the controls
necessary for such evaluation (Guze, 1970).

Over eight hundred studies of outcome in schizophrenia have been reported. Many of these provide important clues to the solutions of these problems (Zubin, 1961). Nevertheless, disagreement and confusion persist (Stromgren, 1961). Two major sources of this confusion are the failure to use comparable diagnostic criteria for schizophrenia and the tendency to use misleading, oversimplified concepts of outcome. These problems hinder interpretation of outcome findings and the comparison of results from different studies.

Problems in Defining Diagnostic Criteria

Since diagnostic criteria vary considerably, in any study of outcome in schizophrenia it is necessary to specify which criteria are used. The more operational the criteria, the more the results can be interpreted and compared. Criteria such as "agreement by two senior staff members" or "hospital discharge diagnosis of schizophrenia" are inadequate. Patient cohorts, thus defined, can, in fact, be quite dissimilar (Kendell, 1971; Kreitman, 1961).

The criteria for the diagnosis of schizophrenia stated in the *Diagnostic and Statistical Manual of Mental Disorders* (1968) are an improvement over mere statements of diagnostic category alone. However, these are not sufficiently operational either to provide a sound basis for defining comparable cohorts of patients. More complete rules for diagnosis are provided by several other commonly used systems — which, however, are complex, only moderately operationalized, and differ considerably among themselves regarding exactly what constitutes the diagnostic criteria for schizophrenia. These systems include the works of Bleuler (1950), Kraepelin (1919), Langfeldt (1969), Leonhard (1961), and Mayer-Gross (1954).

Among the most operational diagnostic criteria are specific symptoms and signs. The first-rank symptoms considered pathognomonic by Kurt Schneider (1959)* provide a set of diagnostic criteria that are particularly clearly defined.

*(1) Hearing voices speaking one's thoughts aloud. (2) Hearing voices arguing or discussing oneself. (3) Hearing voices describing one's actions as they take place. (4) Delusional interpretations of normal perceptions. (5) Feeling one's body sensations as imposed from outside. (6) Experiencing one's thoughts as though they were put in one's mind by an outside force. (7) Experiencing one's thoughts as being removed from one's mind by an outside force. (8) Experiencing one's thoughts as broadcast to other people. (9) Experiencing one's affect as imposed or controlled by an outside force. (10) Experiencing one's impulses as imposed or controlled by an outside force. (11) Experiencing one's actions as imposed or controlled by an outside force.

A major parameter of diagnostic systems is the range of patients which are considered by the systems as schizophrenic. Stephens and Astrup (1965) and others have claimed that narrower definitions of schizophrenia permit more precise prediction of outcome. For example, the diagnostic criteria of Langfeldt (including such symptoms as massive depersonalization and derealization, emotional blunting, and catatonic restlessness or stupor) appear to select a restricted group of patients with similar outcome. Results of several studies suggest that Langfeldt's criteria can be used to discriminate patients who will remit from those who will not (Achté, 1967; Astrup & Noreik, 1966; Eitinger et al., 1958; Langfeldt, 1937; Stephens & Astrup, 1965). Other diagnostic criteria, such as those of Mayer-Gross, Bleuler, and especially the concepts of schizophrenia often used in the United States, include a considerably broader group of patients and may, for that reason alone, have little relation to outcome.

Besides type of symptoms, another factor often included, explicitly or implicitly, as a criterion of diagnosis is the duration of symptoms before the initial evaluation of the patient. This criterion confuses the relationship of diagnosis to chronicity, since it may provide only a nonspecific historical measure of the tendency of symptoms to persist. If duration of symptoms before evaluation is included as a criterion in the diagnosis of schizophrenia, the claim that schizophrenia has a poor outcome may only be a tautology — that symptoms that have lasted a long time tend to persist. Although in some disorders duration of symptoms before evaluation may help to differentiate particular disease entities — for example, in distinguishing pneumococcal pneumonia from pulmonary tuberculosis — in others, duration of symptoms before evaluation is diagnostically nonspecific. This is true, for example, in a number of pulmonary disorders where chronicity of symptoms before evaluation is more related to the individual's general level of health and situational factors than to a particular pathologic entity.

Duration of symptoms before initial evaluation is, indeed, a powerful predictor of chronicity in schizophrenia (Chase & Silverman, 1941; Simon & Wirt, 1961) and in a wide variety of other psychiatric disorders (Ernst, 1959; Goodwin, 1969; Kringlen, 1970; Noreik, 1970; Pollitt, 1957). If chronicity before initial evaluation is wittingly or unwittingly included as a diagnostic criterion of schizophrenia, the finding of poor outcome may add little to an understanding of the nature of the disorder.

315

In some systems for the diagnosis of schizophrenia, duration of illness before diagnosis is an explicit criterion. Faergeman (1963), for example, states that the diagnosis of schizophrenia cannot be made on presenting symptoms alone. Laboucarié and Barres (1954) and Vaillant (1964) support this view. Others, including Bleuler (1950), Kraepelin (1919), Langfeldt (1937), Leonhard (1961), and Schneider (1959) diagnose schizophrenia entirely on the basis of presenting symptoms and signs. However, even outcome studies using only symptom diagnostic criteria may be biased by symptom duration before diagnosis. For example, if diagnostic evaluations are made a month or longer after admission, the more transiently symptomatic patients may have been discharged and automatically excluded from the study. If diagnostic evaluations are made at discharge, the tendency of symptoms to persist during hospitalization may inadvertently influence diagnosis (Astrup & Noreik, 1966).

Some investigators have tried to control chronicity before diagnosis by studying only patients with "recent onset." Eitinger et al. (1958) used such a criterion, but included patients who had onset of symptoms up to four years before their evaluation. Studying only first-admission patients is another method to attempt to eliminate established chronicity before diagnosis. However, our analysis of the data of a study by Achté (1967) demonstrates that first-admission patients had the first appearance of psychotic symptoms an average of fourteen months before their initial hospitalization. First admission is not, therefore, a sufficient criterion to rule out established chronicity.

Because of the predictive power of duration of symptoms before diagnosis and its frequent explicit or implicit inclusion in the diagnostic process, this factor must be considered in all studies of outcome in schizophrenia. A combination of measures, including prior hospitalization, first appearance of psychotic symptoms, and duration of continuous symptoms before hospitalization is probably the best means for accomplishing this.

Characteristics of Outcome

A second major hindrance to understanding the fate of schizophrenic patients arises from inadequate description of the characteristics of outcome. These problems include the selection of outcome criteria, scaling of results, and the evaluation of relationships among different areas of outcome dysfunction.

SELECTION OF OUTCOME CRITERIA

Oversimplified characterization of outcome is a particularly important problem. A common example is the use of a single global measure to describe patients at follow-up as improved, unchanged, or deteriorated. Global measures provide a gross estimate of outcome status, but are difficult to define operationally in an adequate manner since they usually assume a fixed relationship between hospitalization and several areas of function, which is not supported empirically. Such a concept implies that various aspects of a patient's functioning — such as his symptoms, social relationships, ability to work, and length of hospitalization — can be considered as rising and falling together. There is considerable anecdotal and statistical evidence that this assumption is not justified. Kraepelin (1919), Sullivan (1928), and others have described the distinction between clinical and social recovery. Kelly and Sargant (1965) and Brown et al. (1966) have demonstrated with refined methodology that two outcome criteria, work functioning and symptom level, are relatively independent of each other. Other areas of outcome function also appear to co-vary with considerable independence. For example, patients frequently remain hospitalized although they have little evidence of residual psychiatric disorder (Garratt, Lowe, & McKeown, 1957).

Another criterion frequently used as the sole measure of outcome is hospitalization. This measure is appealing because it is easily and reliably obtained on large numbers of patients. Freeman and Simmons (1963) have shown that it does reflect, to some extent, the individual's level of symptoms and ability to function. For more precise evaluation, an outcome index has been devised using a combined measure of both duration of hospitalization and frequency of admission (Burdock & Hardesty, 1961). However, there is evidence demonstrating that hospitalization alone is not a sufficient measure of the pathological process in schizophrenia. In one study (Strauss & Carpenter, 1972), hospitalization correlated to an intermediate degree ($r = .41$, $p < .001$) with the sum of the other outcome variables. Although this correlation is significant, the relationship accounts roughly for only about 17 per cent of the outcome variance.

Hospitalization is affected by many variables not directly related to the patient's psychopathology, such as administrative needs of the hospital (Brooke, 1962); hospital admission and discharge policies (Langsley et al., 1968; Pasamanick et al., 1964); the distance the patient lives from the hospital (Freudenberg et al., 1957; Gruenberg, 1964); the type and availability of rehabilitative or family resources (Brown, 1959; Norris, 1956); the social class of the patient (Myers & Bean, 1968); and the role the individual occupies in his family (Hammer, 1963).

Many patients hospitalized over long periods actually have no marked handicap and would be capable, with some assistance, of living outside the hospital environment (Garratt et al., 1957). Some schizophrenic patients discharged from the hospital lead only a vegetative existence, but are not rehospitalized. Other discharged patients make major attempts at successful social and occupational functioning and often meet stresses that precipitate their return to the hospital, but when discharged again return to high levels of function (Lamb & Goertzel, 1971; Penick & Buonpane, 1971). Finally, there is evidence that long-term hospitalization is not simply the result, but is a cause of deterioration in functioning (Brown & Wing, 1962; Goffman, 1961; Wing, 1962; Wing & Brown, 1961).

It seems apparent that, although hospitalization gives some measure of the need for care, it is affected by too many other variables to be used as the only measure of outcome in schizophrenia.

A more adequate picture of outcome status is provided when several key measures are used simultaneously. Four areas that together provide a comprehensive picture of follow-up status in schizophrenia are: work function, social relationships, symptomatology, and hospitalization. Each of these measures contributes information on a different aspect of the individual's life — each has its value and limitations.

Evaluation of work function gives a measure of the ability to fill one type of role expectation. Duration of employment during the follow-up period can be readily, reliably, and validly evaluated (Brown et al., 1966; Keating et al., 1950). In order for others to interpret the meaning of this measure, the investigator must specify whether he is evaluating total duration of employment over the follow-up period (time in the hospital is then counted as unemployment) or percentage of time employed when out of the hospital, thus separating measures of hospitalization from measures of employment (Monck, 1963).

As with hospitalization, work function as an outcome criterion has limitations, since it can be affected by many variables not directly connected to the individual's psychopathology. Lack of employment opportunities in the community, prejudice against hiring former psychiatric patients, social class, and age of patients (Myers & Bean, 1968) are all variables that influence employment but are not an intrinsic part of the psychopathology. Motivation to return to work, as determined by need and availability of alternate means of support, is another factor not directly related to psychopathology that affects employment measures.

Further complications occur in attempting to evaluate the functioning of housewives or workers in a family business or in protected work programs. In these situations, low levels of function can be concealed by family members or others filling in for an inadequately functioning person (Brown et al., 1966; Cole & Shupe, 1970; Myers & Bean, 1968).

Evaluation of social relationships provides information on an area more directly related to the concept of schizophrenia than measures of hospitalization and employment. However, social relationships are more difficult to evaluate. For example, merely evaluating whether a person has friends or how many friends he has is not a useful measure of social contacts unless an operational definition of friendship is given. Patients at follow-up often include as friends neighbors whose names are unknown and others with whom they have only the briefest contacts. Evaluating the number of social contacts the person has in a week, together with determining the place where these occur and the type of activity undertaken, gives a far more satisfactory record of social relationships. These three kinds of data help to separate, for instance, individuals who only say hello to a neighbor every morning when collecting the mail from someone who goes shopping with a friend or who has coffee at a friend's house. As with hospitalization and employment, social function as an outcome measure is limited, in that it is affected by environmental factors not directly related to psychopathology. These include cultural norms, normal individual variation, and absence of opportunity for social contacts. These factors are especially important in comparing patient cohorts from different cultural backgrounds and different socioeconomic groups.

The fourth area of evaluation necessary for obtaining a comprehensive picture of outcome function is symptomatology. Symptomatology at follow-up is central to the assessment of the chronicity of the schizophrenic process. However, it is the variable least often evaluated, probably because of the effort required to obtain complete and reliable assessments. The problem of obtaining reliable symptom evaluations at follow-up is made especially difficult because even clear-cut psychotic symptoms that may have occurred in the acute state of the illness frequently change over time to vague symptoms and signs such as apathy or lack of personal warmth (Kelly & Sargant, 1965). Semi-structured mental status interview schedules can help improve the reliability of symptom evaluation (Spitzer et al., 1964; WHO, 1973; Wing, 1967), but even these methods will require further development to be made suitable for evaluating the more subtle manifestations of schizophrenia at follow-up.

Together, these four measures of outcome — hospitalization, employment, social relationships, and symptomatology — provide a far more adequate picture of outcome in schizophrenia than any single measure. Still more detailed evaluations can provide greater richness of information. For example, employment data can be enriched by recording promotions and job changes; the evaluation of social relationships by estimating closeness of friendships. Other sources of further valuable detail are provided by obtaining data from several sources (Keniston et al., 1971; May & Tuma, 1964), consideration of pertinent environmental conditions, baseline premorbid function, and variations in the course of illness during the outcome period. A more complete and human component of outcome can be added by evaluation of other areas, such as happiness or fullness of life or detailed accounts of the experiences over time of small numbers of patients. But, for the study of large cohorts of patients, the four basic measures provide a broad, multidimensional picture of outcome.

SCALING OF OUTCOME RATINGS

Many reports of outcome in schizophrenia dichotomize patient function into categories of good or poor. This can give a misleading impression that patients fit into one of two categories, rather than being located somewhere on a continuum between no dysfunction and severe dysfunction. It can also lead to the assumption that there is a group of schizophrenics with "poor" outcome, and another group with "good" outcome. In fact, the frequency distribution of dysfunction severity in schizophrenic outcome is far more complex. To describe both intermediate and extreme levels of dysfunction more adequately, four- or five-point scales of outcome are useful. Even with these scales, however, interpretations regarding the distribution modes are tentative, since the scaling criteria influence the number of patients falling into each scale point. In scales with several rating points, the modality of the results (e.g., into two or three peaks) will be misleading if the scale points do not represent equal intervals. If the midpoint of a three-point scale is very narrow, for example, the distribution of results will be bimodal; if wide, a unimodal distribution may result. Specifying the criteria for each point mitigates this problem somewhat by aiding interpretation regarding the interval widths.

Still another way in which scaling influences results was described by

Levitt (1957), who showed that the more points an outcome rating scale has, the more likely patients will be rated as improved, irrespective of their psychiatric status.

Because of these factors, the ability to interpret and compare outcome findings is greatly enhanced by use of scales with a limited number of points, such as four or five, for which the categories are evenly spread and operationally defined.

Interrelationships of the Areas of Outcome Dysfunction

If one questions the assumption that outcome is a unitary phenomenon, the interrelationships of the component areas become of interest. The degree of relationship or independence among the component areas can be evaluated in terms of their levels of intercorrelation. These give valuable clues regarding the functional relationships among the components and suggest hypotheses about the process of outcome. When interpreting the meaning of intercorrelations, the degree of relationship, not just its statistical significance, must be evaluated (Spitzer & Cohen, 1968).

The features of diagnosis and outcome described above suggest a basic framework for data reporting to facilitate meaningful interpretation and comparison of outcome findings. This framework requires (a) reporting the criteria used for diagnosing schizophrenia and measures of patients' duration of illness before diagnosis; (b) reporting data on the four areas of outcome dysfunction; (c) using scaled data; and (d) describing the interrelationships of the areas of dysfunction.

This framework provides the basis for examining other complex features of outcome. Among these features are: evaluation of the course of illness over time, the degree to which outcome results depend on the duration between onset of illness and time at which outcome is measured, the relationships of premorbid factors and demographic factors to outcome, the evaluation of the relationship of schizophrenic outcome to outcome in other disorders and to normal function, and the difficult problem of whether an individual at some time in follow-up has neither residual dysfunction nor vulnerability to recurrence.

Before these problems can be answered, knowledge must be obtained about the most basic aspects of outcome. Using the framework of diagnostic and outcome criteria described above, what conclusions can be drawn about the fundamental aspects of outcome in schizophrenia?

The Outcome of Schizophrenia

To reach conclusions about outcome in schizophrenia, groups of patients selected by different diagnostic criteria and with different durations of illness before diagnosis should be compared to determine the relationships between these factors and the four areas of outcome. When studies of outcome are compared, certain conclusions can be made about the nature of outcome in schizophrenia; at the same time, areas of particular difficulty in generalizing from outcome studies also become clear. To demonstrate these conclusions and problems, several outcome studies were compared to determine the answers to three major issues: first, the level of outcome dysfunction in schizophrenia; second, the pattern of outcome distribution in schizophrenia (e.g., homogeneous, bimodal, heterogeneous, etc.); and third, the levels of intercorrelation among the four areas of dysfunction.

To describe outcome in these terms, studies of schizophrenia were selected that reported scaled outcome scores with defined scale points. These studies were among the more detailed of over two hundred studies reviewed. Because of their detail they offered the best basis for comparison. Unfortunately, although the selected studies all used scaled outcome criteria and often described diagnostic criteria and duration of symptoms before diagnosis, they did not reach the ideal for comparison, since a global measure was the only outcome criterion that all had in common. Nevertheless, some comparisons were possible, and preliminary conclusions were drawn. Features that hindered comparison and will have to be corrected if future outcome studies are to be more informative were also revealed. The diagnostic criteria used in each study, measures of duration of illness before diagnosis, and source of data where reported are described in Table 1.

Global outcome criteria in four of the studies were reported by the investigators on comparable four-point scales. In the other two cases, we converted the five-point scales used to four-point scales by splitting the middle category, assigning half to each adjacent category. For purposes of analysis, the four points of the outcome scale were given the values 0, 33, 67, 100. Although these adjustments are approximations, they did not appear to distort the data, either clinically or statistically.

THE LEVEL OF OUTCOME DYSFUNCTION IN SCHIZOPHRENIA

Because the selected studies used scaled outcome ratings, it was possible to calculate the mean outcome values for each of the cohorts. The

Table 1. Data Characteristics of Six Outcome Studies of Schizophrenia

Study	Diagnostic Criteria	Source of Diagnostic Data	Data on Previous Illness
Achté	Modified Langfeldt	Diagnosed by author from uncensored hospital records	1st-admission patients (length of time from onset of psychotic symptoms to hospitalization, 14 mo)
Astrup & Noreik	Hospital discharge diagnosis — modified Langfeldt	Hospital records	1st-admission patients (continuous psychotic symptoms before admission, mean 27 mo)
Brown et al.	Mayer-Gross	Diagnosed by author from uncensored hospital records	1st-admission patients; previously admitted patients
Eitinger et al.	Unspecified	Staff diagnosis	No data
Gittelman-Klein & Klein	Langfeldt	Diagnosed by author from uncensored hospital records	"Recent onset" (up to 4-yr duration)
Strauss & Carpenter	U.S. APA DSM II	Diagnosed from standard interview on admission	1st-admission patients (mean duration since first onset of illness, 20 mo); previously admitted patients (mean duration since first onset of illness, 28 mo)

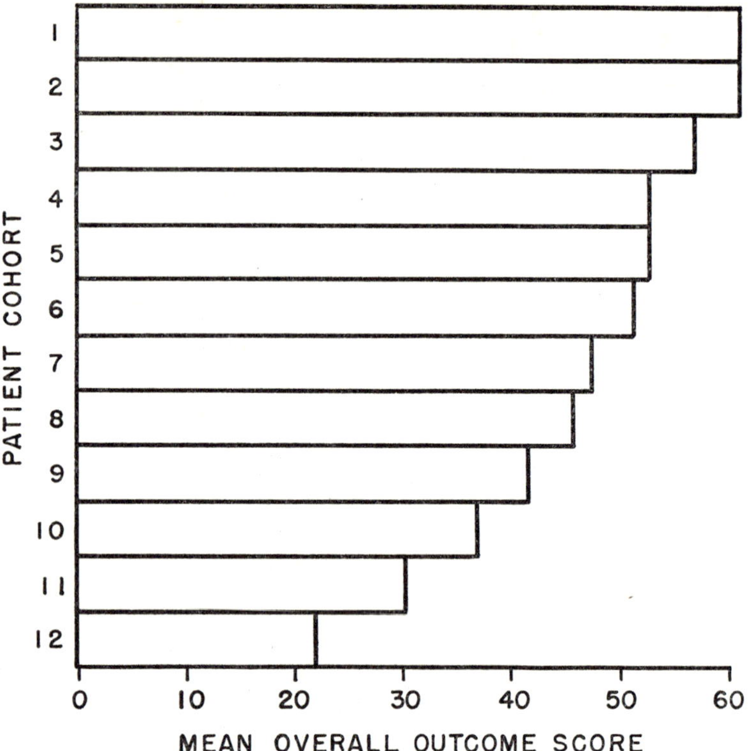

Figure 1. Comparative mean outcomes of several patient cohorts, with mean overall outcome scores ranging from 0 (most impairment) to 80 (least impairment). Patient cohort 1, non-schizophrenics (Strauss & Carpenter); 2, DSM II schizophrenics, first admission (Strauss & Carpenter); 3, Langfeldt Schizophreniform (A); 4, Mayer-Gross schizophrenics, first admission (Brown et al.); 5, DSM II schizophrenics, previous admission (Strauss & Carpenter); 6, "U.S." schizophrenics (Gittelman-Klein & Klein); 7, Langfeldt Schizophreniform (Eitinger et al.); 8, Mayer-Gross schizophrenics, previous admission (Brown et al.); 9, "Reactive psychoses" (Astrup & Noreik); 10, Langfeldt schizophrenics (Astrup & Noreik); 11, Langfeldt schizophrenics (Achté); 12, Langfeldt schizophrenics (Eitinger et al.).

results of this comparison are presented in Figure 1. These data demonstrate the wide variation in the mean levels of outcome found and dispel any notion that there is a uniform outcome for schizophrenia. The disparity among the findings of the different studies is striking. Diagnostic criteria and duration of illness before evaluation both affect results. There is a gradual improvement of mean outcome scores as diagnostic criteria shift from those defined by Langfeldt to the diagnostic criteria of Mayer-

Gross, and those of the *Diagnostic and Statistical Manual*.* More acute patients (for example, first admissions) have better outcome than more chronic patients (those previously admitted to hospitals), but this difference is not so important in predicting outcome as are the diagnostic criteria.

Because of its detailed presentation of raw data, it was possible from one study (Achté, 1967) to evaluate the relationship between duration of illness, outcome, and diagnosis more carefully. Achté used Langfeldt's symptom criteria to diagnose a cohort of first-admission patients as definite schizophrenia, possible schizophrenia, or schizophreniform psychosis. For this analysis, we scaled the diagnoses of the 170 patients studied in keeping with Achté's definitions, giving the diagnosis of schizophreniform psychosis a value of 1, schizophrenia? a value of 2, and certain schizophrenia, a value of 3. Intercorrelations (Kendell's τ) were calculated among outcome, duration, and diagnosis. The results demonstrated that the highest relationship was between schizophrenic diagnosis and duration of illness before evaluation ($\tau = .52, p<.001$). There were lower but significant correlations between duration of illness before evaluation and outcome ($\tau = .33, p<.001$) and between diagnosis and poor outcome ($\tau = .31, p<.001$). To evaluate these interrelationships further, we matched patients from the three diagnostic groups for duration of illness before initial evaluation and calculated the difference in mean outcome scores of these three groups. Using Achté's five-point outcome scale where a score of five signifies worst outcome, we found that the mean outcome of the schizophreniform psychosis group was 2.1, of the intermediate schizophrenia? group was 2.75, and of the schizophrenia group was 3.58. The differences were significant (F $= 9.56, 2/167$ *df*, $p<.001$). The correlation (τ) between diagnosis and outcome for this matched group was significant ($\tau = .40, p<.001$).

The different levels of mean outcome scores from the six studies describe the wide range of outcome characteristics of schizophrenia — from severe to minimal dysfunction. These differences appear to be a function of both diagnostic criteria and duration of symptoms at initial evaluation. Contrasting these studies demonstrates the ability of Langfeldt's diagnostic criteria to predict outcome, apparently irrespective of duration of illness, at least as controlled by first-admission status. Since Langfeldt's was the

---

*Unfortunately, the diagnostic criteria of several of these categories are too complex, with many variables to be weighed and considered, to be presented here. The interested reader is referred to the sources cited.

only diagnostic system of those compared able to do this to an impressive degree, it will be important to investigate the source of this predictive power. Although the diagnostic criteria themselves appear to be the crucial variables, the successful prediction of outcome might have arisen from possible errors in methodology (the Achté diagnoses were made from case records, after the patients had been discharged) or from unrecognized, but important, prognostic factors.

THE FREQUENCY DISTRIBUTION OF OUTCOME SCORES

The frequency distributions of global outcome ratings for several studies are shown in Figure 2. These data demonstrate another way in which it is misleading to describe "the outcome of schizophrenia." They show considerable distribution for each patient cohort, except the Langfeldt schizophrenics, along the entire continuum of outcome dysfunction.

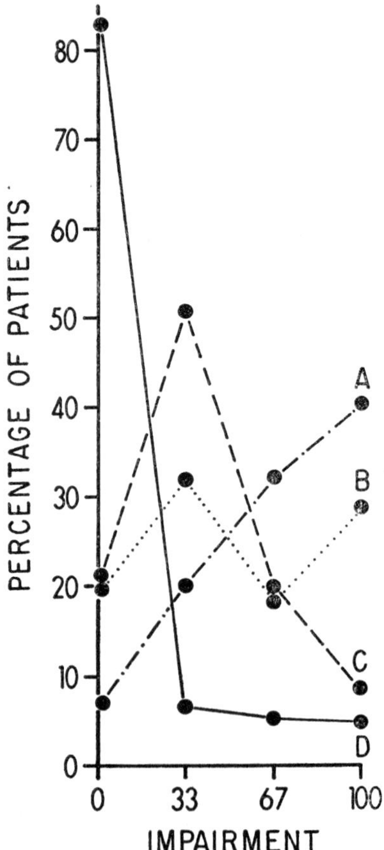

Figure 2. Overall outcome in schizophrenia: a comparison of four studies with different diagnostic criteria, on a scale of 0 (most impairment) to 100 (least impairment). Ss in Study A (Strauss & Carpenter, 1972) were DSM II schizophrenics ($N = 85$); in Study B (Brown et al., 1966), Mayer-Gross schizophrenics, previous admissions ($N = 198$); in Study C (Astrup & Noreik, 1966), schizophrenics ($N = 273$); and in Study D (Eitinger et al., 1958), Langfeldt schizophrenics ($N = 110$).

These distributions suggest that the most accurate description of outcome in most schizophrenic groups is a mean outcome score and a measure of dispersion, rather than a uniform outcome.

The different shapes of these curves also demonstrate the inadequacy of reporting only a mean outcome score and the absence of any consistent modal pattern of outcome. The problems of interpretation of these differences could be greatly reduced if different studies used standardized outcome criteria.

INTERRELATIONSHIP OF THE DIFFERENT AREAS OF DYSFUNCTION

A few outcome studies have reported interrelationships among different areas of outcome dysfunction. Table 2 compares their results. The intercorrelations in all cases are statistically significant. The extent of intercorrelation is modest and variable. Absence of high intercorrelations

Table 2. Relations among Four Outcome Variables (r's)

Outcome Variables	Freeman & Simmons	Turner & Zabo	Gittelman-Klein & Klein	Strauss & Carpenter
Symptoms and nonhospitalization[a]	—.37 (M) —.42 (F)	—.34		—.35
Employment and nonhospitalization	.23		.57	.54
Social relationships and nonhospitalization	.18 (M) .13 (F)		.09	.27
Employment and symptoms				—.52
Employment and social relationships			.20	.52
Social relationships and symptoms				—.63

[a]Time out of hospital during follow-up period.

among outcome measures could be a result of measurement error. This is unlikely, however, since interrater reliabilities of the outcome measures were high. The intermediate levels of the intercorrelations are best interpreted as demonstrating both a significant relationship and relative independence among the outcome variables. This hypothesis is supported by detailed clinical data that suggest reasons for the independence (Strauss & Carpenter, 1972).

327

These findings indicate that each area of dysfunction is related to an intermediate degree with other areas of dysfunction, but is also affected by its own independent system of variables. This suggests that the areas of outcome dysfunction are best considered as open-linked systems. Cumming (1963), Freeman and Simmons (1963), Myers and Bean (1968), and others have begun to map some of the functional links between particular areas of outcome dysfunction. Further clarification of these links will be extremely helpful in providing greater understanding of the nature of outcome disability.

Conclusions

To understand the nature of outcome in schizophrenia, it is essential to consider and report key variables of diagnostic criteria, duration of illness before diagnosis, and outcome dysfunction. Such a consideration could be carried out most effectively by conducting outcome studies following a standardized model that would serve as a common denominator for interpretation and comparison of results. Such a model might include the reporting of:

1. Diagnostic evaluation
   a. Signs and symptoms, including inquiry into the major areas of psychopathology (hallucinations, delusions, depression, elation, etc.), and into characteristic symptoms such as those described by Langfeldt.
   b. Duration of psychopathology before the diagnostic evaluation, including (1) number and total duration of previous psychiatric hospitalizations; (2) an estimate of the continuous duration of psychotic symptoms before diagnostic evaluation; and (3) length of time from first evidence of psychotic symptoms to time of diagnostic evaluation.
2. Evaluation of outcome
   a. Evaluation of outcome dysfunction in at least four areas: employment (percentage of time outside of hospital that the patient is employed); social function; severity of symptomatology; and duration of hospitalization after initial diagnostic evaluation.
   b. Use of a four-point scale with defined scale points for evaluating each area.

Use of this methodology in different centers could provide a basis for more meaningful comparison of findings of outcome studies and eventual understanding of the crucial variables in the outcome of schizophrenia.

Although not reaching this ideal, a comparison of outcome studies that report their findings in adequate detail provides a general picture of the characteristics of outcome in schizophrenia. First, the level of global outcome dysfunction in schizophrenia varies from severe dysfunction to minimal dysfunction depending on the diagnostic criteria used and on the duration of illness before the diagnostic evaluation. Langfeldt's criteria of schizophrenia appear to be the most powerful in predicting a poor mean level of outcome.

Second, the frequency distribution of global outcome dysfunction also varies considerably depending on the diagnostic criteria and duration of illness; but within each cohort, except those diagnosed by Langfeldt's criteria, there is a wide variation of level of dysfunction across patients. Langfeldt's criteria of schizophrenia appear to predict the narrowest distribution of scores.

Third, the four areas of outcome function in schizophrenia appear to represent open-linked systems — each related both to the presence of schizophrenia and to its own system variables.

Most crucially, the comparison of outcome studies demonstrates that outcome is not a thing, it is a group of complex processes. Schizophrenic outcome can be described and understood in a meaningful way only if the complex relationships among the diagnostic criteria, duration of illness, and characteristics of outcome are considered.

COMMENTARY

ZUBIN. There are really three kinds of outcome. There is outcome so far as society is concerned — namely, employment and the expectation that the patient will take his place in society again the way he was before he took sick (if he had a place). Then there is the patient himself — how well he readjusts, how happy he is, and how much enjoyment he gets out of life. Certainly, if he hasn't developed a work ethic, employment wouldn't count much for him personally, although if we regarded him from the point of view of society, he would be a failure. Finally, there is the health delivery outcome — how much service he needs, how much he gets, and so on. Each of these three aspects of outcome have been delineated clearly, and it looks as if in the attempt to relate diagnosis to outcome, you have three options: What is the diagnosis that (a) will give the best relationship to society's demands on the individual; (b) will give the best prognosis with regard to his personal and family adjustment; and (c) will predict the service to give him? It is strange to realize that after all of these years there is no single way of selecting the optimum combination. You have to separate these three options, but the measures, for example, for the internal aspect of his readjustment, his happiness, and so on, are as good as the measure of work adjustment. Our Biometrics Research Unit did develop an outcome index for health services delivery, in which we counted the number of days that the patient spent out of the hospital by a complex formula — the proportion of time spent out of hospital since release, multiplied by the number of readmissions to the cube, divided by the number of releases to the square. With this index, you get three sub-groups of schizophrenics: one that comes in, stays a little while, and never comes back; one that comes in and stays in; and one that oscillates in and out. So it depends on what you want. If you want a criterion based on health delivery, you will take the outcome index. If you want one for society, you will take the employment arrangement. If you want one for the individual himself, you have got to look into the matter further.

But suppose you want a diagnosis of schizophrenia independent of all of these things — true, genuine schizophrenia. How do you go about arriving at that, unencumbered by all of these other aspects, which are socially important, familially important, hospital-important? How do you get free of all of that? That's an interesting idea and raises many interesting questions requiring answers.

Suppose we take the social criterion of earning a living. Lady Barbara Wooton has pointed out the fallacy in utilizing employability as a basis for judging presence of, or outcome of, illness. Suppose, she points out, that employment were taken as a measure of rise and fall in number of one-legged men. In times of prosperity, more one-legged men would find employment. Would that lead to the inference that the number of one-legged men declined? In schizophrenia, the behavior itself is our only criterion, but such behavior may reflect not only the disorder, but the response of society to the disorder and the readiness of society to accept or reject the individual sufferer. That is why the diagnosis of schizophrenia and its outcome is fraught with so much difficulty when social criteria alone are utilized.

If we adopt a genetic criterion for diagnosis, we can test the value of competing diagnostic systems by noting which will give a higher transmission rate in the families of schizophrenics than in the families of normals. It turns out that neither the American "loose" diagnosis, nor the Langfeldtian, continental European "severe" diagnostic procedure, but Essen-Moeller's approach, which is somewhere in between, gives you the highest transmission rate. If you are a devout believer in genetics, that is your answer.

Thus, even though we cannot utilize outcome as the sole basis for diagnosis, we can utilize presumed etiology as a basis. Analogous to the use of genetic transmission as a criteria, we could use criteria based on ecological sources of schizophrenia — developmental, learning, internal environment, and neurophysiology — and perhaps emerge with a set of criteria for different types of schizophrenia.

STIERLIN. I think Strauss's work is important for a number of reasons. Here I can only outline one. He said correctly that assessment of outcome in schizophrenia is tied up with the diagnosis of schizophrenia.

In the past, this has created a problematical situation, first, because diagnoses have remained muddy and complicated and, second, because the criteria for outcome have been rudimentary. Strauss has been working on both ends of the problem. Mainly through his work at WHO and at NIMH, he has refined the diagnosis of schizophrenia and has shown the immense complexities involved. He has now done the same thing for outcome criteria, doing away with existing crude dichotomies and giving us a glimpse of the complexity at hand. What does this mean in terms of our view and treatment of schizophrenia? Here let me briefly reflect. The notion of poor prognosis was from the beginning built into the concept of schizophrenia. Morell asserted this with his concept of dementia praecox, in about 1860, which was then taken over by Kraepelin and Eugen Bleuler, who, in turn, established a European tradition of psychiatry which came to include Kurt Schneider, Langfeldt, Eitinger, and Mayer-Gross, among many others. I became impressed by how much this powerful, though often unconscious, assumption (of poor prognosis) affected the diagnosis and became a factor in the outcome itself. As a student of Kurt Schneider, I observed a number of times how he diagnosed schizophrenic patients (in front of his medical class) on the basis of his first- and second-rank symptoms. This was like declaring a death sentence. It was conveyed to the patient right there and then, as it was conveyed to us students, and to his relatives and family: "This patient is beyond repair. He is schizophrenic." And I realized then that this patient's later life course was probably affected by this powerful professor in the white coat, the authority in psychiatry stepping in and declaring, "This patient is a schizophrenic." We should think about this also in the light of Ricks's paper. Supershrink's gift seems to have prevented a schizophrenic outcome in many of his high-risk cases. One of his qualities was that he, confronted with an immensely difficult and sinister picture, kept his optimism. He conveyed this optimism to the patient and his parents. And this, too, seems to have changed the outcome significantly.

STRAUSS. I was much impressed, too. I agree with Helm about the circular effect of expectation of outcome and what the outcome actually is. That is impressive in Watt's paper, in Rolf's, and, of course, in Rosenthal's works. The expectations of the environment can cause a prediction to be self-fulfilling (Stierlin, 1967). This has certainly occurred in many cases of schizophrenia.

D. KLEIN. The whole area of self-fulfilling prophecies is a tough one. It's easier to tear down than to build up. At Hillside, the ideology was one of marked optimism about schizophrenia. Schizophrenics were considered to have a reversible psychogenic disorder. The belief was that these people would do well given the proper sort of care that we knew how to give. The patients who did badly were the subgroup of schizophrenics who had a history of childhood asociality; 100 per cent of them did badly, regardless of the amount of optimism with which they were treated. There certainly is some degree of truth to your idea of self-fulfilling prophecy, but I think that to make that an overriding symmetrical consideration is also a mistake.

In the kind of follow-up that Kelley (1964) did, treated schizophrenics — who were apparently in complete remission — broke down in spite of the tremendous optimism with which their cure was hailed by the professionals and without relation to family attitude. The findings, over and over again, were that a person who was apparently in complete remission and being treated as in complete remission still broke down and required rehospitalization. It does not require a negative prophecy to break down, and a positive prophecy is not prophylactic.

However, social outcomes are related both to the primary psychopathological processes, whatever they may be, and to a number of sociopsychological secondary effects, which I refer to loosely as demoralization. Demoralization is a state where a person concludes that he is no good and can't manage; he has his own self-fulfilling prophecy, that he can't manage, and therefore he doesn't try. Obviously, poor therapy can contribute to this and good therapy can combat it. Probably a great deal of what passes as psychotherapy is actually combating the secondary demoralization and not combating the primary illness. The entire distinction between good and poor therapists may lie in their ability to deal with secondary effects rather than the primary illness.

STRAUSS. On that first question, at the risk of looking like I am agreeing with everybody, I do agree with you. One of the directions that we are taking actually is to try to look for what there is that seems to be moderately reversible, or fairly easily reversible, about schizophrenia, and what isn't. We're looking at symptoms as compared with premorbid features to see if there are any symptoms, or symptom patterns, that in themselves seem to predict or define a disease process which will then have a downhill course. And the more we look at symptoms alone, using Langfeldt's and other criteria, we are finding what other people have also begun to find — that we cannot come up with any symptom, or any symptom pattern, or any diagnostic criteria that are commonly used that in themselves predict outcome. What does seem to predict outcome is the sort of thing that you were getting at also, the long-term feature, what has happened before. If you look at a person's work function, how he has worked before, that is going to predict how he is going to work in the future. Apparently one of the things that you tap with the childhood situation are these long-term personality patterns, maybe biologically based and maybe not. Those are the things that seem to go beyond the self-fulfilling prophecy, and seem to be something that is in fact really difficult to turn around. But not the symptoms themselves.

REFERENCES

Achté, K. A. *On prognosis and rehabilitation in schizophrenic and paranoid psychoses.* Copenhagen: Munksgaard, 1967.

Astrup, C., & Noreik, K. *Functional psychoses: Diagnostic and prognostic models.* Springfield, Ill.: Thomas, 1966.

Bleuler, E. *Dementia praecox or the group of schizophrenias.* Trans. J. Zinkin. New York: International Universities Press, 1950.

Brooke, E. M. Factors affecting the demand for psychiatric beds. *Lancet,* 1962, 62, 1211–1213.

Brown, G. W. Experiences of discharged chronic schizophrenic patients in various types of living groups. *Millbank Memorial Fund Quarterly,* 1959, 37, 105–131.

Brown, G. W., Bone, M., Dalison, B., & Wing, J. K. *Schizophrenia and social care.* London: Oxford University Press, 1966.

Brown, G. W., & Wing, J. K. A comparative clinical and social survey of three mental hospitals. In P. Halmos (Ed.), *Sociology and medicine, studies within the framework of the British National Health Service.* Keele: University of Keele, 1962.

Burdock, E. I., & Hardesty, A. S. An outcome index for mental hospital patients. *Journal of Abnormal and Social Psychology,* 1961, 63, 666–670.

Chase, L. S., & Silverman, S. Prognostic criteria in schizophrenia. *American Journal of Psychiatry,* 1941, 98, 360–368.

Cole, N. J., Brewer, D. L., Allison, R. B., & Branch, C. H. H. Employment characteristics of discharged schizophrenics. *Archives of General Psychiatry,* 1964, 10, 314–319.

Cole, N. J., & Shupe, D. R. A four-year follow-up of former psychiatric patients in industry. *Archives of General Psychiatry,* 1970, 22, 222–229.

Cumming, J. The inadequacy syndrome. *Psychiatric Quarterly,* 1963, 37, 723–733.

Diagnostic and statistical manual of mental disorders. (2nd ed.) Washington, D.C.: American Psychiatric Association, 1968.

Eitinger, L., Ludv, C., Langfeldt, L., & Langfeldt, G. The prognostic value of the clinical picture and the therapeutic value of physical treatment in schizophrenia and schizophreniform states. *Acta Psychologica et Neurologica Scandinavica,* 1958, 33, 33–53.

Ernst, K. *Die prognose der neurosen.* Berlin: Springer, 1959.

Faergeman, P. M. *Psychogenic psychoses.* London: Butterworth, 1963.

Freeman, H. E., & Simmons, O. *The mental patient comes home.* New York: Wiley, 1963.

Freudenberg, R. K., Bennett, D. H., & May, A. R. Relative importance of physical and community methods in the treatment of schizophrenia. In *Second International Congress for Psychiatry, Report No. 1.* Zurich, 1957.

Garratt, F. N., Lowe, C. R., & McKeown, T. Investigation of the medical and social needs of patients in mental hospitals. 1. Classification of patients according to the type of institution required for their care. *British Journal of Preventive and Social Medicine,* 1957, 2, 165–173.

Gittelman-Klein, R., & Klein, D. Premorbid social adjustment and prognosis in schizophrenia. *Journal of Psychiatric Research,* 1969, 7, 35–53.

Goffman, E. *Asylums.* New York: Doubleday, 1961.

Goodwin, D. W., Guze, S. B., & Robbins, E. Follow-up studies in obsessional neuroses. *Archives of General Psychiatry,* 1969, 20, 182–187.

Gruenberg, E., & Zusman, J. The natural history of schizophrenia. *International Psychiatry Clinics,* 1964, 1, 699–710.

Guze, S. B. The role of follow-up studies: Their contribution to diagnostic classification as applied to hysteria. *Seminars in Psychiatry,* 1970, 2, 392–402.

Hammer, M. Influences of small social networks as factors in mental hospital admission. *Human Organization,* 1963–1964, 22, 243–251.

Keating, E., Patterson, D. G., Stone, C. H. Validity of work histories obtained by interviews. *Journal of Applied Psychology,* 1950, 34, 6–11.

Kelley, F. E. Relative attitude and outcome of schizophrenia. *Archives of General Psychiatry,* 1964, 10, 389–394.

Kelly, D. H. W., & Sargant, W. Present treatment of schizophrenia — a controlled follow-up study. *British Medical Journal*, 1965, 1, 147–150.

Kendell, R. E., Cooper, J. E., Gourlay, A. J., Copeland, J. R. M., Sharpe, L., & Gurland, B. J. Diagnostic criteria of American and British psychiatrists. *Archives of General Psychiatry*, 1971, 25, 123–130.

Keniston, K., Boltax, S., & Almond, R. Multiple criteria of treatment outcome. *Journal of Psychiatric Research*, 1971, 8, 107–118.

Kleist, K. Schizophrenic symptoms and cerebral pathology. *Journal of Mental Science*, 1960, 106, 246–253.

Kraepelin, E. *Dementia praecox*. Trans. R. M. Barclay. Edinburgh: E. S. Livingstone, 1919.

Kreitman, N. The reliability of psychiatric diagnosis. *Journal of Mental Science*, 1961, 107, 876–886.

Kringlen, E. Natural history of obsessional neurosis. *Seminars in Psychiatry*, 1970, 2, 403–419.

Laboucarié, J., & Barres, P. Le pronostic des schizophrenies. *Toulouse Medicine*, 1954, 55, 167–181.

Lamb, H. R., & Goertzel, V. Discharged mental patients — are they really in the community? *Archives of General Psychiatry*, 1971, 24, 29–34.

Langfeldt, G. The prognosis in schizophrenia and the factors influencing the course of the disease. *Acta Psychiatrica Scandinavica*, 1937, Supp. 13.

————. Schizophrenia: Diagnosis and prognosis. *Behavioral Science*, 1969, 14, 173–182.

Langsley, D. G., Pittman, F. S., III, Machotka, P., & Flomenhaft, K. Family crisis therapy — results and implications. *Family Process*, 1968, 7, 145–158.

Leonhard, K. The cycloid psychoses. *Journal of Mental Science*, 1961, 107, 633–648.

Levitt, E. E. The results of psychotherapy with children: An evaluation. *Journal of Consulting Psychology*, 1957, 21, 189–196.

Marks, J., Stauffacher, J. C., & Lyle, C. Predicting outcome in schizophrenia. *Journal of Abnormal and Social Psychology*, 1963, 66, 117–127.

May, P. R. A., & Tuma, A. H. Choice of criteria for the assessment of treatment outcome. *Journal of Psychiatric Research*, 1964, 2, 199–209.

Mayer-Gross, W., Slater, E., Roth, E., & Roth, M. *Clinical psychiatry*. Baltimore: Williams & Wilkins, 1954.

Meyer, A. Constructive formulation of schizophrenia. *American Journal of Psychiatry*, 1922, 78, 354–364.

Monck, E. M. Employment experiences of 127 discharged schizophrenic men in London. *British Journal of Preventive Social Medicine*, 1963, 17, 101–110.

Myers, J. K., & Bean, L. L. *A decade later*. New York: Wiley, 1968.

Noreik, K. A follow-up examination of neuroses. *Acta Psychiatrica Scandinavica*, 1970, 46, 81–95.

Norris, V. A statistical study of the influence of marriage in the hospital care of the mentally sick. *Journal of Mental Science*, 1956, 102, 467–486.

Pasamanick, B., Scarpetti, F. R., Lefton, M., Dinitz, S., Wernert, J. J., & McPheeter, H. Home versus hospital care for schizophrenia. *Journal of the American Medical Association*, 1964, 187, 177–181.

Penick, S. B., Buonpane, N., & Carrier, R. N. Short term acute psychiatric care: A follow-up study. *American Journal of Psychiatry*, 1971, 1626–1630.

Phillips, L. Social competence, the process-reactive distinction, and the nature of mental disorder. In P. H. Hoch & J. Zubin (Eds.), *Psychopathology of schizophrenia*. New York: Grune & Stratton, 1966.

Pollitt, J. Natural history of obsessional states. A study of 150 cases. *British Medical Journal*, 1957, 1, 194–198.

Schneider, K. *Clinical psychopathology*. Trans. M. W. Hamilton. New York: Grune & Stratton, 1959.

Simon, W., & Wirt, R. D. Prognostic factors in schizophrenia. *American Journal of Psychiatry*, 1961, 117, 887–890.

Spitzer, R. L., & Cohen, J. Common errors in quantitative psychiatric research. *International Journal of Psychiatry*, 1968, 6, 109–131.

Spitzer, R. J., Fleiss, J., Burdock, E., & Hardesty, A. The mental status schedule: Rationale, reliability and validity. *Comprehensive Psychiatry*, 1964, 5, 384–395.

Stephens, J. H., & Astrup, C. Treatment outcome in "process" and "non-process" schizophrenics treated by "A" and "B" types of therapists. *Journal of Nervous and Mental Disease*, 1965, 140, 449–456.

Stierlin, H. Bleuler's concept of schizophrenia: A confusing heritage. *American Journal of Psychiatry*, 1967, 123, 996–1001.

Strauss, J., & Carpenter, W. T., Jr. The prediction of outcome in schizophrenia. I. Characteristics of outcome. *Archives of General Psychiatry*, 1972, 27, 739–746.

Stromgren, E. Recent studies of prognosis and outcome in the mental disorders. In P. Hoch & J. Zubin (Eds.), *Comparative epidemiology of the mental disorders*. New York: Grune & Stratton, 1961.

Sullivan, H. S. Tentative criteria of malignancy in schizophrenia. *American Journal of Psychiatry*, 1929, 84, 759–782.

Turner, R. J., Raymond, J., Zabo, L. J., & Diamond, J. Field survey methods in psychiatry: The effects of sampling strategy upon findings in research of schizophrenia. *Journal of Health and Social Behavior*, 1969, 10, 289–297.

Vaillant, G. E. An historical review of the remitting schizophrenics. *Journal of Nervous and Mental Disease*, 1964, 138, 48–56. (a)

———. Prospective prediction of schizophrenic remission. *Archives of General Psychiatry*, 1964, 11, 509–518. (b)

WHO. (Ed). *The international pilot study of schizophrenia*. Vol. 1. In preparation.

Wing, J. K. Institutionalism in mental hospitals. *British Journal of Social and Clinical Psychology*, 1962, 1, 38–51.

———, Birley, L. T., Cooper, J. E., Graham, P., & Isaacs, A. D. Reliability of a procedure of measuring and classifying "present psychiatric states." *British Journal of Psychiatry*, 1967, 113, 499–515.

Wing, J. K., & Brown, G. W. Social treatment of chronic schizophrenia: A comparative survey of three mental hospitals. *Journal of Mental Science*, 1961, 107, 847–861.

Wittman, P. A scale for measuring prognosis in schizophrenic patients. *Elgin State Hospital Papers*, 1941, 4, 20–33.

Zubin, J., Sutton, S., Salzinger, K., Salzinger, S., Burdock, E. I., & Peretz, D. A biometric approach to prognosis in schizophrenia. In P. Hoch & J. Zubin (Eds.), *Comparative epidemiology of the mental disorders*. New York: Grune & Stratton, 1961.

JAMES R. MORRISON]] *Catatonia:*
Results of Treatment

Since the advent of ataractic drugs in the early 1950's, electroconvulsive therapy (ECT) as the primary treatment for schizophrenia has fallen into disuse. However, for a period of 12 to 15 years it was, along with other means of producing convulsions, widely used in many institutions, and has been reported by some (Hamilton & Wall, 1948) to result in a considerable rate of recovery or improvement. Others, however, have found ECT inferior to drugs in alleviating symptoms and in promoting early discharge from hospital (May, 1968).

One of the problems in the evaluation of the treatment of schizophrenia has been a lack of diagnostic consistency. Some authors (Fish, 1962) would argue that the diagnosis "schizophrenia" encompasses many entities, and that studies done on such a group of patients cannot be expected to have much predictive value. One way around this problem is to study only one subtype of schizophrenia and, in particular, one which has as its distinguishing feature behavior which is as readily identifiable as that of catatonia.

Catatonia was described by Kahlbaum in 1874, and although that author regarded the syndrome as a nosologic entity, it was later subsumed under the classification of dementia praecox by Kraepelin, a view which has persisted until the present time. Although it may be legitimately argued that symptoms of catatonia do not constitute an entity (Hearst et al., 1971) they do form a characteristic picture. Thus, if a form of treatment could be delineated which results in a higher rate of improvement for the syndrome of catatonia, which is commonly called schizophrenia today, a step forward will have been taken toward more effective treatment of a sizable group of patients.

In the present study a large group of patients suffering from catatonia has been collected from one institution over a period of half a century, offering the opportunity to compare the history of the illness given only supportive treatment or "milieu" therapy with its course given modern somatic treatments.

MATERIALS AND METHODS

Since the Iowa State Psychopathic Hospital in Iowa City opened its doors in 1920, nearly 20,000 patients have been admitted to the inpatient service. The records of each of these patients have been preserved in original, typewritten form in the hospital archives. A search of these records through the year 1971 revealed 250 patients with the diagnosis of catatonic schizophrenia, catatonic syndrome, or dementia praecox, catatonic type; these records form the material for the present investigation.

Each chart consisted of a workup and progress notes by at least two sets of observers: the psychiatric staff and the social workers assigned to each patient. The information for the social service evaluation, usually obtained from the nearest relative at the time of admission, included a detailed description of the present illness and past history. In addition, it contained a description of all first-degree family members and, during the first 40 years of the study, detailed descriptions of as many grandparents, aunts and uncles, and other more remote relatives as it was possible to obtain, with special reference to the presence of psychiatric illness of any type.

The psychiatrist's history, after restating most of the pertinent information already mentioned, was largely taken up with a lengthy description of the present illness and mental status. Great emphasis has always been placed on phenomenology and diagnosis at this institution, so that mental status examinations would occasionally run to 20 typewritten pages. In addition, all charts contained typed progress notes, and most included verbatim transcripts of interviews with the patient and of discussions among the attending physicians about the diagnosis, treatment, and prognosis.

In general, the diagnosis of schizophrenia rested upon the presence of disturbances of affect and association, ambivalence, and autism as described by Bleuler only nine years before the opening of this hospital. The diagnosis of the subtype "catatonic schizophrenia" has consistently rested upon the demonstration of the motor symptoms of activity (catatonic excitement) or underactivity (catatonic stupor), either one being frequently associated with the symptoms of negativism, mutism, grimacing, posturing, rigidity, or waxy flexibility.

Follow-up information, routinely sought for all discharged patients, was available for most of the subjects of this study. Some had been read-mitted, but the information available for most consisted of letters from relatives written in response to inquiry from the social service department, or letters written by physicians at other hospitals to which our patients had been admitted. This information was diligently sought: the correspondence files often record a half dozen letters sent out by the social service depart-ment before an answer was obtained.

All of the foregoing information was coded and recorded according to prearranged criteria and in a specific order at separate times, so that the family histories were evaluated without knowledge of the patient's symptoms or outcome; the past history and course of the present illness were later evaluated without knowledge of the family history, and blind to the outcome following discharge; and finally, the follow-up information was evaluated blind both to the family history and to the symptomatology. The material was all entered onto IBM punch cards for data processing, which was done by a computer program and counter-sorter. Statistical analyses were made using t test and chi square with Yates's correction.

RESULTS

During the 1920's and 1930's, no effective somatic treatment was available to the patients in this hospital. The patients were given hydro-therapy, "packs," occupational therapy, and psychotherapy of varying persuasions and degrees of intensity. By the late 1930's, however, metra-zole and insulin coma therapies were being utilized to a limited extent, and in July 1940 electroconvulsive therapy was instituted.

In the years since 1940, 58 patients have been treated with ECT alone, and 19 have been treated with ECT plus a major tranquilizer (phenothia-zine or haloperidol). ECT was bilateral, with curare or a synthetic relaxant used as muscle relaxant. Premedication with atropine was used only late in this series (1953); anesthesia was a refinement not instituted until late in this period. The number of treatments, usually given thrice weekly, ranged from 3 to 50 per patient, with a mean of 18. An additional 17 patients were treated with tranquilizers alone. These three groups, plus the 142 patients who received no somatic treatment at all, the "milieu" group, constitute the treatment modalities reported on here. Omitted from this report because of the small numbers are 14 patients who were treated with other combinations of somatic therapy or with insulin coma or metrazole alone.

The accompanying tabulation shows the disposition at discharge for the four major treatment groups; here, institutional discharge includes patients sent to state hospitals, which were generally less treatment-oriented, or in a few cases, to private hospitals and nursing homes. Only slightly over half of the patients who received neither shock treatments nor major tranquilizers were discharged home, whereas nearly three quarters of the ECT group were discharged home ($\chi^2 = 3.9591$, $df = 1$, $p < .05$). An

	Home	Institution
Milieu (N = 142)	54%	46%
ECT (N = 58)	71	29
Drug (N = 17)	88	12
ECT-drug (N = 19)	95	5

even higher rate of discharge home was achieved with the use of drugs, either alone or in addition to ECT. Although the drug alone and ECT-drug groups differed significantly from the milieu group, the difference between the drug and the ECT-drug groups did not attain statistical significance.

At discharge (Table 1), two thirds of the milieu patients were either unimproved or worse, whereas at least two thirds of any of the groups receiving somatic therapy were markedly improved or well. Differences between any of the somatically treated groups and the milieu group are significant at the $p < .001$ level. Drug alone produced improvement in more patients than did ECT alone, but the difference missed significance at the .05 level ($\chi^2 = 3.5789$). Three patients (16 per cent) of the ECT-drug group failed to show more than slight improvement, probably because this group contained more patients who, being more severely ill, were treated with a second modality after the first had failed. In fact, the ECT-drug group spent a significantly longer time (108 days) in the hospital than any of the other three groups: 58 days for the milieu group, 66 days for ECT, and 53 days for the drug group.

Table 1. Condition at Discharge, in Percentage

Treatment	Worse	Same	Mild Improvement	Marked Improvement	Well	Unknown
Milieu (N = 142)	10	56	12	18	3	1
ECT (N = 58)		23	10	64	3	
Drug (N = 17)			6	88	6	
ECT-drug (N = 19)			16	84		

Location of the patients at follow-up is shown in the accompanying tabulation. Over one third of the patients in the milieu group were hospitalized, either continuously or with an interval at home. Of the somatically treated patients, however, only one fifth to one sixth were hospitalized at follow-up, thus differentiating these treatments from milieu at the .05 level.

	Home	*Hospitalized*	*Dead*
Milieu (N = 123)	56%	37%	7%
ECT (N = 58)	78	20	2
Drug (N = 16)	81	19	
ECT-drug (N = 19)	84	16	

Condition at follow-up (Table 2), which was evaluated without knowledge of previous history or treatment during hospitalization or of condition at discharge, was categorized as follows: (A) Complete recovery without relapse — as nearly as could determined, these patients were medically well without defect, and were working at their accustomed trade or profession; housewives and students were back at their usual employment. (B) Complete recovery, followed by at least one recurrence of illness, but again completely recovered at follow-up. (C) Recovery at least once, but ill again at the time of follow-up.

There were three groups of patients who were known never to be well but who had varying degrees of incapacity: (D) Social recovery — patients were back at their usual jobs and living outside the hospital, but still medically ill, having some defect in affect or occasional psychotic symptoms. (E) Never completely recovered, ill at follow-up, and socially unrecovered, but not deteriorated. (F) Unrecovered, and deteriorated at follow-up, as defined by Astrup and Noreik (1966), showing inadequate verbal communication, lack of working capacity, and inability to care for self.

The final two groups included patients for whom the information available was less definite: (G) Patients who were socially recovered but for whom it could not be determined if they were medically well. (H)

Table 2. Condition at Follow-up, in Percentage[a]

Treatment	A	B	C	D	E	F	G	H
Milieu (*N* = 123)	16	7	9	6	28	16	13	5
ECT (*N* = 58)	40	5	5	10	21	3	2	14
Drug (*N* = 16)			19	25	31		19	6
ECT-drug (*N* = 19) ...	27	5	11	16	21	5	11	5

[a]See pages 340–341 for descriptions of categories A–H.

Patients who were outside the hospital but for whom it could not be determined whether they were medically well or socially recovered.

Taken together, categories A, B, and C include those patients who at follow-up had had the best quality of remission, being at some time back to their normal personality and functioning at their premorbid level. Thus defined, the recovery rates for the four treatment groups were: milieu, 32 per cent; ECT, 50 per cent; drug, 19 per cent; and ECT-drug, 42 per cent. Thus, ECT alone was associated with complete recovery significantly more often than either milieu therapy ($\chi^2 = 8.3421$, $df = 1$, $p<.005$) or drug therapy ($\chi^2 = 4.3804$, $df = 1$, $p<.05$) but did not significantly differ from the ECT-drug group.

The sum of categories A, B, D, and G represents all patients known to be socially recovered at follow-up, whether medically well or not. Utilizing this breakdown, ECT alone is still significantly ($p<.020$) better than milieu, 57 per cent of the former group being socially recovered as compared with 41 per cent of the latter. Although fewer of the drug group (44 per cent) were socially recovered at follow-up than of the ECT group, these figures do not differ statistically ($\chi^2 = 1.0968$). All of the somatic treatment groups were associated with a lower percentage of deterioration than was the milieu group, but the figures do not differ statistically.

Of the factors which might have influenced the outcome at follow-up, three seemed especially worthy of further investigation: length of follow-up, presence of affective symptoms in the treatment groups, and the possibility that those patients with the more favorable prognoses were selected for treatment with ECT.

Mean follow-up times for the four treatment groups were: milieu, 3.5 years; ECT, 3.3 years; drug, 1.9 years; and ECT-drug, 2.8 years. Conceivably, if the ECT patients with longer follow-up were eliminated from the study, the two groups might become similar in outcome. Accordingly, all patients with follow-up periods of 7.5 years or longer were discarded from the ECT group, leaving a group of patients with a mean follow-up period of 1.8 years; 53 per cent of this group had had a remission, and the difference from the drug-alone group remained significant ($\chi^2 = 4.4582$, $df = 1$, $p<.05$).

The ECT group also contained 18 patients in whom there were enough symptoms to qualify for the diagnosis of an affective disorder; the milieu group contained 19 such patients; and the drug group only one. With these patients eliminated, 43 per cent of the remaining ECT group had had a recovery, compared with 20 per cent of the drug group

($x^2 = 1.8686$, $df = 1$, $p = $ n.s.). Eliminating both the long follow-ups and the patients with affective symptoms resulted in a recovery rate of 43 per cent for the remaining ECT patients. Thus, the elimination of two major factors, either singly or together, which may have biased the outcome in favor of ECT still left ECT-treated patients with a percentage totally recovered at something over twice that of the drug group alone. Because of the reduced sample size, however, the last two differences were not statistically significant.

To investigate the possibility that only those patients with the more favorable prognoses were treated with ECT, a comparison was made between ECT-treated patients and all other patients admitted during the ECT era (1940–1954) who received no somatic treatment. Of the twelve patients in the latter group, 58 per cent were discharged home, 50 per cent being markedly improved or well at discharge, and on follow-up, 75 per cent were living at home, but only 17 per cent had ever had a complete recovery; 25 per cent had prominent affective symptoms, not significantly different from the treated group. If the patients receiving ECT had been specially selected, one would expect the remaining milieu patients from this era to have had an especially bad outcome at discharge, whereas the actual percentage discharged to another hospital was about the same as that for milieu patients from 1920 to 1940. Further, half of those 12 patients treated with milieu alone were considerably improved at discharge, indicating that it was, if anything, the sicker patients who were being treated with ECT.

DISCUSSION

Because this was not primarily a study of treatment, the interpretation of these results must be tentative. We cannot know the selection criteria which might have been applied for giving ECT: if the treating psychiatrists gave shock therapy only to those patients whom they considered to have a good prognosis, the results of the study would be compromised. However, a comparison of those patients not treated during the ECT period does not reveal striking differences between them and the treated group.

We have no information on whether ECT patients may have received drugs subsequent to discharge from their index admissions, or whether drug-treated patients may subsequently have been given ECT. The latter proposition is less likely than the former, inasmuch as the use of ECT has declined since the introduction of ataractic drugs.

Another source of possible error lies in the follow-up method itself. All follow-ups in this study were based on information contained in the patient's permanent chart, and the quality and diligence with which follow-ups were sought may well have changed over the course of the years. However, follow-up material was available for 92 per cent of the overall patient population, with only 1 per cent of the patients treated with any somatic means lacking follow-up information of any type. Again, eliminating those ECT patients who had long follow-up periods produced little change in outcome. Bias on the part of the rater was substantially reduced in that all follow-up information was evaluated blind to the symptomatology and the type of treatment given, except of course that any patient discharged before 1940 was known to have received no somatic treatment during the hospitalization.

With these warnings in mind, I shall turn to a discussion of the results of this study. The finding that ECT is intermediate to milieu therapy and drug therapy in producing a good outcome at discharge in schizophrenic patients has been reported in several different studies. May (1968) found that patients treated with ECT were hospitalized slightly longer than drug-treated patients, and were rated as slightly less well by therapists at discharge. Findings of the present study are nearly identical, with the drug-treated patients being released slightly earlier and showing a higher percentage either markedly improved or well at discharge than those in the ECT group. In neither study were these differences significant, however. In the present study, all three modalities of somatic treatment were associated with better condition at discharge than milieu alone, and with any form of somatic treatment patients were more likely to be discharged home than to another institution. In a study of catatonics treated with ECT versus nonconvulsive electrical stimulation or Pentobarbital, Miller and Clancy (1953) found that, although all treatment groups had improved to some degree, no differences could be found among the treatment modalities at the end of the treatment period; significant differences might have been found with a higher number of patients in each treatment group, however.

The present study did not include a placebo treatment group; however, it is interesting to note that at release from hospital, 20 per cent of the milieu group were markedly improved or well, very close to the 23 per cent "marked or moderate improvement" of the placebo group of the NIMH collaborative study on schizophrenia (1964) (the two study groups having been hospitalized for similar periods of time). Although it is dangerous to make comparisons between studies done in different hospitals, this remarkable similarity might be interpreted as showing that the improvement of about one fifth of the patients from both studies with hospitalization is a baseline, or essentially the natural history of the illness, and that placebo adds little to the basic effect of hospitalization alone, whatever that may be. With tranquilizer therapy in the NIMH study, over 75 per cent showed marked or moderate improvement after six weeks; this figure is somewhat lower than the 94 per cent who were markedly improved or well at discharge from the drug-alone group of the present study.

Neither May nor the NIMH study included an ECT plus drug group, but other studies have utilized such treatment groups. Smith et al. (1967) noted that although both drug-alone and ECT-drug groups improved significantly with a six-week treatment program, patients who also received ECT improved more rapidly, were discharged sooner, and were readmitted less often than those treated with drug alone. However, there were no differences in global rating and social functioning found at follow-up six months and one year later. In the present study, ECT-drug treatment was associated with a somewhat higher rate of discharge home (though in no better condition) than either of the other two somatic treatment groups. The number of days required for treatment with ECT plus drug was strikingly different, however — that group requiring nearly twice as long in the hospital as either of the other treatment groups or the milieu group.

In a study published before the advent of major tranquilizers, and hence uncontaminated by drug treatment subsequent to discharge, Hamilton and Wall (1948) reported a follow-up of 1½ to 6 years recovery in 43 per cent of 100 female schizophrenics treated with ECT: of the 54 catatonic patients in their study, 76 per cent were at home, and 57 per cent were considered to be recovered. The similarity of these figures to those of the present study is striking, but even more interesting is the finding that a higher percentage of catatonics were reported as well and at home at follow-up than was true of the other diagnostic subcategories, suggesting that ECT may be specifically indicated for catatonia.

Pritchard (1967) has suggested that although drugs may indeed contribute to reduction of psychopathology and rapid discharge, the long-term follow-up of drug-treated patients in terms of readmission rate and duration of stay in hospital may not be so favorable as had first been thought. The results of the present study support this. None of the drug-alone patients could at follow-up be characterized as being completely well, although three of them (19 per cent) had apparently made complete recovery at some time, but were once again ill at the time of follow-up. This percentage compares unfavorably with either the ECT alone or the ECT-drug groups, in both of which over 40 per cent of the patients had at some time experienced a complete recovery. From the tabulation on page 340, however, it is evident that even though fewer of the drug group were completely well, only about 20 per cent of any of the three groups was hospitalized at the time of follow-up. Although tranquilizers are associated with patients remaining in the community, they do not appear to be so closely associated with complete recovery as is ECT, and the possibility exists that if recovery were to occur spontaneously, drugs might mask it. The consistency of this study with some of the other reports in the literature strengthens the argument that ECT, which has largely fallen into disfavor in the treatment of schizophrenia, may actually result in a better quality of improvement than the use of ataractic drugs alone in the treatment of patients with catatonia. The early combined use of drugs plus ECT could result in rapid improvement, early discharge, and optimal recovery rate at follow-up.

Caution should be employed in generalizing these results to other subgroups of schizophrenia: although the patients reported here would nearly all be includable as schizophrenics by the criteria of either May or the NIMH collaborative group, we do not know how many patients in those two studies had catatonia, or how much they improved. Clearly, more care should be taken in the future to differentiate subtypes when reporting treatment studies on schizophrenia.

COMMENTARY

WATT. Do schizo-affective schizophrenics whose families had a higher incidence of affective psychotic disorders tend to have better recoveries than those whose families had schizophrenic but not affective disorders? Could the patient's having a grandmother who also was psychotically depressive influence the psychiatrist in making a judgment about the likelihood of a patient's having depressive elements in the psychotic symptomatology?

MORRISON. I shall attempt to answer that in two parts. The problem of affective symptoms is one that I attempted to deal with carefully because it is very important. Most studies that have considered the problem have shown that patients who are diagnosed as schizophrenic but who have affective symptoms — whether you call them schizo-affective, schizophreniform, atypical psychoses, or what have you — do tend to have a better outcome. I attempted to look at the differences between groups after eliminating the patients so diagnosed, which appeared to make relatively little difference in the percentages of the patients who improved. I started this study with the bias that there really wasn't any such thing as catatonic schizophrenia, and that it was all part and parcel of manic-depressive disorder. I have emerged from reading 250 charts of catatonics with the realization that there is such a thing as catatonic schizophrenia, some of which may be linked with manic-depressive disease. But there is certainly a large number of patients who appear catatonic who are schizophrenic and who remain that way for a good proportion of their lives.

As far as the diagnosis of the grandparents or the parents influencing the diagnosis of the physician at the time of the treatment regimen, I do not think this is necessarily so. There was a great deal of discussion in these charts about what the diagnosis was, and how to make the diagnosis, and what the treatment ought to be. From these verbatim comments made in staff meeting, I got a pretty good idea of how diagnosis was being made in those days. I was somewhat chagrined to note that family history was not mentioned more than once or twice — not only in those 250 charts, but also in 1,000 charts that I have just reviewed for another study.

RICKS. I think Iowa offers you a special advantage for looking at things like this. You have an urban population and a rural population. New York, for instance, produces diagnoses of schizophrenia that don't look like schizophrenics in other parts of the country. Perhaps Iowa is a little more representative. Do the catatonics come from the city or from the country?

MORRISON. They come from both places.

RICKS. There is no regional breakdown?

MORRISON. I don't have figures, at least not yet, breaking down the population during the different eras into how many lived rurally, how many in small towns and how many in large cities (large by comparison — we consider Iowa City to be quite a metropolis at 50,000). I can't tell you whether there are significant differences there, but I can tell you that catatonia is no chooser of locale.

RICKS. You just shot down my hypothesis, which was that catatonics were just people that time had passed by, and they were out in the rural districts.

MORRISON. Not necessarily. Rural patients may not have been brought in for treatment quite so rapidly. I think that people in farming communities tend to tolerate higher degrees of psychopathology than do city dwellers. But I don't think that you could substantiate your statement about time lag.

KNIGHT. Do you have any data on the good and poor premorbidity of your catatonic patients? Garmezy (1967), in his review of process-reactive schizophrenics, reported that catatonics in the Duke studies distributed themselves widely along the "process-reactive continuum." Were your patients distributed this way, and if they were, was premorbidity related to assignment to the various treatment groups? Usually good premorbids have higher affective components. Did this relate to outcome at all?

MORRISON. I am not going to be able to give a very satisfactory answer. I have thousands of bits of information, and I haven't had time to go through them all yet. However, Winokur and I and a couple of others are doing a study now in which we are taking 35-year-old case histories and making diagnoses using extremely hard criteria — I think these criteria would satisfy even Strauss. We have looked at the problem of premorbid personality, and in these cases it split about fifty-fifty. About half of them have a schizoid, or shy, or seclusive premorbid personality, but a good many of them don't. I might add that Iowa is an excellent place for doing follow-ups on patients. We are doing personal follow-ups on 525 patients admitted between 1935 and 1944, and so far 98 per cent of them are traceable to the present or to death.

HUNT. I would agree with Morrison that catatonic schizophrenia exists. And I have even seen a case of cerea flexibilitas, back in 1944. We don't see it around here, but it is reassuring to know that some parts of America are "still intact." I have been struck throughout this volume with the tremendous importance of detail. I think the reason is that life history methods become impossibly difficult and impractical unless one uses a fairly wide or coarse screen. And yet life, looked at behaviorally, often consists of very important junctures which occur only once or twice, and if the person is vulnerable or open to the effects of those junctures when they do occur, tremendous effects can result. In Groeschel's paper, I think, some of the most interesting findings emerged from the detailed examination of exactly what happened at certain junctures in the lives of the children. Details are important. For example, in Morrison's paper we heard a plea for diagnostic specification of different kinds of schizophrenics. In Strauss's paper, again, the importance of specifying certain kinds of symptoms and certain kinds of outcomes in making sense of outcome data in schizophrenia was a major part of the presentation. In connection with self-fulfilling prophecies, those familiar with the literature on hypnosis know that some of the effects of the hypnotists' expectations may be transmitted in extremely subtle ways. If the diagnoser simply believes that the diagnosis of schizophrenia is a serious diagnosis from which there is likely to be no remission, this gloomy expectation somehow may be transmitted to the patient.

What changes when patients improve? Some years ago, we did a before-and-after study at the University of Chicago, using the MMPI on one of the blocks of cases that went through the Counseling Center. Leonard Hersher, now at SUNY Upstate Medical Center in Syracuse, New York, was interested in defensiveness and its relationship to recovery in psychotherapy. He used Hogan's means of analysis, which at that time was a very important way of indexing defensiveness in non-directive therapy. He also used the MMPI as one of the indicators. This was one of the first studies to separate patients who were rated as improved from those rated not improved at the Counseling Center. He found that the improved clients became more defensive, showing higher K scores than unimproved clients on the MMPI. What does a higher K score mean? It means the persons are saying good things, unjustifiably optimistic things about themselves, and that their scores on the clinical scales have been pushed downward by this distortion. When people "fake good" on the MMPI, their K scores go up. Middle-class people who take the test honestly also will tend to have slightly elevated K's. And when middle-class people try to fake good, they often cannot produce much more elevation in K, possibly because of a ceiling effect. Now, I don't know whether that means that denial is necessary for membership in the middle class. It may be. At any rate, these are some of the functional properties of elevations in K.

Hersher found that the improved patients had higher K scores, and this had been interpreted as defensiveness. Then we categorized the items by whether the meaning was obvious or subtle (many years ago Weiner broke the MMPI into two sets of scores, subtle and obvious subscales, for a number of the major clinical scales). In general, the obvious scales all showed drops in score in those cases that improved, but none for those that did not improve. It followed K exactly: K going up as obvious items in the clinical scales went down. The subtle scales remained about as they had been before therapy, both in the improved and the unimproved cases. In view of our earlier discussion, what changed in those people who were improved, in those who said themselves that they were improved, who were considered improved by the therapists, as compared with the others?

REFERENCES

Astrup, C., & Noreik, K. *Functional psychoses.* Springfield, Ill.: Thomas, 1966.

Fish, F. J. *Schizophrenia.* Bristol: John Wright, 1962.

Garmezy, N. Process and reactive schizophrenia: Some conceptions and issues. In M. M. Katz, J. O. Cole, & W. E. Barton (Eds.), *The role and methodology of classification in psychiatry and psychopathology.* PHS Publication No. 1584. Washington, D.C.: GPO, 1967. Pp. 419–460.

Grinspoon, L., Ewalt, J. R., & Shader, R. Psychotherapy and pharmacotherapy in chronic schizophrenia. *American Journal of Psychiatry,* 1968, 124, 1645–1652.

Hamilton, D. M., & Wall, J. H. The hospital treatment of dementia precox. *American Journal of Psychiatry,* 1948, 105, 346–352.

Hearst, E. D., Munoz, R. A., & Tuason, V. B. Catatonia: Its diagnostic validity. *Diseases of the Nervous System,* 1971, 32, 453–456.

May, P. R. A. *Treatment of schizophrenia.* New York: Science House, 1968.

Miller, D. H., & Clancy, J. A comparison between unidirectional current nonconvulsive electrical stimulation given with Reiter's machine, standard alternating current electroshock (Cerletti method), and Pentothal in chronic schizophrenia. *American Journal of Psychiatry,* 1953, 109, 617–620.

NIMH Collaborative Study Group. Phenothiazine treatment in acute schizophrenia. *Archives of General Psychiatry,* 1964, 10, 246–261.

Pritchard, M. Prognosis of schizophrenia before and after pharmacotherapy: I. Short term outcome. *British Journal of Psychiatry*, 1967, 113, 1345–1352.
————. Prognosis of schizophrenia before and after pharmacotherapy: II. Three year follow-up. *British Journal of Psychiatry*, 1967, 113, 1353–1359.
Smith, K., Surphlis, W. R. P., Gynther, M. D., & Shimkunas, A. M. ECT-Chlorapromazine and Chlorapromazine compared in the treatment of schizophrenia. *Journal of Nervous and Mental Disease*, 1967, 144, 284–290.

DAVID F. RICKS *Life History Research:
Retrospect and Prospect 1973*

T HIS BOOK has had three main purposes; to describe children at risk for various kinds of psychopathology, to show some contrasting normal and pathological sequences of development, and to demonstrate some methods for evaluation of intervention. This chapter will look back over the papers reported here and the discussions that followed them in an attempt to say where we have been, where we are now, and where we are going. The chapter will be more speculative than any of the papers have been, trying to extrapolate from them toward some general ideas that they support, and to draw out some of their clinical implications.

A question of importance to every clinician who reads the book is how to apply these research findings in his own work. As a hybrid researcher-clinician myself, I am most interested in research results that have applications. Life history research is a basic natural science that can organize and make coherent the best parts of the applied fields of special education, psychiatry, clinical psychology, social work, and rehabilitation. Since life history research is a field in which basic science and applied work intersect, much of the work is done by research-minded practitioners, and another large segment is done by researchers with a strong clinical interest. We hope this helps us communicate to both scientist and practitioner.

One of the issues the papers address themselves to, for instance, is diagnosis. The diagnostic schemes currently in use were largely invented to solve problems that no longer exist in their original forms, and the diagnostic schemes that will help solve the problems of current practitioners are just coming into being. Strauss provides a model of how to go about refining diagnostic judgments, showing that prognosis is very strongly determined by the narrowness or breadth of the diagnostic criteria one uses. And Lorr shows that diagnosing the varieties of normality may be as complex as diagnosing psychopathology. Such research can refine our clinically derived knowledge, making the general hunches of the practitioners precise and clear. Research can also change our whole perspective on disorder. The most valuable contributions of life history investigations are dynamic descriptions of sequential developmental patterns leading into the different psychopathological syndromes. Such trajectory typologies will gradually replace the overly static descriptions of psychopathologies that still dominate most textbooks. Jordaan and Super show how a career-oriented study of work life has already begun to replace the older static concern with vocational choice in counseling psychology.

As research sifts the received knowledge of each new generation, showing which parts of the conventional wisdom no longer hold true, and which parts need new emphasis, particularly in everyday application, it moves into a new research and development model. Here the role of research is to prepare practice to cope with change, to deal with problems not as they were at some prior time, but as they are now, and as they will be. Increased rates of social change lead to increased need to work with "first-time problems," questions that have not really been encountered before. We have a huge investment, for instance, in a traditional VA system for working with medical and psychiatric diseases. But on visits to VA clinics and hospitals I hear that the biggest problems they now face have to do with the varied types of drug addiction. And pending adequate research, particularly life history research, no one can adequately define their problems. What is a "drug addict" like? How did he get that way? What is the likely prognosis without treatment? Is there a "pan-addict" or are different kinds of drugs differentially attractive to different kinds of people? Here longitudinal research such as that done by Schuckit is necessary if we are to get an adequate conceptual handle on new problems, for which there is no accumulated clinical experience and not enough time in which to accumulate it.

The work reported here has implications for several other crucial clinical issues, such as how to recognize a developing pathological process, how to differentiate it from other processes that it may resemble in some ways, how to intervene, when to intervene, and how to evaluate the effects of different interventions at different life stages. We may also, if we are wise, recognize developing trends toward health and adequacy, and know when to reinforce them or simply to let development take its course, without intervention.

Before considering the papers in this book in detail, I can summarize some of the main results of life history research, and some of the ideas that are still current in clinical work but are increasingly suspect on the basis of research evidence. First the main themes:

a. As students of child development have long known, there is remarkable continuity in development, both within individuals and between generations. We can confidently predict that children will resemble those whose genes they bear, the family that rears them, and those who are socially or self selected to transmit the larger culture to them. The mechanisms of transmission, through genetic codes, early symbiosis and modeling, and later learning, are increasingly understandable. Continuity may be trait specific — in males, aggressiveness observed early predicts aggressiveness later — or it may be a matter of rate of growth — stunting now predicts a more or less permanent lag later. This continuity between generations, and between age-stages in the same individual, allows us to select for study a variety of different kinds of "high risk" for later disorder.

b. Every child, adolescent, or adult syndrome has a sequential developmental course that is open to study through pediatric, child guidance clinic, residential treatment center, or school records as well as through longitudinal direct observation. Chronic and acute disorders differ, not in that chronic disorders have always existed in the same form while acute develop suddenly with no precursors, but in a more subtle way. Chronic and acute schizophrenia, for instance, seem to have somewhat different developmental courses, and one can differentiate them early not in terms of the adult symptoms but in terms of social and academic competence, neurological integration, and goal directedness of activity. Since there are way stations on the road to each of the extreme disorders, we might be able to arrest or reverse the development of psychopathological solutions to life problems at different points along the way, before disorder reaches its adult forms.

c. There are branching patterns of disorder, and for these sets we can look to general early influences. For example, delinquency, criminality, alcoholism, drug addictions, and the various impulse disorders seem to have many common developmental elements, some of which are shared with the cruder forms of hysteria. For such patterns of disorder we might expect many common influences in the genetic backgrounds, family influences, and social pressures on the developing child. Perhaps many mothers of this whole set would be found to be undernourished, relatively ignorant, poorly cared for "ineffective reproducers," and this might account for much of the tendency of these disorders to run in families. Sequences of development are likely to be similar until differentiating influences from peers, school, and jobs occur in adolescence and young adult life. Since most delinquent adolescents go on to law-abiding lives, while a few go on to criminal, addictive, or psychotic episodes, it is important to differentiate the adolescent influences that lead to these contrasting outcomes.

d. Different syndromes develop at different rates. Acting-out patterns are recognizable early and develop fairly consistently. Schizophrenia in girls seems to develop recognizable precursor and premorbid syndromes more rapidly than in boys. Although we lack for most types of disorder the careful description of precursors, premorbid stages, acute stages, and chronic stages that we have for alcoholism (Jellinek, 1952), it is beginning to be possible to develop such longitudinal descriptions for schizophrenia, addictions, depression, and even for the more subtle neuroses.

e. Different interventions are necessary for different age-stages and different types of developing psychopathology. Interventions that can further a child's social competence or peer appeal may be generally valuable, as can tutoring that can help a child catch up or keep up with his school peers. But most forms of intervention will be more effective if they are specifically designed to fit the age, interests, and problems of a particular group of vulnerable children. One of my students, for instance, has developed methods for teaching young autistic children to play with other children, believing that inability to play is one of the main deficits with which these children have to cope. Another student is developing puppet plays for teaching somewhat older children how to recognize and interpret "double-bind" types of adult communications. And a group is hard at work on behavior modification methods for helping hyperactive children develop internal controls and goal directedness. There is no panacea, no one treatment to head off later disorder, and to the extent that practitioners oversell single methods, whether psychodynamic, behavior modification, or educational, they do a disservice to all of the children not helped by their particular method.

f. Clear understanding of a child's developmental course leads to reasonable expectations, and lack of understanding leads to expectations that are too high, and hence frustrating, or even worse, to expectations that are too low and only too likely to be self-fulfilling.

g. In at least one respect, clinical research should follow the example of developmental psychology. We should move from episodic predictions, in which we look for common outcomes to particular events (divorce, loss of a parent through death, early illness, etc.) to developmental models in which we ask how processes get started and what keeps them going. We can no longer believe in the radical environmentalism that says that "traumatic events" cause disorders. Memory sharpens and levels, and traumatic events are often reported to therapists as condensed summaries of long-term developmental influences. Events are clearly related to stress, and stress to psychopathology, but as Birch shows, we not only have to move beyond an episodic to a developmental model, we know how to do it, and in some areas, such as the long-term effects of nutrition, we have already made the switch.

Konrad Lorenz once commented that, "It is a good idea for a research scientist to discard a pet hypothesis every day before breakfast. It keeps him young." In the interests of rejuvenating clinical practice, life history researchers might recommend discarding a number of pet ideas. First among these is the idea that "psychotherapy can't hurt him, so we might as well try it." As Bergin (1971) has demonstrated, there are deterioration effects, and the risk of harm has to be balanced carefully against possible benefits. One psychiatrist has suggested, in a letter responding to Ricks's paper here, that within a few years a university that turns a new psychotherapist loose on the world will have to certify that he has been found to produce few undesirable side effects if taken as directed.

We can also get rid of a lot of misconceptions regarding particular disorders. For schizophrenia, we might stop believing in schizophrenogenic mothers, traumatic events that cause or even precipitate the disorder, intellectual deterioration in the absence of social and stimulus deprivation, and the idea that chronic schizophrenia is a functional disorder with no recognizable organic precursors. We can also throw out the idea that any disorder whatsoever is inherited. There is always interaction between genetic endowment and the prenatal and postnatal environments.

It will help, also, if we never regard normality as a simple, stable, non-developmental state. As presented in the studies reported here, there are more varieties of normality than of psychopathology, and these normal patterns of development are complex patterns of change and adaptation. This has many implications for understanding control groups — and we will be wise to study them developmentally, as Roff did. Suppose we use sibs as the controls for a study of schizophrenics, for example. There is growing evidence in the work of Mednick (1968, 1970), Anthony (1971), and others that the siblings of schizophrenics vary enormously, some making mildly schizoid life adjustments, some continuing a pattern of protest that resembles an adolescent impulse disorder, and some reaching extraordinary levels of creativity and originality. These differences are of interest in their own right, not simply as contrasts to the schizophrenic developmental sequences.

A famous, but somewhat narcissistic, heart surgeon once began a comment, "My clinical experience proves . . ." to be interrupted by an equally famous physiologist in the audience, "Your experience doesn't prove a damn thing. What is the evidence?" To all research workers, the authority resides in the data, not in the man. This lack of respect for authority, together with a lighthearted disregard for precedent and an abiding interest in innovation, make researchers inherently disruptive people. I think clinicians have a right to ask that we balance our disruptions of their work with enough valid new ideas to justify their tolerance. They might ask, for instance, that we take a more active role in helping them invent clinical interventions that will restore disturbed children to normal age–sex-role functions, and in helping them to recognize what those normal functions are. Clinical work, even more than research, is "an art of the possible," and clinicians often have set themselves tasks that are developmentally impossible, or close to it. By specifying some of the varieties of normal life, researchers may help them avoid trying to restore every damaged person to the same level and type of adjustment, and berating themselves when they "fail."

Two projects that have followed the work reported here may illustrate ways in which research can lead to useful clinical innovation. In one of these Jessica Schairer worked with a young boy who was originally considered hyperactive, but unable to benefit from drug treatments because they made it hard for him to sleep at night. The boy fit rather closely the "Puerto Rican apartment syndrome" that Thomas describes, and it was decided to aim therapy at helping his mother become more active and assertive, less depressed, and more able to enjoy her active son without resorting to her usual prohibitions. Two years later, with therapy still in full swing, this boy seems to be doing well in school, is no longer considered hyperactive, and the mother, in addition to taking him out to the movies and allowing the estranged father to take him out, is a member of a women's consciousness-raising group. Of all of the ideas useful in the treatment of this boy, the central one has been Thomas's idea that a constitutionally active child needs a chance to do things, and if such chances are found or made for him, other types of irritating behavior may be modified.

In the other project, Father Groeschel has worked with a group of people concerned about his finding that black adolescents tend to have poor outcomes even when they have good records of involvement at Children's Village and good prognoses at the time of discharge. On the basis of his research evidence that this relates to returning to a community in which neither parents nor the larger society provides much support, they have set up family-like halfway houses in the inner city of New York. This work is still under way, and later volumes in this series might have a report on whether the work succeeds, and with which boys.

As Chess has indicated, learning how and when to intervene may require independent investigation, but knowing how a disorder develops — how it starts and what maintains its developmental course — will usually provide the best clues to what might change the pattern. In Schairer's case, it was clear that the boy's initial hyperactivity and the mother's initial depression exacerbated each other, so that intervention could proceed on the basis of modifying either or both together.

Clinical intervention still concerns itself largely with the problem presented to the clinical worker, problems apparent at the time of referral. Life history research is concerned with such problems, but also with later outcomes. At the time he is in Children's Village, for example, a "prepsychotic" child may be seen as having a more severe problem than a child more given to active or passive aggression. Groeschel's follow-up work indicates, however, that children judged prepsychotic tend to make quiet, nondisruptive, marginally adequate social adjustments after discharge, but the prognosis for actively aggressive boys is not so benign. This suggests that special efforts be made with actively aggressive boys. More generally, we can consider it more important to arrest a downward spiral in any child, thereby heading off a later pathological outcome, than to refine still further already adequate social adjustments in young, attractive, verbal, intelligent, sensitive adults, an enterprise that occupies a surprising amount of clinical time and energy.

It would be interesting to utilize all of the reports in this and previous volumes in the series to develop a study of children at "highest risk" for schizophrenia, or adult character disorder, or addiction. For schizophrenia, the study might include one or more schizophrenic parents, living together in an emotional divorce situation, the mother dull and poorly nourished during her own development, with no adequate medical supervision of diet during her pregnancy. The parents should be poor and members of a minority group, existing in a social situation that provides few services for the mother or child and subjects the family to multiple social stresses. The child should be born prematurely, be low in birth weight, and manifest many non-localizing signs of neurological disorder. His sickliness should further a symbiotic union between his mother and himself. Infants picked on these criteria could be followed up until school, and sometime during school age we might refine the group, moving out of the "highest risk" category all those children who did not show high anxiety, with a jump to still higher anxiety levels when stimulated, scattered attention, and a tendency to quick habituation and overgeneralization. Later in childhood we might refine the group still further, removing from "highest risk" all those who did not show serious maladjustment in school, low popularity with peers, fear of everything new, and the sorts of school problems that Watt and Rolf describe. What would be the risk for schizophrenia in the group that remained? My own guess would be about 50 to 60 per cent. There are still many influences toward schizophrenia or toward health that are poorly understood, and these, together with the ambiguity and unreliability of the adult schizophrenic diagnoses, would lower our predictive power.

Some people might ask whether groups of such multiply handicapped children do in fact exist. I am sure that many such children can be found. The group I have described as "highest risk" would not be too different from the everyday populations of many residential treatment centers. So long as America continues to produce its current rate of poor, stupid, and pregnant girls, such children will continue to be born.

It would be especially interesting to discover any environmental influences common to "highest risk" children who did not become schizophrenic. We might find especially helpful teachers, relatives, summer camps, residential schools, or psychotherapists who had deflected these children from schizophrenic outcomes. Birch said that he was obsessed with one issue: not all children at risk turn out badly — some children show all of the effects of early malnutrition and still turn out well. Why? This sounds like one of the healthiest obsessions available. We might discover these influences in a study of Mednick's and Anthony's control groups, looking at the roughly nine tenths of children born to schizophrenic mothers, or two thirds of those born to two schizophrenic parents, who do not become schizophrenic.

There are two intriguing parallels between Birch's work on malnutrition and current research on schizophrenia. The first is that in malnutrition research, as in studies of schizophrenia, we have to look at the state of the organism at the time an influence is operating in order to understand the effect of that influence. Starvation has transitory and reversible effects on a developed organism, but it can be devastating and irreversible in its effect on an organism in its early stages of development. Symbiotic attachments can be healthy and beneficial in the early life of an infant, but devastating in adolescence and young adult life, preventing the developmental achievements of moving out of the home, finding a job that provides an independent income, and so forth that Jordaan and Levinson describe.

A second parallel relates to a set of symptoms that look like *outcomes* of early malnutrition and *precursors* to adult psychosis. "The first consequence of malnutrition is a change in behavior. The child becomes apathetic, he becomes irritable, he becomes environmentally unresponsive, he becomes an organism who is incapable of profiting from the environment that surrounds him." The numbers of malnourished children are immense, so that if this condition even slightly raises the risk for schizophrenia it would result in a large increase in the absolute number of schizophrenics. What to do about such children is also clear — feed them, and see that girls who are likely to be mothers get adequate nutrition. This simple program of feeding mothers and children should lower, to a marked degree, the later incidence of those forms of irritable apathy and environmental unresponsiveness that we call schizophrenia.

We might also suspect that the kinds of early neurological damage studied by Hertzig and by Stewart are predictive of poor outcomes. Mednick and Shulsinger (1970) have reported finding more birth complications in children who break down than in those who do not. Minimal brain damage seems to be a relatively general predictor of later poor outcomes, but the follow-up research to establish this has as yet not been done. When it is done, it will be well to keep in mind the role of parental and social expectations in labeling an activity level as normal or hyperactive (Thomas) and to see whether the hyperactivity, when it does exist, is accompanied by other forms of behavioral or cognitive deficit (Stewart).

From these reports it would also seem that we should be looking into the factors in psychotic mothers that lead to birth complications and early neurological symptoms in some children and not in others. Are these current poor nutrition, lack of exercise, chronic tension, or relayed effects from the mother's earlier poor nutrition?

The Aberdeen findings for mental subnormality — that extremely low IQ, below 50, is no respecter of social class, whereas mild retardation is heavily related to low social class, and is in turn related to low birth weight and mothers who were themselves stunted — provide yet another parallel to psychotic outcomes. It appears that infantile autism, or severe atypical development, is not related to social class. But schizophrenia definitely is, and like mild retardation, it is most frequent in people who are in the down-and-out end of the social class scale. Can this also be a matter of a socially transmitted deficiency disease, and if so can we do something about it? Nothing seems quite so unfair as damning a child to a high risk for mental deficiency or schizophrenia before he has had a chance to get out of the womb and utter his first yell of protest.

A new wave of social Darwinism is going through the social sciences, and a quietistic, "nothing can be done about it anyway" influence is apparent in the new emphasis on heredity in the thought of Jensen, Banfield, and others. Birch's interpretation of Scarr-Salapatek's data provides a useful dash of skepticism here. In optimal environments hereditary influences are large, but in environments that stunt populations, such as the environments that we have provided for many people in our urban and rural slums, family resemblance coefficients drop to near zero.

A reviewer of the first volume whose own IQ did not appear to be very high took us to task for overemphasizing IQ in our reports on the precursors of schizophrenia. In this volume we run the risk of offending people who do not like schools. Much of the most important information we can report about a person, though, relates to how well he does in school, what teachers think of him, and how he gets along with peers. One major advantage of this work, in contrast to the intensive but time-limited material available from hospitals and clinics, is that the school system is likely to be in contact with a child for twelve years or so. In Watt's data we can see a particular value in this long contact, a beginning picture of change over time, so that we do not see the pre-schizophrenic boy or girl only at adolescence but also going through the transitions of the school years. The need for this kind of careful developmental description was one of the points that Roff emphasized in launching this series.

Our diagnostic terms tend to overlook sex differences, although anyone who has ever worked on a men's ward and a women's ward can remember many marked differences in noise level, patient-staff relationships, and so on. Watt's data support a point made before (e.g., Gardner, 1967), that boys grow up to be men and girls grow up to be women, and the two lines of development are not parallel at every point. The pre-schizophrenic girls studied by Watt seem to have substantial areas of resemblance to adult schizophrenic women — insecure, maladjusted, and unsociable — although they are quiet, which adult schizophrenic women often are not. The pre-schizophrenic boys, particularly in adolescence, are disagreeable and unstable, but they are not shy or withdrawn. The girls are different from other girls by the grade school years, but the pre-schizophrenic boys are not distinguishable from other boys before junior high and high school, roughly grades 7–12. Whether the differences are a matter of personality only, or aspects of a developing disease process that is distinguishable from personality, is open to debate. Zubin holds for separate consideration of personality and disease process, Lorr for unity.

The source of data during the school years can be the child himself, his teachers, or peers. Rolf validates once more Roff's conclusion that peers can be sharper and more critical observers of some kinds of psychopathological behavior than teachers are.

Roff's results indicate that we can differentiate children who are headed for bad conduct episodes early, by the age of 9 or 10, on the basis of either the child's own behavior or the behavior of the parents. A mother who did not want the child, and whose handling of him features neglect, inadequate control, a wish to be rid of him, physical cruelty, and abandonment, is going to produce a child with a high risk for adult bad conduct. This research finding fits well with Groeschel's data and with the clinical experience of psychotherapists who work in prisons. One psychiatrist who works with violent criminals has described to me the extreme panic, and often murderous rage, that some of his patients have felt as they approached in psychotherapy an insight that their mother never wanted them, loved them, or valued their continued existence. By contrast, he said, the kind of anxiety involved in homosexual panic was mild indeed. Perhaps the increased use of contraceptive methods and permissiveness about abortion that have developed within the last decade will do more to prevent adult bad conduct than any more direct applications of law and order. As Roff says, "repressive measures applied late will not substitute for earlier affection and adequate care." Affection and care are likely to be given to wanted babies.

One of Schuckit's conclusions has comparable importance for practice. "Most students avoided certain drugs because of their perceived medical or psychologic consequences, such as gene damage, habituation, or the precipitation of a psychosis. Only a minority of students gave legal dangers as a reason for abstention, an indication that programs designed to decrease student drug use should concentrate on real medical dangers and avoid legalistic or moral arguments." Like Roff's conclusion, this suggests that punishment is likely to be an ineffective control, and that early intervention, in this instance educational, is likely to be more effective.

Schuckit's study also illustrates one of the values of designing studies in a prospective, longitudinal way. He can study the order, or sequence, in which different kinds of symptoms and behaviors appear. In some of Thomas's longitudinal research, he found that symptoms long thought to be the result of earlier anxiety states actually preceded anxiety developmentally. In Schuckit's study we can look at drug use and psychiatric symptoms longitudinally, seeing which precedes the other (drug use generally, but it also occurs in many students with no later psychiatric symptoms) and seeing in which students some vulnerability exists that either independently or in combination with drug usage relates to the later symptoms. Klein's comments remind us that the degree of the problem is important, and that there may be more difference between occasional drug users and "heads" than between non-users and occasional users.

Finally, drug use, like alcohol use, seems to be transmitted primarily through peer groups, and if we want to develop methods of control (in the event that drug use is harmful, which is not yet demonstrated for some of the most common drugs), we ought to concentrate on the sociology and epidemiology of drug use.

In sections 2 and 3 some of the most exciting current work of counseling psychology, psychiatry, social psychology, and sociology come together to describe the stages and the stresses of adult life. Here we move into the world of work and the legal, educational, medical, and other strains of life as an adult.

Jordaan's report illustrates the methodological advances that occurred when counseling psychology moved from its static focus of the past, vocational choice, into a dynamic longitudinal concern with career development. In the generation of progress or change measures, this work on occupational movement is well ahead of clinical research, which has largely confined itself to static measures of diagnosis, symptoms, or subjective distress at one or two particular points in time.

The points of intersection between prospective studies of developing psychopathology and prospective studies of developing social and vocational competence are practically endless, but those relating to life stages and sequential coping or failing to cope with developmental tasks seem most important. In studying psychopathology, as in studying career development, we need to look at the rate of development (lags or developmental precocity), at organized stages of development (the strain toward some kind of consistency of personality at each step), and at the determinants of development. As we compare many studies, we can sort out those variables that are predictive from those that may be equally interesting at a given point in time, but have no predictive significance. Perhaps by some technique such as path analysis, as Schooler points out, we can get beyond strictly correlational handling of the data, and a correlational interpretation of relationships, into causal data analysis and interpretation.

Where a variable has played a part in both studies of psychopathology and studies of career development, we can study relative importance. Intelligence, as measured by IQ, has proved to predict a variety of types of psychopathological development — criminals, schizophrenics, and alcoholics, for instance, frequently have had low IQ scores in childhood, relative to classmates, their sibs, and so on. The fact that the predictive power of the IQ is higher than that of other, clinically more central, variables is partly a matter of the quality of its measurement. In predictive studies IQ is not always the most relevant variable, but it is often the best measured and most reliable predictor. As peer relations, moral development, and Piagetian aspects of cognitive development have come to be reliably measured, they have also proved to be good predictors. When we turn to the prediction of career development, IQ becomes less important, not because its validity shrinks, but because other variables, such as school achievement and avocational activities, which are also reliably measured if the work is done carefully, become even more powerful predictors.

Like all prediction in complex fields, career development requires the investigator to relate many predictors to many criteria. Factor analysis can reduce the complexity of both domains, and stepwise multiple regression analysis (done with some care as to its assumptions) can deal with the areas of interrelationship among predictors. These methods are not new, but their use in predicting psychopathological outcomes has lagged behind their use in educational and vocational research. Students of psychopathology need to ask, as Jordaan does here: How good are the predictions? Which criteria can be predicted best? and Which are the best predictors? In the field of psychopathology, we would have to conclude (Kohlberg, LaCross, & Ricks, 1972) that the predictions are as yet not very impressive. But data such as Roff reports show that bad conduct can be predicted rather well, and we might guess that addictions and impulse disorders are also predictable at a fairly high level, and psychoses fairly well, while neurotic outcomes are relatively hard to predict. The search for the best predictors has occupied many of the papers in the three volumes of this series, and has led people to look at genetic variables, families, peer relationships, school behavior, early emotional life, and so on. At the moment it would seem that the best predictors of later psychopathological outcomes are: (a) low IQ and related forms of poor cognitive development, (b) moral development, and (c) peer relationships. This search for early predictors has led many of us to a new concern with early neurological characteristics of the sort that Hertzig, Birch, Stewart, and Thomas have been concerned with. In time these may prove to be the most powerful predictors we have.

As Birch would have expected ("Get away from episodic predictions and into developmental"), Vaillant finds that particular time-limited stresses and losses can be compensated by later experiences, but long-term stress predicts mental distress in later years, together with relative inability to enjoy life in play and close supportive relationships with other people. The long-term stresses are similar to those found earlier in data from child guidance clinics: destructive relationships with disturbed parents, inability to get along with a sib, and so on. There is special value in the perspective that a psychiatrist can bring to the study of health, and Vaillant's data show this.

Levinson and Lorr both point out the complexity of "normal" adult life. After Levinson's paper had received a thoughtful popularization (Wolfe, 1972), a good many of the male readers of *New York* magazine discovered that they were having a mid-life crisis. And even more frequently, their wives discovered that this was why the family had suddenly had to move from California, go off to Afghanistan, or go through some otherwise inexplicable uprooting. I would like to pick out just two aspects of this rich paper for comment.

The first relates to leaving the family as a developmental task of the years somewhere between 16–18 at the lower end and 20–24 at the upper. This is of course the peak period for first diagnoses of schizophrenia. How many cases of schizophrenia might best be understood as complex failures of individuation and leave taking? A good Ph.D. thesis might be done on a comparison of leave taking in schizophrenics and their sibs. Some of the quotes from various parents that come to mind are: "You must be crazy to want to go way out there," "What kind of person are you to be so ungrateful to your father?" "If he stays here his mother will have a heart attack," "That boy [a suitor] represents everything that is wrong with the world today." Perhaps the saddest was one mother who had never heard of Oedipus, yet told her daughter, "Why don't you marry someone like your father," and then followed with, "After all we have done for you, you want to marry a stranger." From the side of the separating nascent adult we hear themes like: "I will die if I don't get out of here," "This whole family is nuts," and so on. One of the girls in the Judge Baker studies had said at 12 that, "I don't need any friends, my mother is the best friend a girl could have." At 20 she tried to kill her mother, believing this was the only way she could achieve independence.

A second theme relates to the mid-life transition. How many depressions are belatedly honest attempts to come to terms with one's own depressed, disowned, less adequate under side? During the early stages of my own mid-life transition I worked with a great mentor, Abraham Maslow. One day, musing about Abe and his theoretical emphasis on peak experiences, which contrasted strongly with a persistent depressed quality in many of our conversations together, I decided that he would never reach his true potentials if he kept concentrating on peak experiences rather than looking into, and theorizing about, his own and other people's depressed depths. This struck me as a basic insight, and I drove along bathed in the sense of having come to a very important new understanding of a person who meant a lot to me — until it struck me to ask, "Why am I using Abe as a vehicle to think about this? Whose depressions do I have to understand anyway?"

We might hope that the new set of ideas developed by Jordaan, Levinson, and Vaillant will be as productive for thinking about the stages of adult life as Erikson's and Piaget's ideas have been for thinking about earlier stages and transitions. This work also provides a link with the sophisticated understanding of human development now coming out of the work of Havighurst, Neugarten, and people they have influenced.

Probably the most serious block to really understanding psychopathology is the primitive mechanism of separating the world into us and them, in group and out group, acceptable people and rejects. Lorr's report contains the good news that most of the people we meet in prisons and in outpatient clinics are going to have interpersonal styles much like those of the sets of people we know in the "normal" world. As Governor Reagan said, in another context, they are not "criminals at heart." Lorr's work also illustrates another theme of life history research. Lives are complex, and if we are to deal with them adequately, we have to use comprehensive models. Multivariate statistics provide one of these models.

In their comments on early papers in the book, Zubin and Birch call for careful measurement of environment, comparable in precision to the types of scaling we can do with physiological measures or with degrees of genetic relatedness. Myers shows how this kind of social scaling might be done. Perhaps because his variables are so carefully scaled, his results are beautifully unequivocal — the more events that happen in a given period of life, the more psychiatric disability there will be, while decrease in the number of events is accompanied by a decrease in symptoms.

Myers also throws light on an argument that never comes up at scientific meetings, but that has often marred professional or trade union discussions between psychologists and psychiatrists. This is the claim that emotional or psychological problems often have a medical base, and so are best diagnosed by a medically trained person. Myers's results indicate that the psychiatrically relevant stressful events are most often legal, interpersonal, educational, and financial, not crises of health. Neither psychiatrists nor psychologists are currently well trained in evaluating such types of stress, and more humility on the part of both camps might be in order.

In the last section, Groeschel develops further a theme that was introduced by Thomas and elaborated by Myers: the group in which a person lives helps determine the kinds of events that happen to him, and these, in turn, help shape the kinds of social difficulties and psychological disabilities into which he moves. Thomas reports that the New York Puerto Rican family is protective to the point of restricting children from the kinds of random play we expect of active young boys. Coming on other Puerto Rican families later, in Groeschel's report, we find that they remain loving, protective, and accepting even when the boy has caused them and himself a lot of trouble. Groeschel reports that Caucasian boys who "make it" often do so because they have access to social agencies, remedial help, and so on which make up for earlier parental and neighborhood influences toward disturbance. One of the things that the unusually able therapist described by Ricks was able to do was to put boys in touch with such helping agencies. A therapist working today should probably plan to know intimately all of the resources available in his community, particularly to minority group children and youth. When a particular resource is not available, but clearly needed, he might follow Groeschel's example and invent it.

It would be interesting to look at boys such as those Groeschel studied in the light of Jordaan's descriptions of vocational development. Massimo and Shore (1964) have demonstrated some of the values for delinquent boys of a form of psychotherapy built around vocational counseling. Perhaps in his next study, Groeschel (or someone else interested in such boys) might scale each boy at the time he entered an institution such as Children's Village on all of the vocational maturity and other measures in the Jordaan report. If this were also done at the time of discharge, and on follow-up, we might have a particularly sensitive indicator of the degree to which an institution helped to get its graduates back onto the paths of modal adult development.

We cannot shy away from the seamy side of American life that Groeschel uncovers. Participants in the conference may remember a certain shock when Groeschel, in some off-the-cuff comments, attempted to distinguish between antisocial mothers and respectable prostitutes who sought to supplement the inadequate family support provided by ADC with some discreet personal saleswomanship. If simply being black has such a devastating influence on adult outcome in what has often been considered the most liberal of Northern cities, what kind of society are we? In commenting on Groeschel's results, Thomas describes the biggest scandal in clinical work. The children most likely to have a lifetime of trouble are poor, acting out, and low in an IQ measure that reflects middle-class values and middle-class kinds of school learning. Yet these are the children who are most often rejected for treatment, and many clinicians see this as entirely reasonable — "They are not responsive, will not come for appointment hours, won't talk, don't want to change, etc., etc." This is like saying, in the midst of a cholera epidemic, "I only treat acne."

One of the reasons for the bewildering variety of contradictory findings in psychotherapy research is that most researchers have proceeded in a vacuum of information about naturally occurring antecedents and consequents of the different forms of disorder. Without base-line kinds of information we cannot reliably evaluate any kind of intervention. Those research workers who like to keep science in the laboratory might ponder the wisdom of one of the medium high priests of measurement theory on naturalistic method. "The method, for its part, can study what man has not learned to control, or can never learn to control. Nature has been experimenting since the beginning of time, with a boldness and complexity far beyond the resources of science. The mission is to observe and organize the data from nature's experiments" (Cronbach, 1957).

Balkin follows Strupp in looking beyond all of the parochial schools of psychotherapy and their esoteric criteria for evaluating outcomes, and asking simply why people come for therapy. Children may be in therapy for a variety of reasons having to do with their effects on parents, peers, and teachers, but adults who come for therapy generally offer internal, emotional reasons. They feel lousy, unhappy, dissatisfied, tired, angry, and so on, and they hope that therapy will help them feel better. Balkin's data indicate that therapy does seem to result in good feelings, emotional levels that put a post-therapy group on levels of happiness, energy, and sociability about the same as a group that had never sought psychotherapy and far above the emotional levels of those who are applying for psychotherapy. The paper provoked a vigorous discussion, and it would be hard to disagree with some of the criticisms. Clearly, the next step is a longitudinal, before-during-after follow-up design, in which moods are measured over the whole course of applying for, getting, and moving beyond psychotherapy. But I think we have to accept Balkin's main point, that the best way to go about evaluating psychotherapy is to ask what people come for, and whether they get it.

Another theme that runs through all of these papers, but is most explicit in Strauss's, is the necessity of making our criteria specific, operational, and long term.

Arranging a conference is a time-consuming, frustrating, far from tidy undertaking, even in a benign environment such as Teachers College. We might ask whether the give and take is worth it, or whether we might all learn as much by simply reading what the others have to say. I cannot speak for all authors, but I know that if I had had a chance to hear Strauss, and to consult with him, my own follow-up studies of schizophrenics after hospitalization would have been done with far greater specificity as to what we were looking for. I also suspect that having heard Jordaan, Strauss might be able to be far more specific about the dimensions of adequate work function that he uses as one of the four main dimensions of outcome.

Klein's comment on Strauss's paper raises another issue about which we have much to learn from talking together. If duration of illness is a strong predictor of later outcome, when do we say the illness started? Take a modal schizophrenic career. Johnny was ill in the first week after birth, and had a series of days with high temperature. He was a hyperactive child from about 2 to 8, and from 9 to 12 he was quiet and fearful, sought to avoid contact with other children, and did poorly in school. At about 12 he began stealing, and his school reported that he was touchy, irritable, had no friends, and was often picked on by other boys. After high school he drifted for a while, got into the drug scene, and then settled down into a routine job that demanded little of his ability. In his early twenties he offered a girl he worked with a box of candy, and when she refused it, he attempted suicide. Brought to the hospital, he said that he was being followed by the FBI and the Mafia, because he had certain secrets they wanted. He was dull and apathetic on the ward, but could be assaultive if other patients or staff irritated him. Now, when did the "schizophrenia" begin? Klein's comments suggest that it began with the childhood asociality. And behind that we can see easily recognizable neurological symptoms, with their own etiology. Certainly we cannot consider duration of illness as dating only from the first clearly psychotic thoughts or acts.

In his comments on "Supershrink" Stierlin suggests that careful monitoring of psychotherapy outcomes might find many therapists like this man. It might be worthwhile to study such therapists in Levinson's framework, as early mentors, and see what sorts of models they provide to young people. Evaluative research is not particularly welcomed by clinical workers, who are already overburdened with problems that families and schools have given up on. If this research is seen as not just a way of weeding out or re-educating the incompetent, but of finding and celebrating especially helpful therapists, research may be more welcome. There must be many exceptionally helpful people, but unless one happens to see a patient who is a writer, and so gets immortalized in fiction, or is found and studied by research such as this, his or her therapeutic skills may not be transmitted to the next generation.

In the absence of research, the methods of therapy most applied are those advanced by the most charismatic therapist, or those that have most recently come into use and so have a transitory faddish appeal. Morrison's paper shows that older methods of somatic therapy, properly evaluated, continue to have a place in the therapeutic program.

The book presents the beginnings of some integrative conceptions that can help us organize life histories, but it must be admitted that we still have a set of studies that resembles one of Bruner's not yet focused images instead of a smoothly integrated pattern. Each of us tends, in his institutional setting, to deal with a different age group and with a different set of problems. And if we are good clinicians, "the method we use is conditioned by the problems that confront us" (Bettelheim, 1950). Coming together, and talking together, is a way of working toward that general integration and cross-population robustness of results that we all seek.

A common misconception puts all of innovation and invention into science, with clinical work only application: "the clinical psychologist takes knowledge accumulated in one place, scientific psychology, and applies it to the solution of problems that emerge in another place, the lives of people. Therefore the clinical psychologist must be familiar with the source of knowledge, which is research, but he must also be familiar with the situations in which he plans to apply the knowledge, where real people have real problems" (Swensen, 1968). In life history research there has never been such a neat one way flow. Kraepelin's emphasis on outcomes, and Freud's on origins, gave clinical work a life history orientation well before academic theorists were willing to grapple with such complexity. The routes of influence and learning continue to be open both ways, and life histories continue to be a topic on which clinicians and research workers can talk to, and learn from, each other.

REFERENCES

Anthony, E. J. A clinical evaluation of children with psychotic parents. In R. Cancro (Ed.), *The schizophrenic syndrome*. New York: Brunner-Mazel, 1971. Pp. 244–256.

Bettelheim, B. *Love is not enough*. New York: Free Press, 1950.

Bergin, A. E. The evaluation of therapeutic outcomes. In A. E. Bergin & S. L. Garfield, *Handbook of psychotherapy and behavior change*. New York: Wiley, 1971. Pp. 217–270.

Cronbach, L. J. The two disciplines of scientific psychology. *American Psychologist*, 1957, 12, 671–684.

Gardner, G. The relationship between childhood neurotic symptomatology and later schizophrenia in males and females. *Journal of Nervous and Mental Disease*, 1967, 144 (no. 2), 97–100.

Jellinek, E. M. Phases of alcohol addiction. *Quarterly Journal of Studies on Alcohol*, 1952, 13, 673–684.

Kohlberg, L., LaCross, J., & Ricks, D. F. The predictability of adult mental health from childhood behavior. In B. B. Wolman (Ed.), *Manual of child psychopathology*. New York: McGraw-Hill, 1972.

Massimo, J. L., & Shore, M. F. Job focused treatment for anti-social youth. *Children*, 1964, 11, 143–147.

Mednick, S. A., & Schulsinger, F. Some premorbid characteristics related to breakdown in children with schizophrenic mothers. In D. Rosenthal & S. S. Kety, *The transmission of schizophrenia*. Oxford: Pergamon, 1968. Pp. 267–291.

———. Factors related to breakdown in children at high risk for schizophrenia. In M. Roff & D. F. Ricks (Eds.), *Life history research in psychopathology*. Vol. 1. Minneapolis: University of Minnesota Press, 1970. Pp. 51–93.

Swensen, C. J., Jr. Revision of a clinical training program: Integrated diversity. *Clinical Psychologist*, 1968, 21, 73–75.

Wolfe, L. A time of change. *New York Magazine*, June 5, 1972, 68–69.

LIST OF CONTRIBUTORS AND PARTICIPANTS

<h1 style="text-align:right">❧ List of Contributors
and Participants</h1>

George W. Albee, Department of Psychology, University of Vermont, Burlington, Vermont 05401

Joseph Balkin, Department of Psychology, John Jay College of Criminal Justice, City College of the City University of New York, New York, New York 10019

Victor Bergenn, Department of Psychology, Teachers College, Columbia University, New York, New York 10027

Allen Bergin, 118 FOB, Department of Psychology, Brigham Young University, Provo, Utah 84602

Herbert G. Birch, Department of Pediatrics, Albert Einstein College of Medicine, 1300 Morris Park Avenue, Bronx, New York 10461. Dr. Birch died February 4, 1973.

William T. Carpenter, Jr., Psychiatric Assessment Section, Adult Psychiatry Branch, National Institute of Mental Health, 9000 Rockville Pike, Bethesda, Maryland 20014

Stella Chess, Department of Psychiatry, New York University Medical Center, 550 First Avenue, New York, New York 10016

Charlotte M. Darrow, Department of Psychiatry, Yale University, 34 Park Street, New Haven, Connecticut 06519

William Fremouw, Department of Psychology, University of Massachusetts, Amherst, Massachusetts 01002

Norman Garmezy, Department of Psychology, University of Minnesota, Minneapolis, Minnesota 55455

Rachel Gittelman-Klein, Director, Child Development Clinic, Hillside Hospital, 75–59 263rd Street, Glen Oaks, New York 11004

Benedict J. Groeschel, Children's Village, Dobbs Ferry, New York 10522

James A. Halikas, Department of Psychiatry, Washington University School of Medicine, St. Louis, Missouri 63110

Margaret E. Hertzig, Rockland Children's Psychiatric Hospital, Convent Road, Orangeburg, New York 10962, and Department of Psychiatry, New York University School of Medicine

Howard F. Hunt, New York State Psychiatric Institute, Columbia University, 722 West 168th Street, New York, New York 10032

Jean Pierre Jordaan, Department of Psychology and Education, Teachers College, Columbia University, New York, New York 10027

Donald F. Klein, Director (Evaluation), Department of Psychiatry, Long Island Jewish–Hillside Medical Center, P.O. Box 38, Glen Oaks, New York 11004

Edward B. Klein, Department of Psychiatry, Yale University, 501 George Street, New Haven, Connecticut 06519

Ruth B. Klein, 200 East 17th Street, Brooklyn, New York 11226

Ray Knight, Department of Psychology, Brandeis University, Waltham, Massachusetts 02154

Daniel J. Levinson, Department of Psychiatry, Yale University, 34 Park Street, New Haven, Connecticut 06519

Maria H. Levinson, Department of Psychiatry, Yale University, 34 Park Street, New Haven, Connecticut 06519

Jacob J. Lindenthal, Department of Sociology, Rutgers University, New Brunswick, New Jersey 07102

Maurice Lorr, Department of Psychology, The Catholic University of America, Washington, D.C. 20017

James McClure, Department of Psychiatry, Washington University School of Medicine, St. Louis, Missouri 63110

Ronald D. Mack, Department of Psychiatry, Cornell University, Ithaca, New York 14850

Braxton McKee, Department of Psychology, Yale University, 58 Trumbull Street, New Haven, Connecticut 06519

Olga Mendez, Department of Psychiatry, New York University Medical Center, 550 First Avenue, New York, New York 10016

Ray Miller, School District of Webster Groves, Webster Groves, Missouri 63119

James R. Morrison, Department of Psychiatry, University of California, San Diego, P. O. Box 109, La Jolla, California 92037

Jerome K. Myers, Department of Sociology, Yale University, New Haven, Connecticut 06520

Helen Palkes, Department of Pediatrics, Washington University, St. Louis, Missouri 63110

Max P. Pepper, Department of Community Medicine, St. Louis University School of Medicine, St. Louis, Missouri 63104

David F. Ricks, The Psychological Center, City College of the City University of New York, Convent Avenue at 138th Street, New York, New York 10031

David J. Ricks, 15 Rectory Lane, Scarsdale, New York 10583

Ronald O. Rieder, Laboratory of Psychology, National Institute of Mental Health, 9000 Rockville Pike, Bethesda, Maryland 20014

John Rimmer, Department of Psychiatry, Washington University School of Medicine, St. Louis, Missouri 63110

Merrill Roff, Institute of Child Development, University of Minnesota, Minneapolis, Minnesota 55455

Jon E. Rolf, Department of Psychology, University of Vermont, Burlington, Vermont 05401

David Rosenthal, Laboratory of Psychology, National Institute of Mental Health, 9000 Rockville Pike, Bethesda, Maryland 20014

Jessica G. Schairer, Clinical Psychology Program, City College of the City University of New York, New York, New York 10031

Carmi Schooler, Laboratory of Socio-environmental Studies, National Institute of Mental Health, 9000 Rockville Pike, Bldg. 10, Rm. 3D41, Bethesda, Maryland 20014

Judith J. Schuckit, Department of Psychiatry, Medical School, University of California, San Diego, La Jolla, California 92037

Marc A. Schuckit, Department of Psychiatry, Medical School, University of California, San Diego, La Jolla, California 92037, presently serving as LCDR, MC, USNR, with the Navy Medical Neuropsychiatric Research Unit, San Diego, California 92152

Janet Sillen, Department of Psychiatry, New York University Medical Center, 550 First Avenue, New York, New York 10016

Mark A. Stewart, Child Psychiatry Service, University of Iowa School of Medicine, Iowa City, Iowa 52240

CONTRIBUTORS AND PARTICIPANTS

Helm Stierlin, Family Studies Section, Adult Psychiatry Branch, National Institute of Mental Health, 9000 Rockville Pike, Bethesda, Maryland 20014

John S. Strauss, Department of Psychiatry, University of Rochester School of Medicine and Dentistry, Rochester, New York 14642

Donald E. Super, Department of Psychology and Education, Teachers College, Columbia University, New York, New York 10027

Alexander Thomas, Department of Psychiatry, New York University Medical Center, 550 First Avenue, New York, New York 10016

George E. Vaillant, The Cambridge Hospital, 1493 Cambridge Street, Cambridge, Massachusetts 02139

Norman F. Watt, Department of Psychology, University of Massachusetts, Amherst, Massachusetts 01002

Zela Welner, Department of Psychiatry, Washington University, St. Louis, Missouri 63110

Robert D. Wirt, Division of Health Care Psychology, University of Minnesota, Minneapolis, Minnesota 55455

Carol Young, Department of Pediatrics, Washington University, St. Louis, Missouri 63110

Richard P. Youniss, Department of Psychology, The Catholic University of America, Washington, D.C. 20017

Joseph Zubin, Biometrics Research, State of New York Department of Mental Hygiene, 722 West 168th Street, New York 10032

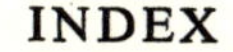

INDEX

<h1 style="text-align:center">❧ Index</h1>

Heritability coefficient: effect of sub-optimal environment on, 18

Hidden Figures Test, 70

High-risk method: in schizophrenia research, 25–41; degree of risk in, 28, 356–357; criteria of, 29, 31, 79, 87; design problems in, 29, 32–34; and age at initial study, 36–37; and longitudinal follow-up, 38; and perinatal conditions of risk, 42–43; and academic achievement, 87–107; comparison of, with follow-up and follow-back methods, 195; and childhood intervention, 279–284, 290, 350; good outcomes of, 357

Hyperactivity: and prematurity, 45–47; and restriction, 61–63, 84–85; and minimal brain dysfunction, 63, 68–70; and intelligence, 70–76; prevalence of, 72–73; and schizophrenia, 79, 80; intervention in, 355

Identity: in adolescent transition, 245–246

Intelligence: in hyperactive children, 70–71; and malnutrition, 80; in pre-schizophrenics, 99–100, 203; in childhood of neurotic and bad conduct adults, 137; in case history outline, 140; in school records, 197; and Kuhlmann-Anderson Test, 197; and Otis Test, 197; and high achievement, 239; and outcome of residential treatment, 264; and psychopathology, 363

Interpersonal style: of neurotics, 179–180, 187; of prison inmates, 180, 187–188; of normals, 183, 186; in personality trait ratings of pre-schizophrenics, 197–199, 202–203

Interpersonal Style Inventory (ISI), 179

Intimacy: predicting adult capacity for, 236–237; and transition to adult world, 247

Jastak Wide Range Achievement Test, 70

Kuhlmann-Anderson Test, 197

Learning disabilities: and hyperkinesis, 69; and neurosis, 274

Life events: connected with psychiatric symptoms, 212–213, 220; and areas of social activity, 219–220; entrance-related and exit-related, 220–221;

desirable and undesirable, 221; degree of uncertainty in, 222; training for understanding of, 365

Life history: stages and tasks, 109–111; major types of events in, 220; psycho-social stages in adult, 243–256; perspective on treatment, 275; continuity in, 352; developmental course in, 352; patterns of disorder in, 352–353; rate of development in, 353; age-related interventions in, 353; reasonable expectations in, 353

Malnutrition: in adults, 4; in children, 4–17; effects of, on behavior, 4; acute and chronic, 5–6, 15; and neuro-integrative capacities, 7–8; and growth retardation, 7–9; as result of inadequate stimulus, 9–10; in sibling comparisons, 10–11; and marasmus, 12; and kwashiorkor, 12; and school behavior, 13; effect of, on intrauterine environment, 22–23; and schizophrenia, 358

Marital history: categories for analysis of, 149; as antecedent to neurosis and bad conduct, 149–151; and mental status, 220, 223; relationship of, to career adjustment and maturity of defenses, 235

Mental status: and screening tests, 215; and life events, 217–221

Mentor: in adult psychosocial development, 251–253, 257; therapist as, 289, 296, 368; in apprenticeship and role models, 295–296

Minnesota Multiphasic Personality Inventory (MMPI): lack of family items in, 134

Mother: effect of malnourishment in, on intrauterine environment, 22–23; schizophrenia of, 26, 36, 37, 87; separation from, as high-risk indicator, 32; illness of, during pregnancy, 48; depression of, 89, 103; and neglect of offspring, 132, 135; in Categories of Case Abstracts, 140; role of, in neurotic and bad conduct cases, 145–146, 150; relationship of, with child, 232; in ethnocultural groups, 262, 268; relationship of, to acceptance and outcome, 265–266

Neonate: condition of premature, 44; antenatal and postnatal conditions of, 49